AF556879

THE YEAR IN UROLOGY

VOLUME 3

THE YEAR IN UROLOGY

VOLUME 3

EDITED BY

JOHN L PROBERT, HARTWIG SCHWAIBOLD

CLINICAL PUBLISHING

OXFORD

Clinical Publishing

an imprint of Atlas Medical Publishing Ltd

Oxford Centre for Innovation
Mill Street, Oxford OX2 0JX, UK

Tel: +44 1865 811116
Fax: +44 1865 251550
E mail: info@clinicalpublishing.co.uk
Web: www.clinicalpublishing.co.uk

Distributed by:
Marston Book Services Ltd
PO Box 269
Abingdon
Oxon OX14 4YN, UK
Tel: +44 1235 465500
Fax: +44 1235 465555
E mail: trade.orders@marston.co.uk

First published 2006

A catalogue record for this book is available from the British Library

ISBN 1 904392 82 2
ISSN 1479-5353

Project Manager: Rosemary Osmond, Helimetrics Ltd, Chipping Norton, Oxon, UK
Typeset by Hope Services (Abingdon) Ltd, Abingdon, Oxon, UK
Printed and bound in Great Britain by Biddles Ltd, King's Lynn, Norfolk

Contents

Part III

Non-malignant conditions of the lower urinary tract

Part IV

New techniques and experimental developments

Editors

John L Probert, BMedSci, DM, FRCS(Urol)
Consultant Urological Surgeon and Senior Clinical Lecturer in Surgery, Department of Urology, Western General Hospital, Weston super-Mare, Somerset, UK

Hartwig Schwaibold, MD
Head of Urology Department, Kreiskliniken Reutlingen GmbH, Klinikum am Steinenberg, Reutlingen Teaching Hospital, University of Tübingen, Tübingen, Germany

Contributors

Paul Abrams, MD, FRCS
Professor of Urology, Bristol Urological Institute, Southmead Hospital, Westbury-on-Trym, Bristol, UK

Omar Al-Salihi, BSc, MRCP, FRCR
Locum Consultant Clinical Oncology, Meyerstein Institute of Oncology, University College London Hospitals, London, UK

Conor J Corr, FRCSI, FRCR
Specialist Registrar Radiology, Department of Radiology, Bristol Urological Institute, Southmead Hospital, Westbury-on-Trym, Bristol, UK

Paul Crow, MD
Specialist Registrar, Torbay Hospital, Torquay, Devon, UK

Malcolm C Crundwell, MA, MD, FRCS(Urol)
Consultant Urologist, Department Urology, Royal Devon and Exeter NHS Hospital, Exeter, UK

Oliver Gee, MBChB, MRCS
Specialist Registrar in Paediatric Urology, Bristol Royal Hospital for Children, Bristol, UK

Hashim Hashim MBBS, MRCS
Urology Specialist Registrar, Bristol Urological Institute, Southmead Hospital, Westbury-on-Trym, Bristol, UK

Kieran P Jefferson, MA, FRCS(Urol)
Locum Consultant Urologist, Department of Urology, North Bristol NHS Trust, Southmead Hospital, Westbury-on-Trym, Bristol, UK

Katherine P Kennedy, MBChB, MRCS(Edin), DTMH
Research Registrar, Department of Urology, Taunton and Somerset Hospital, Musgrove Park, Taunton, Somerset, UK

Anthony Koupparis, BSc, MD, MRCS
Specialist Registrar in Urology, Royal United Hospital, Bath, UK

Chi-Ying Li, MB BS, MRCS(Eng)
Clinical Research Fellow, Institute of Urology, St Peter's Andrology Centre, London, UK

Evangelos N Liatsikos, MD, PhD
Lecturer of Urology, Department of Urology, University of Patras Medical School Rio, Patras, Greece

Ruaraidh P MacDonagh, MBBS, FRCS, MD
Consultant Urologist, Department of Urology, Taunton and Somerset Hospital, Musgrove Park, Taunton, Somerset, UK

Guy Nicholls, BSc, MD, FRCS(Paeds)
Consultant Paediatric Urological Surgeon, Department of Paediatric Urology, Bristol Royal Hospital for Sick Children, Bristol, UK

Jonathan R Osborn, MBChB, MSc, MRCS
Research Fellow, Bristol Urological Institute, Southmead Hospital, Westbury-on-Trym, Bristol, UK

Jon D Oxley, BSc, MD, MRCPath
Consultant Histopathologist, Department of Cellular Pathology, North Bristol NHS Trust, Southmead Hospital, Westbury-on-Trym, Bristol, UK

Tobias Page, MBBS, BSc, MRCS, PhD
Specialist Registrar, James Cook University Hospital, Middlesbrough, UK

Heather Payne, MD
Consultant in Clinical Oncology, Meyerstein Institute of Oncology, University College London Hospitals, London, UK

John L Probert, BMedSci, DM, FRCSUrol
Consultant Urological Surgeon and Senior Clinical Lecturer in Surgery, Department of Urology, Western General Hospital, Weston super-Mare, Somerset, UK

David Ralph, BSc, MS, FRCS(Urol)
Consultant Andrological Surgeon, Institute of Urology, St Peter's Andrology Centre, London, UK

Hartwig Schwaibold, MD
Head of Urology Department, Kreiskliniken Reutlingen GmbH, Klinikum am Steinenberg, Reutlingen Teaching Hospital, University of Tübingen, Tübingen, Germany

Mahmood Shafei, MCh, FRCSI
Specialist Registrar in Urology, Department of Urology, Royal Gwent Hospital, Cardiff Road, Newport, UK

Sivaprakasam Sivalingam, MB, BCh, BAO, BMedSci, MRCS
Research Registrar, Bristol Urological Institute, Southmead Hospital, Westbury-on-Trym, Bristol, UK

Jens-Uwe Stolzenberg, MD, PhD
Associate Professor, Department of Urology, University of Leipzig, Leipzig, Germany

Mark Stott, MD, FRCS
Consultant Urologist, Royal Devon and Exeter NHS Hospital, Exeter, UK

Marto Sugiono, MBChB, FRCS
Specialist Registrar, Royal Devon and Exeter NHS Hospital, Barrack Road, Exeter, UK

Alun W Thomas, FRCS
Specialist Registrar in Urology, Bristol Urological Institute, Southmead Hospital, Westbury-on-Trym, Bristol; Department of Urology, Royal Gwent Hospital, Newport, UK

Mark J Thornton, MRCP, FRCR
Consultant Radiologist, Department of Radiology, Bristol Urological Institute, Southmead Hospital, Westbury-on-Trym, Bristol, UK

Steve Williams, MRCS
Research Registrar, Department of Urology, Southmead Hospital, Westbury-on-Trym, Bristol, UK

Ulrich K Fr Witzsch, MD
Department of Urology and Paediatric Urology, Krankenhaus Nordwest der Stiftung Hospital zum Heiligen Geist, Frankfurt/Main, Germany

Mark N Woodward, MD, FRCS(Paed)
Consultant Paediatric Urologist, Department of Paediatric Urology, Bristol Royal Hospital for Sick Children, Bristol, UK

Foreword

PAUL ABRAMS, MD, FRCS

Professor of Urology
Bristol Urological Institute
Southmead Hospital
Westbury-on-Trym
Bristol, UK

Welcome to the third volume of *The Year in Urology*.

Each of the volumes produced so far in this series has reviewed what the editors of each individual chapter consider to be the best, most pertinent and most interesting papers published in the academic urological literature during the year. The contents list has deliberately been varied from volume to volume. In some years more papers are published on a particular topic than in others; if this series were to have identical chapter headings each time, then there would be the danger of material becoming repetitive. This is why stone disease has not been included this time, but there are chapters on Quality of Life and Phytotherapy, topics which have not been covered before but which are increasingly becoming recognised as important in the field of urology, with a considerable quantity of good quality research appearing in the literature to reflect this.

The first part of the book also includes reviews by the regular expert contributors in the fields of paediatric urology, radiology and uropathology. As well as dealing with phytotherapy, the uro-oncological section provides updates on bladder cancer, renal cell carcinoma and prostate cancer, including a review of the treatment options in advanced disease.

The third part of the book covers a similar brief to the previous volume, with chapters on urinary incontinence, lower urinary tract symptoms with specific reference to benign prostatic hyperplasia, trauma and reconstruction, and andrology.

Finally, the 'New Techniques' section once again takes a look at the disparate world of the basic sciences in the investigative urology chapter, and the more complex world of molecular oncology in a chapter devoted to new developments in this field.

Cryotherapy was a subject touched upon last year in a brief chapter that also dealt with radiofrequency ablation and photodynamic therapy. This current volume is rounded out by a chapter devoted entirely to cryotherapy that covers the literature dealing with the use of this technique in treating both prostate and renal tumours.

The aim of this series of books is to provide an up-to-date review of the latest developments and findings in the world of urology, and the authors hope that they are also giving the reader a taste as to which of these are going to be of greater importance in the years to come. Only time will tell. The feedback for this series of books has been excellent, and if anyone has any comments or has anything they feel deserves greater coverage in future volumes, then the editors would be more than happy to hear from them via the publisher.

Part I

Diagnostic and general urology

1

Paediatric urology

OLIVER GEE, GUY NICHOLLS, MARK WOODWARD

Introduction

A key systematic review concerning the role of circumcision in preventing urinary tract infection (UTI) has been published among other papers. The late David Gough was senior author on an important paper that looked objectively at the results of hypospadias surgery. A series of papers looking at multicystic dysplastic kidney (MCDK), the risk of hypertension and the outcome of nephrectomy for renally mediated hypertension have also been considered. Finally, a number of key papers on the undescended testis, varicocele and intersex are reviewed.

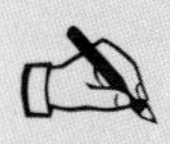

Circumcision for the prevention of urinary tract infection in boys: a systematic review of randomised trials and observational studies

Sing-Grewal D, Macclessi J, Craig J. *Arch Dis Child* 2005; **90**: 853–8

BACKGROUND. Circumcision remains the commonest surgical procedure carried out on boys worldwide. Although the absolute indications for circumcision are limited, a number of urologists recommend circumcision to prevent UTI. This important systematic review compared the rate of UTI in circumcised and uncircumcised boys.

INTERPRETATION. A total of 402 908 children, with 1953 separate UTI episodes, were identified from the 12 studies analysed (one randomized control trial [RCT], four cohort studies and seven case–control studies). Circumcision was associated with a significantly reduced risk of UTI (odds ratio [OR] 0.13; 95% confidence interval [CI] 0.08–0.20; P <0.001) with the same odds ratio (0.13) for all three types of study design. The authors identified weaknesses in this review: its reliance on observational studies of variable quality, the single small RCT failed to achieve significance, and the majority of studies measuring UTI episodes rather than number of patients experiencing UTI. The authors used the risk ratio with estimates of UTI incidence and circumcision complication rate to construct a harm-vs-benefits table (Table 1.1). They concluded that circumcision should be considered in those boys with recurrent UTI or significantly increased risk of UTI.

Table 1.1 Benefit versus harm for circumcision in preventing urinary tract infection in boys at different levels of risk for UTI per 1000 boys, assuming a complication rate of 2% and odds ratio of 0.13

Patient group	Risk of UTI (%)	UTI in uncircumcised (*n*)	UTI in circumcised (*n*)	UTI prevented by circumcision (*n*)	Complications of circumstances (*n*)
Normal	1	10	1	9	20
Past UTI	10	100	13	87	20
High-grade VUR	30	300	39	261	20

UTI, urinary tract infection; VUR, vesicoureteric reflux.
Source: Sing-Grewal *et al.* (2005).

Comment

Circumcision, as a prophylactic measure for 'medical conditions', remains controversial. This stringent and well-structured review finds that circumcision leads to a decreased rate of urinary tract infections in boys. The authors acknowledge that it is let down by the poor quality of the studies analysed, but few would disagree with the paper's findings. The interpretation of these findings, and how this should influence clinical practice, is a more interesting topic.

This is well demonstrated by the conflicting perspectives published with the article. Schoen's |**1**| interpretation, a US author, is that this study backs routine newborn circumcision for all boys, suggesting that the author's summary is 'analogous to postponing immunization of an infant until the child is exposed to the pathogen or is diagnosed with the disease'. In contrast, Malone |**2**|, a UK author, agrees with Sing-Grewal *et al.* that circumcision should be reserved for those boys with recurrent UTI or those at increased risk of UTI.

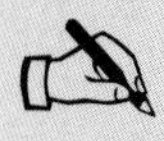

Inguinal hernia in female infants: a cue to check the sex chromosomes?

Deeb A, Hughes IA. *BJU Int* 2005; **96**: 401–3

BACKGROUND. Complete androgen insensitivity syndrome (CAIS) arises from target tissue androgen resistance and results in a female phenotype in a genotypical XY male. This study reviews the clinical presentation of CAIS and assesses the current practice of considering this diagnosis in female infants presenting with an inguinal hernia.

INTERPRETATION. Patients were identified from the Cambridge Intersex Database, and details of presentation, presence of hernia, hernial contents and family history of CAIS were recorded. A questionnaire considering the diagnosis of CAIS, in female infants with a hernia, was distributed to paediatric surgeons and endocrinologists. The intersex database identified 120 cases of CAIS, and the presentation mode is shown in Fig. 1.1.

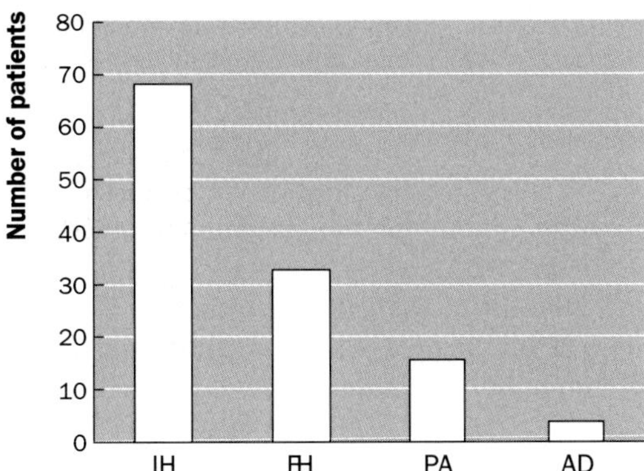

Fig. 1.1 The mode of clinical presentation of CAIS. IH, inguinal hernia; FH, positive family history of CAIS; PA, primary amenorrhoea; AD, antenatal diagnosis. Percentages of total number in each category are shown on the bars. Source: Deeb and Hughes (2005).

There was an equal distribution of hernia side and half were bilateral. Gonads were palpable in the hernial sac in a third of cases. The questionnaire response is shown in Table 1.2, with most considering the diagnosis of CAIS in any female patient presenting with inguinal hernia. The authors conclude that, as an inguinal hernia is the commonest presentation of CAIS, it should be considered in all females with inguinal swellings. They

Table 1.2 Response to the questionnaire

	Response, *n*	
CAIS should be considered in: options	**Surgeons (87)**	**Endocrinologists (64)**
1 All female infants presenting with an inguinal hernia	54	52
2 Only in female infants with bilateral inguinal hernias	5	
3 Only for inguinal hernias containing gonads	6	4
4 In female infants with a family history of inguinal hernias (female sibling/cousin)	0	0
5 In infants with a family history of CAIS (female sibling/cousin)	6	
2 and 5	4	8
3 and 5	6	
Other options chosen by surgeons:		
Inspection of gonads and internal genitalia	4	
CAIS diagnosis not worth considering as association with hernia presentation is low	2	

Source: Deeb and Hughes (2005).

felt investigation was justifiable, but the method should be decided upon by the individual clinician.

Comment

This study reaffirms that CAIS should be considered in all girls who present with inguinal hernias. The options of assessment by gonadal inspection, gonadal biopsy, ultrasound and karotyping are all considered, without reaching any real conclusion or suggestions. Common practice is to attempt to visualize the ovary or fallopian tube in all females undergoing inguinal herniotomy. If this is not possible, blood would be routinely sent intra-operatively for a subsequent karyotype to be performed.

An objective assessment of the results of hypospadias surgery

Ververidis M, Dickson AP, Gough DCS. *BJU Int 2005*; **96**: 135–9

BACKGROUND. A number of different hypospadias repairs are used by paediatric urologists worldwide. Recently, the Snodgrass repair has gained widespread acceptance as it is reputed to have an excellent cosmetic outcome. However, there are very few published reports of objective cosmetic outcome data, which was the purpose of this paper.

INTERPRETATION. Five independent heath professionals used post-repair photographs to compare the cosmesis of different hypospadias repair techniques. The Snodgrass technique was used for both distal (10) and proximal (6) hypospadias by one surgeon. A second surgeon performed the Mathieu repair for distal hypospadias (10) and an onlay preputial island flap for proximal hypospadias (6). Cosmesis was graded as poor, unsatisfactory, satisfactory or very good (1–4) for different aspects of penile appearance: meatus, glans, shaft and overall appearance. One author assessed the incidence of a vertical slit-like meatus.

The mean assessment score of the panel for each cosmetic variable is shown in Table 1.3. The score for any aspect of cosmesis was significantly higher for the

Table 1.3 The mean assessment scores for the S and M/D groups

	Meatus		**Glans**		**Shaft**		**Overall**	
Assessor	**S**	**M/D**	**S**	**M/D**	**S**	**M/D**	**S**	**M/D**
1	3.56	2.94	3.43	2.88	3.38	2.88	3.44	2.88
2	3.00	2.44	3.13	2.69	2.81	2.67	3.06	2.88
3	3.38	2.38	3.25	2.56	2.94	2.38	3.06	2.38
4	2.81	2.25	2.94	2.31	2.88	2.60	2.88	2.31
5	3.63	2.56	3.63	2.56	3.53	2.87	3.64	2.57

Source: Ververidis *et al.* (2005).

Table 1.4 Comparison between the S and M/D onlay techniques

Feature	Mean difference (95% CI) (SD)	*P*
Meatus	0.76 (0.45–1.10) (0.25)	0.002
Glans	0.67 (0.38–0.97) (0.24)	0.003
Shaft	0.42 (0.16–0.69) (0.21)	0.01
Overall	0.62 (0.24–1.00) (0.30)	0.01

Source: Ververidis *et al.* (2005).

Snodgrass technique (Table 1.4). The incidence of vertically orientated meatus was significantly higher for the Snodgrass repair (88%) than for the other technique group (38%), $P = 0.009$. The horizontally orientated meatus, reported previously with the Mathieu repair, was not found, and this technique could reproduce a vertical meatus with minor modification. The authors note that this is a method for assessing the outcome of hypospadias repair techniques by healthcare professionals. However, they comment that this does not always equate with the patient's or parents' own perceptions.

Comment

This interesting study strengthens the evidence that the Snodgrass repair can produce a very good cosmetic result, perhaps even better than other techniques. This study's strength lies in the use of independent assessors, blinded to surgical technique, to objectively evaluate cosmesis. However, this is only one facet in the evaluation of penile appearance post hypospadias repair. A complete assessment would include complication rates and, ideally, the patient's own assessment of the appearance. Most of the children undergoing this surgery would have been circumcised as part of the repair, and there was no discussion as to the potential role of the foreskin in cosmetic outcome. As the authors conclude, an ideal study to compare cosmesis would be a multicentre, randomized, prospective trial involving several surgeons, which is probably not feasible.

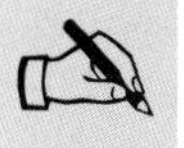

Predictive factors of ultrasonographic involution of prenatally detected multicystic dysplastic kidney

Rabelo EAS, Oliveira EA, Silva GS, Pezzuti IL, Tatsuo ES. *BJU Int* 2005; **95**: 868–71

BACKGROUND. Antenatal ultrasound (US) has resulted in a substantial increase in the detection of asymptomatic MCDK. The authors of this study aimed to evaluate possible predictive factors for the involution or disappearance of MCDK.

INTERPRETATION. Forty-five children with prenatally detected unilateral MCDK were managed conservatively. US was performed 6-monthly for the first 2 years and yearly thereafter. Variables analysed were: gender, affected side, palpability at first examination, initial MCDK length (US) and contralateral kidney length. The mean (range) follow-up was 50 (12–167) months with a mean of six ultrasounds per patient (3–10). US showed partial involution in 30 (67%) children and complete involution in nine (20%). The mean (95% CI) time to complete involution was 121 months (99–142). Twenty-two (49%) were reduced by half the initial renal length, with a mean (95% CI) time of 76 (62–92) months. The MCDK length remained unchanged in six (13%) children. The only factor predictive of complete involution was a renal length at diagnosis <62 mm (hazard ratio 8; 95% CI 0.98–68; $P = 0.05$). Two children (4.5%) developed hypertension during follow-up.

Comment

There is an increasing incidence of diagnosis of many conditions, such as MCDK, by antenatal US, and it is therefore important to understand the natural history of such conditions. This study has shown similar rates of complete involution of MCDK to those reported previously, although at a slower rate. The only factor apparently predictive of involution was length at diagnosis, but this finding needs to be reproduced in larger studies if it is going to be used to counsel parents more effectively.

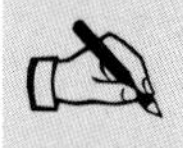

Risk of hypertension with multicystic kidney disease: a systematic review

Narchi H. *Arch Dis Child* 2005; **90**: 921–4

Background. Children with MCDK are usually managed conservatively in the first few years of life. Blood pressure is monitored, as a number of reports have highlighted a risk of hypertension, even after apparently complete MCDK involution. The authors have conducted a systematic review of all published cohort studies, in order to estimate the probability of a child with a conservatively treated unilateral MCDK developing hypertension.

Interpretation. In the follow-up period, six out of 1115 eligible children from 29 studies developed persisting hypertension (excluding four patients who developed transient hypertension). The mean probability of a child with unilateral MCDK developing hypertension was therefore 5.4 per 1000 (95% CI estimated at 1.9–11.7 per 1000). The follow-up period, in the 15 studies in which it was stated, varied between 0.2 and 13 years (range of means 3–5.3 years). The authors commented on weaknesses in their review: hypertension was not uniformly defined and the older studies would have missed antenatal diagnosis.

Comment

This study demonstrates that the risk of developing hypertension in childhood secondary to MCDK is low, at approximately 1 in 200. This figure can be used for counselling parents if an MCDK fails to involute in infancy. However, the available data do not indicate whether MCDK involution is associated with a reduced risk of hypertension, and further longer-term studies are vital to quantify the risk of hypertension in adulthood.

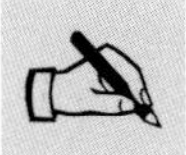

The role of unilateral nephrectomy in the treatment of nephrogenic hypertension in children

Johal NS, Kraklau D, Cuckow PM. *BJU Int* 2005; **95**(1): 140–2

BACKGROUND. Paediatric hypertension is most commonly secondary to renal disease, with a prevalence in children of 0.5–1.5%. This study aimed to define the efficacy of unilateral nephrectomy in patients presenting with benign renal disease and hypertension and a normal contralateral kidney.

INTERPRETATION. Twenty-one children undergoing nephrectomy for hypertension (defined as a systemic blood pressure [BP] >95th centile for age and height) between 1968 and 2003 were reviewed retrospectively. Blood pressure and medication requirements were compared before and after surgery.

The median age at presentation was 5 years (birth–12 years) with all patients having persistent hypertension, despite treatment with between two and four anti-hypertensives. The time from diagnosis to surgery was 11 (0–105) months, with a follow-up of 39 (1–169) months. After nephrectomy, 76% (16/21) stopped anti-hypertensives and became normotensive. Four patients were able to reduce the number of anti-hypertensives, and only one patient had no response to nephrectomy. The median time to BP normalization was 7 (1–120) days, which varied with different histological groups.

Comment

Paediatric hypertension secondary to unilateral renal disease occurs reasonably frequently, and lifelong medical treatment is potentially necessary. The authors concluded that nephrectomy is successful in normalizing nephrogenic hypertension in most cases, and that children may benefit from early nephrectomy to reduce the potential morbidity from this condition.

Apoptosis and proliferation in human undescended testes

Ofordeme KG, Aslan AR, Nazir TM, Hayner-Buchan A, Kogan BA. *BJU Int* 2005; **96**: 634–8

BACKGROUND. Cryptorchidism is associated with decreased fertility and reduced sperm counts. Animal data suggest that this may arise as a result of a decrease in germ cell proliferation or an increase in apoptosis. In this study, testicular biopsies taken at orchidopexy from a consecutive series of patients were studied using immunohistological techniques.

Table 1.5 Apoptosis rates according to age at orchidopexy and testicular location at operation

	Testicular location at operation		**Mean (SD) no. of apoptotic cells**
	Inguinal (n = 83)	**Abdominal (n = 18)**	
Orchidopexy <1 year (n = 29)	25	4	1.35 (1.56)
Orchidopexy >1 year (n = 72)	58	14	0.68 (1.40)
Mean (SD) no. of apoptotic cells	**0.71 (1.31)**	**1.63 (1.95)**	

Source: Ofordeme *et al.* (2005).

INTERPRETATION. Biopsies were taken from 101 undescended testes from children between 2 months and 15 years of age (median age 23 months). The numbers of cells undergoing apoptosis or proliferation, per 50 seminiferous tubules, was recorded. Five testicular biopsies from autopsy cases were used as controls (age range 26–156 months).

Apoptosis was identified in all specimens (Table 1.5). Rates were generally low, but were higher in the controls (mean [SD] 10.6 [1.34] per 50 seminiferous tubules). There was less apoptosis in children >1 year than in children <1 year (P <0.03), and in the inguinal testes compared with the intra-abdominal testes (P <0.02). Proliferation was very limited in all the biopsies and again more common in the autopsy controls, although no data were supplied in the paper.

Comment

This study showed that the reduced fertility associated with undescended testes cannot be explained by either reduced proliferation or increased apoptosis of testicular germ cells at the time of surgical intervention. It remains possible that the testis simply has fewer germ cells, or that abnormalities in germ cell turnover occur before 6 months of age.

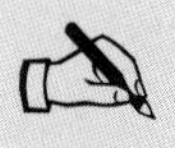

Managing varicoceles in children: results with microsurgical varicocelectomy

Schiff J, Kelly C, Goldstein M, Schelgel P, Poppas D. *BJU Int* 2005; **95**: 399–402

BACKGROUND. Varicocele in childhood may be associated with symptoms or growth arrest of the ipsilateral developing testis. A number of different surgical procedures are used, with the majority of surgeons favouring the Palomo procedure. The authors in this retrospective study describe their experience of microsurgical varicocelectomy (MSV) in boys <18 years old, over a 4-year period in a single institution.

INTERPRETATION. Subinguinal varicocelectomies were performed assisted by an operating microscope (×10–15). The technique involves mobilizing the spermatic cord at the superficial inguinal ring. All testicular veins, vas-associated veins >2.5 mm and large gubernacular veins were ligated. Seventy-four boys (mean age 14.7 years) underwent 97 MSVs. The mean operative duration was 65 min for unilateral and 112 min for bilateral MSVs. The mean follow-up was 10.1 months, during which time four (5%) complications were identified: two hydroceles (one resolving spontaneously after 4 months), one orchalgia (resolving after 8 months) and one hypertrophic scar. During the follow-up period, no orchitis, infection, haematoma, recurrence of varicocele, or testicular atrophy was identified.

Comment

This technique provides another good approach for the surgical management of varicocele, with a low incidence of complication. However, the technique is technically challenging, relatively slow, and the data are of course from a single centre, which has both the equipment necessary and the experience to perform MSV.

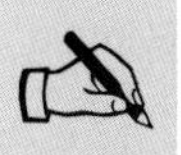

A new classification for genital ambiguity and urogenital sinus anomalies

Rink RC, Adams MC, Misseri R. *BJU Int* 2005; **95**: 638–42

BACKGROUND. Currently, ambiguous genitalia and urogenital sinus anomalies tend to be described by the degree of masculinization (Prader's classification) and by describing the urogenital sinus as simply high or low. This system is often too subjective and can fail adequately to describe the wide spectrum of these complex anomalies. The authors of this study describe a new classification system that allows for more detailed and anatomically precise description.

INTERPRETATION. The PVE classification system includes phallic size (P), the true location of vaginal confluence in relation to the bladder neck and perineal meatus (V) and external genital appearance (E). The phallic measurement ($P_{e,w}$) is the maximal extension (P_e) of the phallus (cm), from the pubis to the glans tip, and the phallic width (P_w). $V_{b,m}$ is measured cystoscopically, using a calibrated catheter, and records the distance from the bladder neck to the confluence of the urogenital sinus (V_b) and from the confluence to the perineal meatus (V_m). The original 1–5 Prader designations are used for the 'E' component, with the addition of 0 for normal external genitalia and 6 for rare variants (Fig. 1.2).

Comment

This new classification system allows a more detailed and reproducible description of the spectrum of anomalies seen. This should allow better planning and more accurate comparison between techniques, ultimately aimed at improving the outcome in these complex conditions.

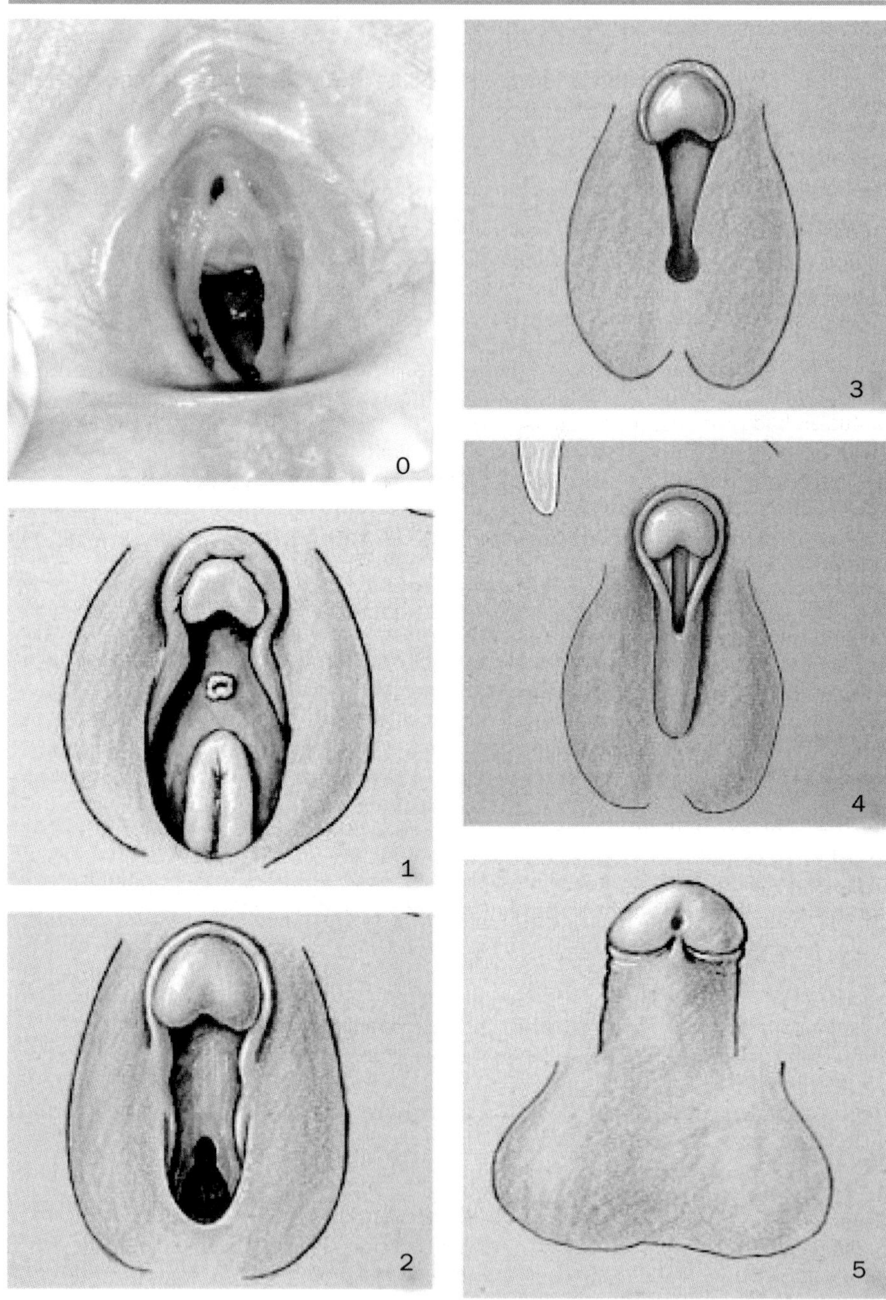
0
1
2
3
4
5

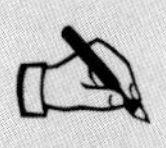

Trying to predict 'dangerous' bladders in children: the 'area under the curve' concept

Hashim H, Ellis-Jones J, Swithinbank L, *et al.* *J Pediatr Urol* 2005; **1**: 343–7

Background. Bladder compliance, using conventional urodynamic studies, is determined from initial and end detrusor pressures compared with the fill volume. In children with neuropathic bladders, high-pressure detrusor overactivity may occur throughout the study. This limited study introduced the concept of the area under the detrusor pressure curve (AUC) as a potential predictor of an unsafe bladder.

Interpretation. AUC was determined using computer software. Only 11% (15/130) of patients had analysable data because of various technical problems: 33 studies had recording problems; 66 studies had not been stored; 31 studies were too big to download between software packages (limited by a DOS-based system). There was no reported correlation between the AUC and predicting 'dangerous' bladders.

Comment

This preliminary study introduced an interesting concept, but was unable to draw any conclusions. Further work is clearly necessary to determine whether AUC has any role in predicting risk of upper tract deterioration.

Conclusion

The systematic review from Sing-Grewal *et al.* is one of the most important papers published recently. Not surprisingly, the interpretation of the results is greatly influenced by the nationality of the reader. US urologists conclude that the data support routine newborn circumcision, whereas UK urologists would generally reserve circumcision for those boys with recurrent or significant risk of UTI, e.g. in vesicoureteric reflux or with posterior urethral valves. Deeb and Hughes' paper is interesting as it raises awareness of the possibility of androgen insensitivity presenting with an inguinal hernia in a phenotypically normal female, and David Gough's team's paper should be applauded as one of the first objective reports documenting cosmetic outcome following hypospadias surgery.

Fig. 1.2 (*opposite*) Prader classification 1–5 (1, female external genitalia with clitoromegaly; 2, clitoromegaly with partial labial fusion forming a funnel-shaped urogenital sinus; 3, increased phallic size with complete labioscrotal fusion forming a urogenital sinus with a single opening; 4, complete scrotal fusion with the opening of the urogenital sinus at the base of the phallus; 5, normal male external genitalia) and the added classes of 0 to represent normal anatomy and 6 to represent variants difficult to categorize. Source: Rink *et al.* (2005).

The series of papers looking at MCDK, hypertension and nephrectomy has provided us with some useful information. Rabelo *et al.*'s data would suggest that an initial renal length <62 mm is associated with complete MCDK involution, but the numbers in this study were small and, more data are needed before this is used in discussions with parents. Narchi *et al.*'s paper has demonstrated that the risk of hypertension developing in childhood secondary to MCDK is approximately 1 in 200, and Johal *et al.* showed that blood pressure should return to normal in approximately 80% of children undergoing nephrectomy for unilateral renal disease.

Animal data suggest that abnormalities in germ cell turnover explain the reduced fertility associated with undescended testes. Ofordeme *et al.* looked at germ cell proliferation and apoptosis in children undergoing orchidopexy and found no evidence of disorder of either. Of course, surgery was only performed after 6 months of age, so it remains possible that abnormalities could have existed prior to surgery, but this will prove difficult to confirm.

Schiff *et al.*'s paper reports excellent results following microsurgical varicocelectomy. This is clearly a technically challenging procedure requiring access to an operating microscope, so it is likely that the laparoscopic Palomo will remain the procedure of choice for most paediatric urologists. Rink *et al.* published an extremely important new classification system for urogenital sinus anomalies. This system provides an objective reproducible method of description of the anatomical abnormalities seen, which should allow various centres to compare data properly and therefore learn from each other. Finally, the concept of 'area under the curve' was introduced by Paul Abram's unit as a possible predictor of 'dangerous bladders'. The data from this small study were limited, and further reports are awaited with interest.

References

1. Schoen EJ. Circumcision for preventing urinary tract infections in boys: North American view. *Arch Dis Child* 2005; **90**: 772–3.
2. Malone PSJ. Circumcision for preventing urinary tract infection in boys: European view. *Arch Dis Child* 2005; **90**: 773–4.

2

Advances in uroradiological imaging

CONOR CORR, MARK THORNTON

Introduction

As the technology of cross-sectional imaging modalities increases, the potential clinical applications of these modalities will inevitably expand, often with a corresponding decrease in the usage of more traditional techniques. Predictably, there is a large body of literature regarding the increasing role of both computed tomography (CT) and magnetic resonance imaging (MRI) in many areas of uroradiology.

This section aims to review some of the best recent papers which demonstrate the increasing role of cross-sectional techniques in uroradiology. There is also a paper that adds further evidence to the importance of image-guided ablation of renal tumours.

The three main sections in this chapter relate to renal tumours, bladder cancer and CT urography (CTU) and pyelography. The roles of CT and MRI in diagnosing, staging and guiding treatment in bladder and renal cancers are discussed. The increasingly accepted role of CTU, despite the potentially large radiation dose, in imaging the collecting system and ureters for both urolithiasis and urothelial tumours is the other main topic.

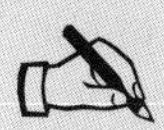

MRI for preoperative staging of renal cell carcinoma using the 1997 TNM classification: comparison with surgical and pathologic staging

Ergen FB, Hussain HK, Caoili EM, *et al. AJR Am J Roentgenol* 2004; **182**: 217–25

BACKGROUND. With the advent of conservative approaches to surgery for renal cell carcinoma, accurate pre-operative staging is increasingly important. This study was planned to determine the accuracy of MRI staging, using surgical pathological staging for comparison.

Interpretation. MRI was a good technique for staging (81–86% accuracy), and very good for tumour thrombus demonstration (93%). It was poor for nodal staging, however, with most of the pathologically involved nodes understaged, as well as 16% of the N0 (Node 0) tumours being overstaged. It also has poor coverage and missed one of the two distant metastases.

Comment

This study shows that MRI can have a role in the staging of renal cell carcinoma, but it does not indicate that it should replace CT as the primary mode of staging. CT is the standard method for staging at present, as it gives similar local staging accuracy when compared with MRI |**1–3**|, but also stages the chest on the same examination. With modern multislice CT scanners, good staging information can also be gained from the bones. As stated by the authors, this study looked mainly at symptomatic tumours, whereas renal cancers commonly present as small incidental tumours.

The MRI findings were compared with the pathological findings, but the important factor is whether it is a better staging tool than CT, and this was not discussed. Even in this study, the patients needed a CT of their chest, as well as the MRI.

Without data comparing CT and MRI, it is difficult to recommend MRI over CT at present as the standard staging tool, especially as CT of the chest is still required. A study by Hallsteidt *et al.* (2004) |**4**| did, however, do a comparison and showed CT and MRI to have similar accuracy in staging renal carcinoma. In this study, Ergen *et al.* have also shown that MRI is an accurate way of staging renal cell carcinoma locally, particularly vena cava spread |**1,2,5**|, and it may be a useful adjunct to CT in difficult cases. Further study is required before it can become the first-choice local staging tool for renal cell carcinoma.

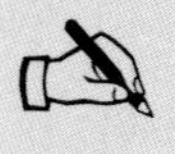

Evaluation of cystic renal masses: comparison of CT and MR imaging by using the Bosniak classification system

Israel GM, Hindman N, Bosniak MA. *Radiology* 2004; **231**: 365–71

Background. The Bosniak classification is an accepted way of stratifying the risk of malignancy in cystic renal masses on CT |6,7|. It has been in use for several years and is based on certain characteristics of the cyst—number and thickness of septa, presence of solid components, presence of calcification and enhancement pattern. MRI is a useful tool in imaging renal lesions |8,9|, especially those with contraindications to iodinated contrast and also in young patients in whom repeated high doses of radiation in CT should be avoided. This study aims to compare the efficacy of MRI with that of CT.

Interpretation. Findings on MRI and CT were similar in 56 out of 69 (81%) cystic renal lesions. In 7 of the remaining 13 cases, the differences were enough to grade the lesions differently, using the same criteria for CT and MRI. MRI tended to show more septa and thicker septa, leading to a tendency to upgrade the lesion. The authors concluded that MRI is a useful tool in characterizing renal cystic lesions, but in borderline cases, CT correlation should be given.

Comment

The Bosniak classification is based on CT findings. Therefore, if MRI was used to characterize cystic renal lesions using Bosniak, the results may be spurious, as these imaging modalities may give different information on similar lesions. Before using MRI, it should be shown that it gives similar information to CT.

This study showed that, in 62 out of 69 cases, the classification would have been the same on CT as on MRI. However, the other seven cases would have been upgraded if MRI was used. The conclusion is that MRI is a useful tool in evaluating cystic renal lesions as it gives similar information to CT. However, in borderline cases, CT correlation is advised. The Bosniak classification using CT is still the most robust system available. This study does not recommend that MRI should replace CT in evaluating cystic tumours, but it can be used successfully in certain circumstances.

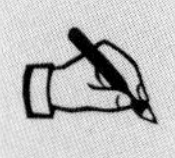

Percutaneous CT-guided radiofrequency ablation of renal neoplasms: factors influencing success

Zagoria RJ, Hawkins AD, Clark PE, *et al. AJR Am J Roentgenol* 2004; **183**(1): 201–7

BACKGROUND. Percutaneous radiofrequency ablation (RFA) is a relatively new but promising method of treating several types of tumour. For it to become an established part of treatment algorithms for particular tumours, its efficacy and safety must be proven. There are several studies which demonstrate that RFA is effective in treating small renal tumours |10–13|. This paper attempts to add further evidence that RFA is a safe and effective method of treating small renal tumours that are not suitable for surgery. It also discusses features that predict the success of the procedure.

INTERPRETATION. The results from the RFA for renal cell carcinoma in this study were very promising, in line with other studies. There were good results for immediate ablation and recurrence, with low complications. Although there were only 22 patients involved, it still adds valuable evidence to the belief that RFA is an important method of treating small renal cell carcinoma where surgery is not considered ideal.

Comment

Twenty-seven RFA sessions were performed in 24 tumours in 22 patients. Twenty out of 22 patients had no demonstrable tumour on follow-up. Most patients required only one session. There were several minor complications, such as small haemotomas and pain, but no major complication. The factors that correlated with success in one session were small tumour size (<3 cm) and performing an immediate contrast-enhanced CT of the area before the end of the session. This allowed the operator to ablate any enhancing area before finishing. Follow-up was 1–35 months.

Many patients are not ideally suited for surgery because of a comorbid condition or lack of functioning renal tissue. A technique that easily allows for treatment of small tumours is very valuable. Interpreted with other similar studies, this study gives further useful evidence for the efficacy of this technique. It indicates that those tumours <3 cm are the most likely to be treated successfully in one session, although tumours up to 7 cm were treated successfully, and that contrast-enhanced CT should be performed before finishing, if possible.

Overall, this was a useful study that adds further evidence that RFA is a useful modality in the treatment of small renal cell carcinomas when surgery is not suitable. Further study will be required to demonstrate whether it will become the treatment of choice for small renal tumours in all patients.

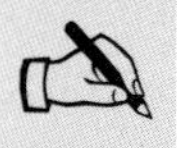

Patient radiation dose at CT urography and conventional urography

Nawfel RD, Judy PF, Schleipman AR. *Radiology* 2004; **232**: 126–32

BACKGROUND. CT urography is an accurate modality in diagnosing many renal tract abnormalities. It provides images of the kidneys, ureters and bladder, and pathologies outside the urinary tract. This makes it a very attractive alternative to the conventional intravenous pyelogramme (IVP), and it is advocated by many that it should completely replace the IVP |14–16|. However, there are concerns about the potentially high radiation doses of CTU. This study was designed to compare the dose of CTU and IVPs.

INTERPRETATION. The study showed that CTU had on average 1.5 (15 mSv [milliSeiverts] vs 10 mSv) times the radiation dose of the standard IVP. However, the IVP protocol used in the study included several tomograms and oblique views, which is not typical of an IVP in the UK (typical IVP here 2.4 mSv |**17**|). Therefore, CTU would be a much greater dose than a standard IVP in the UK, possibly up to six times the dose. However, the CTU dose could also be reduced if the number of acquisitions were reduced to target specific conditions.

Comment

The standard IVP is still a useful test but is often suboptimal for many technical factors. Even a technically perfect IVP gives limited information on renal parenchymal lesions and lesions compressing the urinary tract. CTU would go a long way to solving these problems if it could be performed at safe dose levels.

A full CT urogram includes:

- pre-contrast scan of the renal tract, mainly looking for calculi;
- venous phase scans of the kidneys for assessment of renal parenchymal lesions;
- delayed images to image the pelvicaliceal system, ureters and bladder, primarily looking for obstructive level and urothelial lesions.

The paper notes that one or more of these acquisitions can be dropped, depending on the indication for the scan. Also, single acquisition can be performed after two separate contrast boluses |**16**|, one after 2 min and one after approximately 10–15 min, which gives the venous and delayed phases in one scan. Another way of reducing the dose was to tailor the radiographic parameters when possible to the size of the patient.

The paper reaches a sensible conclusion, in that CTU may replace the IVP because of the increased diagnostic information, but that the dose should not be forgotten. Efforts should be made only to perform the acquisitions that are necessary, and stringent dose monitoring should be in place so that the maximum information can be gained with the smallest possible dose.

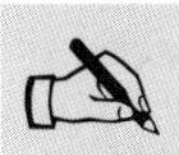

Multislice CT urography: state of the art

Noroozian M, Cohan RH, Caoili EM, Cowan NC, Ellis JH. *Br J Radiol* 2004; **77**: S74–86

Background. There are several imaging investigations for diseases of the urinary tract—ultrasound (US), IVP, CT, MRI and nuclear medicine. Often, a patient will have several investigations. A single examination that could effectively and safely examine the whole urinary tract in a majority of cases would be desirable in terms of clinical usefulness, cost and convenience. CTU promises to be such an examination. This paper examines the evidence for using CTU in examining the whole urinary tract, including imaging for renal masses, urolithiasis and urothelial lesions.

Interpretation. CTU is a very promising test with several advantages over conventional investigations. It can investigate urolithiasis, renal cancer and urothelial lesions with higher levels of accuracy than conventional methods, and also give diagnostic information for non-urinary structures in the abdomen. However, the radiation dose is high, as discussed previously and, although the diagnostic accuracy in all aspects of using CTU is very promising, further data are needed so that the role of this high-dose examination can be fully defined.

Comment

As discussed previously, the radiation dose of CTU is high. This is due to the fact that thin slices are used and there are multiple acquisitions. The dose can, however, be reduced by targeting the examination to each patient, thus possibly allowing one acquisition to be dropped. Also, a split bolus technique can be used, which allows for examination in the nephrographic phase and excretory phase in a single acquisition.

All the data on CTU are very promising |**14,15,18**|. It is accepted as superior to IVP and US in renal masses and urolithiasis. Now several studies show it to be accurate in detecting upper tract lesions, with one study showing it to be more sensitive than retrograde pyelography.

As the resolution of CT scanners increases, the use of CTU is inevitably going to increase, with many feeling that it will replace the IVP. As experience increases and the technique is refined, this may happen within the next several years.

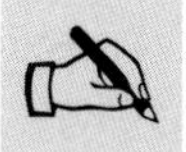

Antegrade MDCT pyelography for the evaluation of patients with obstructed urinary tract

Ghersin E, Brook OR, Meretik S, *et al.* *AJR Am J Roentgenol* 2004; **183**: 1691–6

BACKGROUND. Patients with obstructed urinary tracts may be easily diagnosed by unenhanced CT or IVP. However, especially when the cause is not urolithiasis, other investigations are often needed. Also, IVP is often contraindicated because of impaired renal function. This paper aims to show that antegrade multidetector CT (MDCT) is an accurate method for diagnosing the cause of obstruction that can also be used safely in patients with renal impairment.

INTERPRETATION. In patients with high-grade urinary tract obstruction, antegrade multislice CT pyelography accurately diagnosed the site and cause of the obstruction in all 21 patients. It was performed in patients whose diagnosis was equivocal on conventional imaging (usually conventional antegrade pyelography). This may be a helpful method of diagnosing the cause of urinary tract obstruction in difficult cases, especially those who have a nephrostomy *in situ*.

Comment

Prone unenhanced computed tomographic scanning of the renal tract (CTKUB) often gives the diagnosis in obstructed patients, but there are still patients whose diagnosis is equivocal after CTKUB, and in whom IVP or CTU is unsuitable on account of renal failure. Direct injection of contrast into the dilated pelvicaliceal, i.e. conventional antegrade pyelography (nephrostogram if nephrostomy *in situ*), can be the next step.

This study shows that antegrade pyelography using MDCT was more accurate than conventional antegrade pyelography in giving the cause of the obstruction. The causes included urolithiasis, transitional cell carcinomas (TCCs) of bladder and ureter, ureteric stricture, external compression by nodes and retroperitoneal fibrosis.

Although the study was small, it indicates that MDCT antegrade pyelography is a good way of diagnosing the cause of urinary tract obstruction when the initial investigations are equivocal. It can be used in renal failure and would be particularly useful in those patients with nephrostomies already in place.

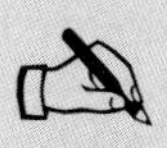

Bladder cancer: analysis of multidetector row helical CT enhancement pattern and accuracy in tumor detection and perivesical staging

Kim JK, Park SY, Ahn HJ, Kim CS, Cho KS. *Radiology* 2004; **231**: 725–31

BACKGROUND. Clinical staging of bladder carcinoma is often inaccurate, and a reliable radiological method of locally staging this tumour would be helpful in planning treatment. MRI and CT have both been used in bladder cancer staging, and there has been disagreement as to which is most effective |19,20|. The recent advent of multislice CT technology has allowed for higher resolution scanning, with possibly increasing accuracy. The authors of this paper attempt to show that CT is an accurate tool in detecting and staging bladder carcinoma.

INTERPRETATION. CT had sensitivity and positive predictive value of 97% and 95%, respectively, in detecting bladder cancers. This increased to 100% if the CT was left for >7 days post transurethral resection of bladder tumour (TURBT). For perivesical staging, the sensitivity, specificity and accuracy were 89%, 95% and 93%, respectively. The optimal time delay post-contrast was 60–80 s. CT was felt to be an accurate tool in detecting and locally staging advanced TCC of the bladder if a dedicated multislice CT examination was performed.

Comment

Initially, 20 patients had multiphase post-contrast scans of their bladders pre TURBT. This was in order to see which phase gave most enhancement, so that this could then be used in the subsequent patients in the study. A period of 60–80 s was found to be the optimal phase of enhancement. A further 67 patients underwent CT after TURBT for proven cancer, then had radical cystectomy. Their CT and histology results were compared. All patients were scanned with a full bladder.

Seventy-five out of 77 lesions found on histological examination of the cystectomy specimens were correctly identified on CT. There were four false positives. Eleven of the 13 <1 cm cancers were detected. All cancers above 1 cm were seen on CT. The missed cancers were in CTs performed <7 days post TURBT. Sixteen tumours had histologically proven perivesical invasion. CT had one false positive and one false negative.

Note, however, as acknowledged by the authors, that there was a bias in the patient population, as only patients deemed suitable for cystectomy post TURBT were included. Those with superficial, small or low-grade cancers not requiring cystectomy were excluded.

These results are better than those obtained previously with CT, and they compare favourably with previous studies using contrast-enhanced MRI |**19–21**|. This study was slightly less sensitive but more specific for perivesical invasion than previous MRI studies, and cancer detection rates were similar. The improved results for CT in this study were felt to result from using multislice CT with optimal scan delay time after contrast.

CT performed optimally with a multislice CT is an accurate tool for detection and local staging of advanced TCC of the bladder. A scan delay of 60–80 s is ideal. The accuracy increases if the CT is left for 7 days, although the numbers involved were small.

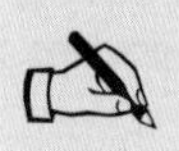

Urinary bladder cancer: preoperative nodal staging with ferumoxtran-10-enhanced MR imaging

Deserno WM, Harisinghani MG, Taupitz M, *et al. Radiology* 2004; **233**: 449–56

Background. Lymph node involvement is an important factor in formulating management plans in patients with bladder cancer. In patients considered for radical cystectomy, lymph node positivity would mean that adjuvant chemotherapy was required, or that surgery was not appropriate if the lymph node involvement was widespread. Also, removal of all involved lymph nodes is said to improve survival |22,23|. At present, pre-operative staging using CT or unenhanced MRI is insensitive. A more sensitive technique would help in pre-operative planning.

Interpretation. In 58 patients, 172 nodes imaged with MRI before and after ferumoxtran were compared with histological findings. Fifty were malignant, and 122 were benign. The sensitivity was 96% for post-ferumoxtran and 76% for the non-contrast scans, which was statistically significant. The negative predictive value was 98% versus 91% for before and after contrast, again significant. Thus, post-ferumoxtran MRI is a more sensitive method for detecting malignant lymph nodes in bladder cancer, and potentially improves the accuracy of lymph node dissection by giving the surgeon an accurate map of positively involved lymph nodes.

Comment

The attraction of using iron particles in scanning for malignant lymph nodes is that it may demonstrate involvement in normal-sized nodes. Conventionally, lymph node size has been relied upon, but this is inaccurate. Normal lymph nodes have been shown to take up iron particles uniformly, thus having a diffuse drop in signal on gradient echo T2 scans (T2*). If the gland is involved, the signal drop will be absent or heterogeneous |**24–28**|.

In this study, patients considered for surgery had pre- and post-contrast scans. Lymph nodes were regarded as malignant if they were oval and >10 mm or round and >8 mm on the pre-contrast scan. On the post-contrast scan, lymph nodes were considered to be malignant if the signal drop was absent or heterogeneous. There were no significant complications of ferumoxtran, but it was slightly cumbersome in that it needs to be infused over 30 min and scanned the next day.

The post-contrast scans were significantly more sensitive, but very slightly less specific (not significant). The clinical effect of the lower sensitivity is low, as it leads only to dissection of a few extra lymph nodes. All positive lymph nodes on MRI, before or after contrast, were confirmed via lymph node dissection or image-guided biopsy.

The clinical effect was to direct the surgeon to perform a slightly wider lymph node dissection in 9 of the 50 patients. Further study is required on how this imaging technique can alter overall management decisions and surgical technique. This study does, however, indicate that post-ferumoxtran MRI is more sensitive in detecting positive lymph nodes in bladder cancer than conventional MRI, which may improve the accuracy of pre-operative staging and surgical resection.

Conclusion

These papers continue the trend of emphasizing the increasing clinical usefulness of cross-sectional techniques in uroradiology, in keeping with similar changes in most other radiological sub-specialities. The increasing resolution of multislice CT scanners has led to the expansion of the indications for their use.

CT can be used successfully to image the kidneys and collecting systems in one examination for renal and urothelial lesions and urolithiasis. CT is also an accurate way of staging and localizing bladder tumours. It is still uncertain as to whether CT or MRI is superior in staging renal and bladder tumours, but both modalities can play important roles. Radiation dose considerations are still important but, as techniques are being refined, the dose burden of CT can be decreased. With the use of iron oxide contrast, MRI can be used to detect metastatic bladder cancer in small lymph nodes. This may become part of the standard staging protocol, but further study is needed to confirm its clinical usefulness.

Another paper relating to the success of percutaneous RFA for renal tumours was discussed. This is now established as a successful technique in treating small tumours in patients unsuitable for surgery. The next step may be that it becomes the first-line therapy for all patients with small renal tumours.

References

1. Hallscheidt P, Stolte E, Roeren T, Pomer S, Drehmer I, Kauffmann GW. [The staging of renal-cell carcinomas in MRT and CT—a prospective histologically controlled study.] *Rofo* 1998; **168**(2): 165–70.
2. Torricelli P, Puviani M, De Santis M, Nasi G, Pollastri C. [Magnetic resonance in the staging of renal carcinoma. The results compared with computed tomography in 42 cases.] *Radiol Med (Torino)* 1992; **84**(1–2): 85–91.

3. Heidenreich A, Ravery V; European Society of Oncological Urology. Preoperative imaging in renal cell cancer. *World J Urol* 2004; **22**(5): 307–15.

4. Hallscheidt PJ, Bock M, Riedasch G, Zuna I, Schoenberg SO, Autschbach F, Soder M, Noeldge G. Diagnostic accuracy of staging renal cell carcinomas using multidetector-row computed tomography and magnetic resonance imaging: a prospective study with histopathologic correlation. *J Comput Assist Tomogr* 2004; **28**(3): 333–9.

5. Hallscheidt P, Pomer S, Roeren T, Kauffmann GW, Staehler G. [Preoperative staging of renal cell carcinoma with caval thrombus: is staging in MRI justified? Prospective histopathological correlated study.] *Urologe A* 2000; **39**(1): 36–40.

6. Koga S, Nishikido M, Inuzuka S, Sakamoto I, Hayashi T, Hayashi K, Saito Y, Kanetake H. An evaluation of Bosniak's radiological classification of cystic renal masses. *BJU Int* 2000; **86**(6): 607–9.

7. Aronson S, Frazier HA, Baluch JD, Hartman DS, Christenson PJ. Cystic renal masses: usefulness of the Bosniak classification. *Urol Radiol* 1991; **13**(2): 83–90.

8. Ho VB, Choyke PL. MR evaluation of solid renal masses. *Magn Reson Imaging Clin N Am* 2004; **12**(3): 413–27.

9. Israel GM, Bosniak MA. MR imaging of cystic renal masses. *Magn Reson Imaging Clin N Am* 2004; **12**(3): 403–12.

10. Johnson DB, Cadeddu JA. Radiofrequency ablation of small renal tumors. *Expert Rev Anticancer Ther* 2004; **4**(1): 77–83.

11. Lui KW, Gervais DA, Arellano RA, Mueller PR. Radiofrequency ablation of renal cell carcinoma. *Clin Radiol* 2003; **58**(12): 905–13.

12. Chiou YY, Hwang JI, Chou YH, Wang JH, Chiang JH, Chang CY. Percutaneous radiofrequency ablation of renal cell carcinoma. *J Chinese Med Assoc* 2005; **68**(5): 221–5.

13. Mahnken AH, Gunther RW, Tacke J. Radiofrequency ablation of renal tumors. *Eur Radiol* 2004; **14**(8): 1449–55.

14. Lin WC, Wang JH, Wei CJ, Chang CY. Assessment of CT urography in the diagnosis of urinary tract abnormalities. *J Chinese Med Assoc* 2004; **67**(2): 73–8.

15. Akbar SA, Mortele KJ, Baeyens K, Kekelidze M, Silverman SG. Multidetector CT urography: techniques, clinical applications, and pitfalls. *Semin Ultrasound CT MR* 2004; **25**(1): 41–54.

16. Noroozian M, Cohan RH, Caoili EM, Cowan NC, Ellis JH. Multislice CT urography: state of the art. *Br J Radiol* 2004; **77**(Spec No 1): S74–86.

17. Royal College of Radiologists. *Making the best use of a department of clinical radiology*, 5th edn. London: Royal College of Radiologists, 2003.

18. Caoili EM, Inampudi P, Cohan RH, Ellis JH. Optimization of multidetector row CT urography: effect of compression, saline administration, and prolongation of acquisition delay. *Radiology* 1005; **235**(1): 116–23.

19. Barentsz JO, Jager GJ, Witjes JA, Ruijs JH. Primary staging of urinary bladder carcinoma: the role of MRI and a comparison with CT. *Eur Radiol* 1006; **6**(2): 129–33.

20. Husband JE, Olliff JF, Williams MP, Heron CW, Cherryman GR. Bladder cancer: staging with CT and MR imaging. *Radiology* 1989; **173**(2): 435–40.

21. Tekes A, Kamel I, Imam K, Szarf G, Schoenberg M, Nasir K, Thompson R, Bluemke D. Dynamic MRI of bladder cancer: evaluation of staging accuracy. *AJR Am J Roentgenol* 2005; **184**(1): 121–7.

22. Herr HW. Extent of surgery and pathology evaluation has an impact on bladder cancer outcomes after radical cystectomy. *Urology* 2003; **61**: 105–8.

23. Leissner J, Allhoff EP, Hohenfellner R, Wolf HK. [Significance of pelvic lymphadenectomy for the prognosis after radical cystectomy.] *Zentralbl Chir* 2002; **127**: 315–21.

24. Anzai Y, Piccoli CW, Outwater EK, Stanford W, Bluemke DA, Nurenberg P, Saini S, Maravilla KR, Feldman DE, Schmiedl UP, Brunberg JA, Francis IR, Harms SE, Som PM, Tempany CM. Evaluation of neck and body metastases to nodes with ferumoxtran 10-enhanced MR imaging: phase III safety and efficacy study. *Radiology* 2003; **228**(3): 777–88.

25. Rockall Ag, Sohaib SA, Harisinghani MG, Babar SA, Singh N, Jeyarajah AR, Oram DH, Jacobs IJ, Shepherd JH, Reznek RH. Diagnostic performance of nanoparticle-enhanced magnetic resonance imaging in the diagnosis of lymph node metastases in patients with endometrial and cervical cancer. *J Clin Oncol* 2005; **23**(12): 2813–21.

26. Harisinghani MG, Dixon WT, Saksena MA, Brachtel E, Belzek DJ, Dhawale PJ, Torabi M, Hahn PF. MR lymphangiography: imaging strategies to optimize the imaging of lymph nodes with ferumoxtran-10. *RadioGraphics* 2004; **24**(3): 867–78.

27. Bellin MF, Lebleu L, Meric JB. Evaluation of retroperitoneal and pelvic lymph node metastases with MRI and MR lymphangiography. *Abdom Imaging* 2003; **28**(2): 155–63.

28. Harisinghani MG, Saini S, Weissleder R, Hahn PF, Yantiss RK, Tempany C, Wood BJ, Mueller PR. MR lymphangiography using ultrasmall superparamagnetic iron oxide in patients with primary abdominal and pelvic malignancies: radiographic–pathologic correlation. *AJR Am J Roentgenol* 1999; **172**(5): 1347–51.

3

Quality of life

KATHERINE KENNEDY, RUARAIDH MACDONAGH

Introduction

In 1948, the World Health Organization defined health as 'a state of complete physical, mental and social well-being and not merely the absence of disease or infirmity'. This definition is fundamental to medical practice and highlights the importance of the holistic approach to patient care. Historically, disease has been viewed in terms of a biomedical model, with the outcome of treatment measured only in terms of death, disability or cure [1]. Over recent years, however, the concept of Quality of Life (QoL) has gained increasing significance, with huge expansion in research in this field. QoL has been defined as 'an individual's overall satisfaction with life and their general sense of well being' [2]. It is undoubtedly a complex and subjective issue and is related not only to the physical, functional, psychological and social health of an individual, but also to their cultural expectations. Figure 3.1 summarizes this concept.

Over the last 10 years, urologists have embraced the importance of QoL, as illustrated by the large number of papers published on this topic. The papers chosen for this chapter come from study centres around the world, and cover a range of urological conditions, displaying the importance of QoL across our whole speciality. The papers included demonstrate the use of a selection of QoL questionnaires, some generic (e.g. the Short Form 36 questionnaire (SF-36)) and some disease specific (e.g. the European Organisation for Research into the Treatment of Cancer QoL questionnaire (EORTC QLQ-C30)). As research into QoL increases, so does the development of questionnaires to assess it. The development of a new QoL questionnaire is a complex process that should follow well-established methodology. Questionnaires should demonstrate three important criteria: validity (the degree to which the measure reflects what it is intended to measure rather than something else); reliability (the ability of the measure to produce consistent results); and responsiveness (the sensitivity of the measure to detect clinically significant change). The majority of papers reviewed in this chapter use questionnaires that have been appropriately psychometrically validated.

The following chapter includes a review of ten papers that demonstrate the importance of QoL in both benign and malignant urological conditions. It also

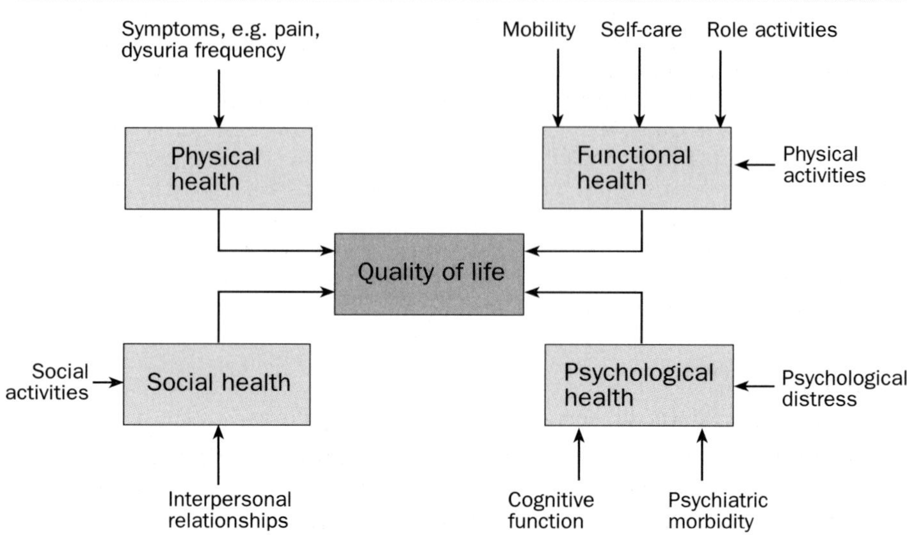

Fig. 3.1 The multidimensional concept of Quality of Life. Source: MacDonagh (1996) |**1**|.

highlights the importance of assessing QoL in addition to other outcome measures when targeting treatment to the individual patient.

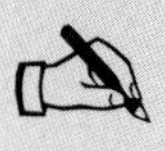

Combination treatment with an alpha-blocker plus an anticholinergic for bladder outlet obstruction: a prospective, randomized, controlled study

Athanasopoulos A, Gyftopoulos K, Giannitsas K, Fisfis J, Perimensis P, Barbalias G. *J Urol* 2003; **169**: 2253–6

BACKGROUND. Benign prostatic hyperplasia (BPH) is a common condition, affecting as many as 70% of men over 60. Patients may suffer from 'voiding' or 'storage' symptoms or, commonly, a combination of both. Historically, clinicians have prescribed medication to alleviate the predominating symptom complex, i.e. anticholinergics for storage symptoms and alpha-blockers for voiding symptoms. In their study, Athanasopoulos *et al.* aimed to assess the effect of tolterodine combined with tamsulosin on QoL in men with urodynamically proven mild or moderate bladder outflow obstruction and concomitant detrusor instability. Fifty patients were recruited after urodynamics and asked to complete the 'UROLIFE'™ BPH QoL questionnaire. All patients initially took 0.4 mg of tamsulosin orally once daily for one week. Patients were then randomly allocated to group 1, tamsulosin alone (i.e. control group); or group 2, tamsulosin plus tolterodine 2 mg orally twice a day. At 3 months, urodynamics and questionnaires were repeated.

Interpretation. At 3 months from baseline, there was a statistically significant ($P = 0.0003$) improvement in QoL score in patients in group 2 (combination treatment) with mean QoL scores before and after treatment of 525 and 628, respectively, as demonstrated in Fig. 3.2. There was also no increase in the incidence of acute urinary retention (AUR) in this group. There was no significant improvement in QoL in group 1 patients (tamsulosin alone). Detailed analysis revealed that the improvement in QoL in group 2 was due to improvement in items 1–6 in the questionnaire (related to urinary symptoms and general life). Interestingly, there was no improvement in items 7–9 (related to sexual function) in either group. Both groups showed a significant improvement in maximum flow rate and volume at first contraction, although this was not enough to cause an improvement in QoL in group 1 patients.

Comment

This prospective randomized study demonstrates good design, using a matched control group and urodynamically proven disease. However, patients in this study had low baseline post-void residual volumes, and those with severe obstruction were excluded from the trial. Caution should therefore be used if applying these results to the general population, especially those with high post-void residual volumes who may be at risk of retention with administration of anticholinergics. Of note, the authors had expected an improvement in sexual function domains, secondary to general improvements in lower urinary tract symptoms (LUTS) and thus overall well-being. Although this did not occur, it may have been due to the

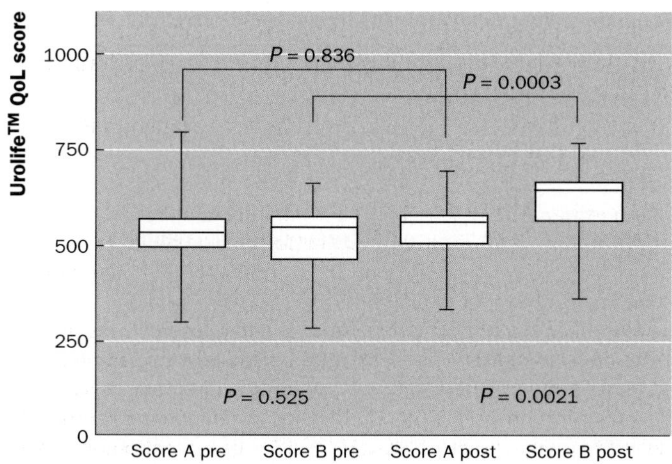

Fig. 3.2 Differences in QoL scores from baseline and between groups before and after treatment. Top *P*-values indicate differences within groups, and bottom *P*-values indicate differences between groups before and after treatment. Source: Athanasopoulos *et al.* (2003).

short follow-up time of the study. Storage symptoms are mainly attributable to detrusor instability, which is thought to occur in 40–60% of patients with benign prostatic obstruction or bladder outlet obstruction. This study suggests that, for these patients, combination therapy may be the key to maximal symptom reduction and maximum improvement in QoL. If applied, this study could change practice for the majority of urologists.

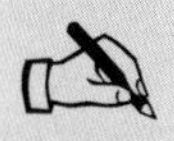

Acute urinary retention: what is the impact on patients' quality of life?

Thomas K, Oades G, Taylor-Hay C, Kirby R. *BJU Int* 2005; **95**(1): 72–6

BACKGROUND. The risk of an episode of AUR has been identified as 1.6% at 5 years for men aged 40–49 and 10% at 70–79 years |3|. This condition is rarely life threatening and is often treated with less importance, and perhaps less compassion, than other 'emergency' admissions. Patients are, however, often in severe pain until catheterized. In this paper, Thomas *et al.* aimed to assess the impact of AUR on patients' Health-Related Quality of Life (HRQoL) compared with the impact of admission for elective surgery for BPH and renal colic (RC). The study consisted of three patient groups: group 1, men aged over 50 presenting to Accident and Emergency (A&E) with AUR (*n* = 43); group 2, men aged over 50 admitted for elective surgery for BPH (*n* = 35); and group 3, men aged over 40 presenting to A&E with RC (*n* = 17). A questionnaire was completed within 72 hours of the first admission and again at 1, 2, 3 and 6 months. This consisted of a combination of elements from several existing HRQoL and health economic questionnaires, as shown in Table 3.1.

INTERPRETATION. Patients in group 1 underwent more investigations than patients in the other groups, had more attendances at A&E and more hospital admissions during the study period. Analysis of the Visual Analogue Pain Score (0 representing no pain, 10 representing most severe pain) revealed that group 3 had the worst mean pain score with a value of 8.3. Interestingly, group 1 also reported high pain scores with a mean value of 7.7. Patients in group 1 were also significantly more concerned about inability to

Table 3.1 The HRQoL instruments used to form the present questionnaire

Instrument	Domain measured
AUR pain and discomfort	Pain and discomfort
International Prostate Symptom Score (IPSS)	Frequency of urinary symptoms
BPH impact index	Impact of urinary problems
BPH symptom interference assessment	Impact of urinary problems
Urinary-specific worries and concerns	Worry, concern and embarrassment
Hospital Anxiety and Depression Score	Anxiety and depression
Euro-QoL	General health
Health utilization questionnaire	Use of healthcare resources
Medical Outcome Study Short-Form 12	General health

Source: Thomas *et al.* (2005).

urinate than patients in group 2. Fifteen per cent of group 1 patients reported the need to pay someone for home help after their admission compared with 0% in group 3 and 6% in group 2. The average amount paid for this care during the course of the study was £403, £82 and £0 for groups 1–3 respectively. Group 1 patients also needed prolonged help from relatives and friends compared with patients in the other two groups.

Comment

This study does suffer from some methodological flaws. Patient groups were not age-matched and the study had a considerable withdrawal rate (33%). Also, the study questionnaire was a combination of parts of other questionnaires, and it is unclear whether this was validated. Despite these flaws, however, the conclusions are important and clinically relevant. AUR impacts significantly on HRQoL, an issue that is often underestimated by clinicians. Not only did patients with AUR experience considerable pain and worry, but the inconvenience of multiple hospital admissions and the financial burden of the requirement for subsequent home help were also important factors. The results of this study should be taken into account when planning healthcare services and resource allocation. Patient care could be improved by either a fast-track method of admission to hospital or, alternatively, protocol-driven policies for catheterization in the community. These suggestions would speed the 'patient journey' and help to relieve the suffering that men experience while waiting to be catheterized in a busy surgical unit. Additionally, the negative impact on HRQoL demonstrated in this study would support the use of combination therapy with an α-blocker and 5α-reductase inhibitors to prevent AUR, as previously suggested by the Medical Therapy of Prostatic Symptoms (MTOPS) study [4].

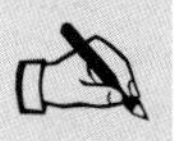

ICIQ: a brief and robust measure for evaluating the symptoms and impact of urinary incontinence

Avery K, Donovan J, Peters TJ, Shaw C, Gotoh M, Abrams P. *Neurourol Urodyn* 2004; **23**: 322–30

Background. Urinary incontinence is a common and distressing condition. Consequently, many questionnaires have been developed to assess incontinence. However, most are condition and gender specific and therefore less applicable to everyday use and less valuable in comparative studies. More importantly, few have addressed the impact of incontinence on QoL. This effect varies enormously, depending on factors such as employment, religion, psychological well-being and personality. In this paper, Avery *et al.* describe the development and validation of the ICIQ (International Consultation on Incontinence Questionnaire), a short questionnaire to assess urinary incontinence (its frequency and amount) and its effect on QoL.

Interpretation. Issues related to incontinence and QoL were collected from systematic literature review and expert opinion. A prototype questionnaire was created using this information and was subsequently assessed at in-depth interviews with patients with incontinence or LUTS. At interview, 63 patients were observed completing the questionnaire and asked if they understood the questions. From the results of these interviews, a developmental questionnaire with nine items (dICIQ) was produced and psychometrically tested. Repetitive or non-discriminative questions were then removed to create a manageable final questionnaire containing three scored items and an unscored self-diagnostic item, as shown in Fig. 3.3. QoL was subsequently assessed using this questionnaire in a population undergoing either conservative or surgical intervention for urinary incontinence. The questionnaire showed good reliability and was able to detect reduction in symptoms post intervention (conservative or surgical).

Comment

In order to plan patient care appropriately, knowledge of the impact of incontinence on QoL is essential. Such information can be obtained from the ICIQ. The questionnaire shows good validity, reliability and responsiveness. The ICIQ is able to discriminate between community and urology clinic patients and is also able to detect differences in QoL between those with urge and stress incontinence. The ICIQ is available in 35 languages, and is not specific to gender, age, patient group, setting or category of incontinence. It is also user friendly on account of its briefness and easy scoring system. The development of a new QoL questionnaire is a complex process that should follow well-established quantitative and qualitative methodology in order to ensure that the resulting measure is clinically appropriate and that its results are interpretable. The ICIQ displays these properties and should therefore be useful in clinical practice and research fields. Although widely used in research, its use in everyday clinical practice is unfortunately less extensive. The key to improving the management of incontinence is the universal use of standardized measures such as the ICIQ, in conjunction with functional measures of incontinence, in order to understand better the effect of incontinence on QoL and thus target treatment appropriately.

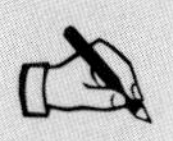

Impact of superficial bladder cancer and transurethral resection on general health-related quality of life

Yoshimura K, Utsunomiya N, Ichioka K, Matsui Y, Terai A, Arai Y. *Urology* 2005; **65**(2): 290–4

BACKGROUND. Superficial bladder cancers are rarely associated with mortality. As such, it is often assumed that their impact on QoL is minimal. Until now, there has been little research on the effect of recurrent superficial cancers requiring frequent transurethral resection (TUR) on patients' QoL. The authors conducted a prospective study to determine the impact of superficial bladder cancer and repeat TUR on patients' QoL. One hundred and thirty-three patients with superficial bladder cancer were recruited. These patients underwent 178 TURs and were asked to complete the SF-36 before each TUR. The SF-36 assesses eight domains of QoL: general health, bodily pain, physical function, role limitations – physical, role limitations – emotional,

Many people leak urine some of the time. We are trying to find out how many people leak urine, and how much this bothers them. We would be grateful if you could answer the following questions, thinking about how you have been, on average, over the PAST FOUR WEEKS.

1. How often do you leak urine? (*tick one box*)

never	☐	0
about once a week or less often	☐	1
two or three times a week	☐	2
about once a day	☐	3
several times a day	☐	4
all the time	☐	5

We would like to know how much **you think** leaks.
2. How much urine do you **usually** leak (whether you wear protection or not)? (*tick one box*)

none	☐	0
a small amount	☐	2
a moderate amount	☐	4
a large amount	☐	6

3. Overall, how much does leaking urine interfere with your everyday life?
Please ring a number between 0 (not at all) and 10 (a great deal)

0 1 3 4 5 6 7 8 9 10
not at all a great deal

ICIQ score: sum scores 1+2+3 ☐ ☐

4. When does urine leak? (*please tick all that apply to you*)

- never – urine does not leak ☐
- leaks before you can get to the toilet ☐
- leaks when you cough or sneeze ☐
- leaks when you are asleep ☐
- leaks when you are physically active/exercising ☐
- leaks when you have finished urinating and are dressed ☐
- leaks for no obvious reason ☐
- leaks all the time ☐

Items in the ICIQ.

Fig. 3.3 Items in the ICIQ. Source: Avery *et al.* (2004).

vitality, mental health and social functioning. It also assesses two summary scores: physical component summary and mental component summary. A higher score represents a better QoL. The SF-36 scores of study participants were compared with age- and sex-matched Japanese control subjects. Comparison was also made between the SF-36 of scores at first, second, third, fourth or later TUR for the study group.

Interpretation. Compared with age- and sex-matched control subjects, patients in the study group had a significantly worse perception of general health throughout follow-up. Also, at first TUR, there was significant role limitation and deterioration in mental health compared with the control group. This change, however, became non-significant over time. The diagnosis of cancer is probably part of the reason for the initial impairment in mental health, but the symptoms of early bladder cancer may also contribute. Physical functioning, role limitations because of physical and emotional health problems and social functioning were most impaired at second or third TUR. However, these domains returned to normal if the patient underwent four or more TURs. Only two domains of the SF-36 questionnaire (bodily pain and vitality) were not adversely affected by the diagnosis and treatment of the superficial bladder cancer.

Comment

This paper is clinically relevant because it demonstrates that, despite carrying low mortality, superficial bladder cancer may have a greater effect on QoL than previously acknowledged. This study is supported by Miyakawa *et al.*, who reported that superficial bladder cancer significantly impaired patients' working status and sexual life [5]. As clinicians, there is a feeling of relief at cystoscopy to discover a superficial tumour rather than one that is invasive. However, for patients, this is a diagnosis of cancer and is distressing. This study highlights the need for better communication between clinicians and patients regarding the diagnosis of superficial bladder cancer and the effect it may have on QoL. It is interesting to note that several domains of the SF-36 questionnaire returned to near baseline after the fourth TUR. Perhaps patients begin to accept the disease as part of their daily lives and suffer less. Alternatively, perhaps they adapt, change their goals and lower their expectations. This may be explained by the emerging concept of response shift, which is defined as 'a change in the meaning of one's self-evaluation of QoL' [6]. Although well validated, the SF-36 (which is a non-disease-specific questionnaire) has been criticised for poorly identifying bladder and bowel symptoms. The application of a disease-specific questionnaire such as the EORTC QLQ-C30 may have improved the power of this study. In summary, further research is needed to assess how clinicians can improve the management of patients with superficial bladder tumours, perhaps utilizing the skills of specialist nurses to provide support and counselling for these patients, especially at the time of diagnosis.

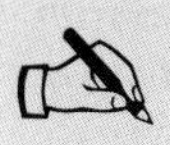

Health-related quality of life following modified ureterosigmoidostomy (Mainz Pouch II) as a continent urinary diversion

Bastian PJ, Albers P, Hanitzsch H, *et al. Eur Urol* 2004; **46**: 591–7

BACKGROUND. Today, cancer treatment no longer implies only the cure and control of disease. The effect on psychological, functional, social and economic well-being must also be acknowledged. Previous studies have shown that, in generic terms, those who survive surgery for muscle-invasive bladder cancer have a very good QoL with little differences found in QoL between different diversion techniques. There has, however, been little investigation into HRQoL in patients following modified ureterosigmoidostomy (Mainz II Pouch). In this study, Bastian *et al.* aimed to assess the HRQoL of patients following Mainz Pouch II urinary diversion. Forty-one patients were recruited from two centres (Bonn, Germany, and Pesaro, Italy). Patients completed the validated EORTC QLQ-C30 questionnaire at a mean follow-up interval of 24.4 months after Mainz II diversion. Results were compared with reference data for the QoL questionnaire EORTC QLQ-C30 in the general German population, i.e. the German population was used as a control. Thirty-one of the German patients also completed a newly designed, non-validated questionnaire assessing the effect of the urinary diversion on urinary frequency and continence, changes in eating, dressing or sexual habits, social life, daily activities or work, marital status and whether the patient would undergo this type of diversion again. This questionnaire is shown in Table 3.2.

INTERPRETATION. At 1 year post surgery, there was no statistically significant difference in overall HRQoL (as measured by the EORTC QLQ-C30) between the treatment group and the control population. There was also no statistically significant difference in HRQoL scores between patients from Italy and Germany, and no difference in QoL and functional or symptom scores between men and women. Of all the scales, diarrhoea was the only condition that was significantly worse in the study population compared with the control population. Results of the non-validated urinary diversion questionnaire revealed that 100% of the patients had daytime continence and none experienced incontinence with flatulence. One-third of the patients had to urinate more than three times during the night. Nevertheless, this was not reported to be bothersome. Outcome in terms of sexual function was, however, significantly worse, with 93% of patients reporting a negative change in sexuality following surgery.

Comment

This retrospective, non-randomized study did not record baseline data for HRQoL and used a non-validated questionnaire for part of the study. Despite these flaws, the study is clinically relevant as it reveals that patients do experience a good QoL after cystectomy and Mainz Pouch II urinary diversion. Ureterosigmoidostomy was first introduced as a continent urinary diversion in 1852 and gained popularity during the first half of the 20th century. Its modification, using detubularization

Table 3.2 Results of the self-developed questionnaire used in 31 of the 41 evaluated patients (%)

Voiding frequency	**Daytime**	**Night-time**
0–1	0	1 (3)
1–3	7 (23)	19 (61)
3–6	13 (45)	9 (29)
>6	11 (35)	2 (7)
Continence	31 (100)	31 (100)

Changes in habits	
Eating habits	9 (29)
Dressing habits	3 (10)
Sexual habits	29 (93.5)
Sexual activity after diversion	6 (19.4)
Impacts on	
Daily activities	27 (87)
Social life	27 (87)
Work life	27 (87)
Marital status	
Married/partner	30 (97)
Widow	1 (3)
Employment	
Active	9 (29)
Retired	22 (71)
Grade of education	
Higher	27 (87)
Lower	4 (13)
Patients who would undergo Mainz Pouch II diversion again	30 (97)

Source: Bastian *et al.* (2004).

(Mainz Pouch II), is a safe and acceptable technique, as demonstrated by this study and supported by previously published research |**7**|. Historically, clinicians in the UK have underused device-free rectal augmentation procedures, favouring bladder reconstruction. Mainz Pouch II is a feasible alternative to other forms of continent urinary diversion in selected patients in terms of both operative technique and HRQoL. Its use is appropriate, not only in the developed world, especially for younger or sexually active patients in whom a stoma may cause a negative impact on self-esteem and body image |**8**|, but also in the developing world where equipment such as stoma bags is often unaffordable and impractical. A prospective, randomized, longitudinal study, adjusting for covariants, is needed to assess fully the effect on HRQoL in patients undergoing different types of urinary diversion, to corroborate the results of this study.

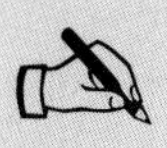

Sexual functioning and quality of life after prostate cancer treatment: considering sexual desire

Dahn J, Penedo F, Gonzalez J, *et al.* *Urology* 2004; **63**(2): 273–7

BACKGROUND. As more and more patients undergo potentially curative treatment for localized prostate cancer, important long-term follow-up data regarding side effects and QoL after treatment have been recorded. Curative treatments for localized prostate cancer are associated with erectile dysfunction and impairment of QoL |9|, specifically sexual interest and desire, relationship quality, perceptions of body image and masculinity, and self-esteem. In their paper, Dahn *et al.* aimed to evaluate the relationship between sexual desire, sexual functioning and QoL in men who had undergone treatment for localized prostate cancer. Study criteria included being in a relationship with a spouse or partner and taking no current adjuvant treatment for prostate cancer. Ninety-one patients were recruited; 29 had undergone radiotherapy and 62 had had radical prostatectomy, all within the preceding 18 months. Socio-demographic and comorbidity data were recorded as well as the frequency of use of sexual aids. Patients were asked to complete the Functional Assessment of Cancer Therapy—General Module (FACT-G) and also items of the University of California, Los Angeles—Prostate Cancer Index (UCLA-PCI) and the Expanded Prostate Cancer Index Composite (EPCIC) questionnaires.

INTERPRETATION. Quality of life was not significantly related to treatment procedure (i.e. radiotherapy or surgery), time since diagnosis or age. It was, however, affected by education, income and Charlson comorbidity score. These variables were therefore controlled in further analysis. Only 24% of the patients had made any attempt to improve erectile functioning via the use of medication or vacuum pump. Mean score for sexual desire correlated to a response of 'fair', whereas the mean level of sexual functioning was reported as 'poor'. In regression models controlling for covariants, there was a statistically significant relationship between sexual functioning and QoL. The interaction of sexual functioning and desire also showed a statistically significant correlation with QoL. For men with low sexual functioning, a greater sexual desire was significantly associated with lower QoL, and less sexual desire was associated with a higher QoL. An opposite trend was found for men with higher sexual functioning scores. In these men, a higher sexual desire was associated with a higher QoL, and a lower sexual desire was associated with a lower QoL.

Comment

The results of this study must be evaluated in light of the lack of pre-treatment data and the absence of comparison with a control group. In addition to this, it is unclear whether the questionnaire, created from items of the UCLA-PCI and the EPCIC, was validated. Despite these shortcomings, this study is important as it reveals an insight into the correlation between variables of sexuality. The relationship between sexual desire and QoL is moderated by the level of sexual functioning. The authors found that men with discordance (e.g. high sexual desire/low sexual functioning) had significantly lower QoL scores compared with those with concordant factors (e.g. low desire/low functioning). This study is relevant to clinical practice as it highlights the fact that not only sexual functioning, but also sexual desire, may be affected by treatment for prostate cancer, and that it is essential to warn patients of this pre-operatively. It is also important to use standardized measures to assess sexuality post-operatively, in order to target treatment or counselling to those who are most likely to benefit from it. Interventions to improve erectile dysfunction will only be of benefit to QoL if the patient has a corresponding sexual desire. An understanding of this desire, and the factors that affect it, is therefore essential.

Quality of life compared during pharmacological treatments and clinical monitoring for non-localized prostate cancer: a randomized control trial

Green H, Pakenham K, Headley B, *et al*. *BJU Int* 2004; **93**(7): 975–9

Background. Prostate cancer is a leading cause of cancer death in men. Treatment goals for men with advanced prostate cancer include prolonging survival, preventing or delaying symptoms due to disease progression, improving and maintaining QoL and reducing treatment-related morbidity. Androgen suppression therapy (AST) is considered the mainstay of treatment for men with advanced prostate cancer; however, there is debate over its benefit on overall QoL. Da Silva *et al.* reported improvement in urinary function, pain and QoL with AST |10|, while Herr *et al.* reported the converse to be true, with poorer emotional, physical and sexual function in those on AST |11|. Luteinizing hormone releasing hormone (LHRH) analogues have also been associated with self-reported memory decline in females |12|. In this study, Green *et al.* investigated the effect of different treatment regimens for non-localized prostate cancer on QoL and cognitive function. Eighty-two men with non-localized prostate cancer were recruited to the study. None had symptoms requiring immediate therapy. Patients were randomized to one of four treatment arms: leuprorelin, goserelin, cyproterone acetate (CPA) or close clinical monitoring. A community comparison group of 20 men of the same age with no prostate cancer were recruited as control subjects. Participants completed well-validated QoL questionnaires and underwent established cognitive and psychosocial assessment at enrolment (1 week before 'treatment') and 6 months and 12 months after treatment.

Interpretation. Analysis of the results at 1 year revealed evidence of an adverse effect of leuprorelin, goserelin and CPA on cognitive function. Word recall was significantly worse in men on hormone therapy compared with those on close monitoring. Over the 1-year study period, sexual dysfunction increased for patients on AST. This was consistent with previous studies |**13**|. Increased sexual difficulties were particularly pronounced for men prescribed goserelin. There was no significant sexual deterioration in men on clinical monitoring or community participants. Emotional distress increased in those assigned to CPA or close clinical monitoring, but not in those assigned to the other groups. Overall, there was no clear HRQoL advantage to active treatments compared with clinical monitoring.

Comment

A recent Cochrane review found that early AST for men with non-localized prostate cancer or asymptomatic metastasis reduces disease progression and complications due to progression when compared with delayed AST. Early AST may also provide a small but statistically significant improvement in overall survival at 10 years. There was no statistically significant difference in prostate cancer-specific survival, but a clinically important difference could not be excluded |**14**|. These improvements must, however, be balanced against the cost of AST, the time spent administering the drug and also the considerable side effects, as highlighted by this well-planned, randomized control study. This study is clinically relevant, as a decline in cognitive function in those on AST for non-localized prostate cancer is not previously well documented. Although clinicians commonly discuss the sexual side effects of AST, the effects on cognitive function are rarely mentioned, despite their significant impact on QoL. Better communication of the risks of AST is therefore essential in order to help patients to make informed choices regarding treatment options. The results of this study also support the use of intermittent therapy to reduce side effects of AST by decreasing the time that men receive the active drug. Additional studies are required to evaluate more definitively the efficacy and adverse effects of AST in men with prostate cancer. It would also be interesting to assess whether newer anti-androgens such as casodex have an equally negative impact on cognitive function.

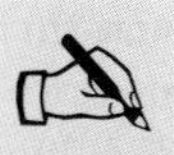

Watchful waiting and health-related quality of life for patients with localized prostate cancer: data from CaPSURE

Arredondo S, Downs T, Lubeck D, *et al. J Urol* 2004; **172**: 1830–4

BACKGROUND. Current UK guidelines suggest that radical treatment for localized prostate cancer should only be offered to patients with a life expectancy of more than 10 years. Watchful waiting (WW) is an alternative for men with a poor prognosis, because of age or comorbidity, or for men with low-risk prostate cancer. In this study, Arredondo *et al.* assessed how HRQoL changed over time in men who selected WW. Data were obtained from 310 patients who were undergoing WW for localized prostate cancer, from the CaPSURE registry (Cancer of the Prostate Strategic Urological Research Endeavor). This is a longitudinal observational disease registry in the USA. The UCLA-PCI and SF-36 questionnaires were completed at enrolment and approximately every 6 months after commencing WW. HRQoL was assessed for up to 5 years after diagnosis. The changes in HRQoL for the study group were compared with changes that would be expected to occur from the ageing process alone.

INTERPRETATION. In the WW group, seven of the eight domains of the SF-36 deteriorated over time. Although role emotional and physical component summary declined over time, this decline was not found to be significantly different from that which might occur as a result of ageing alone. The deterioration in the remaining SF-36 domains was, however, found to be significantly greater than would be expected from ageing alone. The decline was most significant for physical function and role physical. Only mental health remained unchanged with no significant decline in mental component summary over time. There was also a significant deterioration over time in four of the six domains of the UCLA-PCI. The decline was most significant for the sexual function domain, being significantly greater in the prostate cancer group than would be expected from ageing alone. Urinary bother and bowel function were the only domains to remain stable during this study.

Comment

The results of this study provide information on the natural history of the HRQoL changes experienced by men with localized prostate cancer who chose WW. The study also highlights the important issue that patients on WW may experience deterioration in their HRQoL in numerous domains and, although small, this deterioration is greater than would be expected from the ageing process alone. Patients should be informed of this when making treatment decisions. They should also undergo regular review, perhaps by a nurse specialist, to assess factors that have a negative effect on their individual QoL, so that they receive appropriate treatment and counselling if necessary.

The deterioration in HRQoL reported in this study may have been due to the fact that patients had an underlying pathological condition for which they were not receiving treatment. The decline may therefore reflect disease progression. Alternatively, the decline in HRQoL may have been due to newly emerging or progressive comorbidities during the study period. Although comorbidity was taken into account at the initial assessment, it was not followed up over time. This study therefore ignored factors that could have adversely affected HRQoL and thus acted as confounding variables. Lubeck *et al.* |**15**| reported less significant differences than those discovered by this study, which may have been because of shorter follow-up in the Lubeck study (1 year), or because of Arredondo's absence of adjustment for comorbidity, as described above. Although this study detected no deterioration in mental health, this may have been because most of the patients in the study group had low-risk prostate cancer and thus worried less than those with high-risk disease who are more likely to have chosen curative therapies |**16**|.

Despite its drawbacks, this is an important study as it provides information to aid decision-making by clinicians and patients in the management of localized prostate cancer. The risk of disease progression and consequences of WW must be weighed up against the side effects of potentially curative therapies. Further prospective studies with baseline data are therefore required to compare the effect of WW versus prostatectomy, radiotherapy and brachytherapy on long-term QoL.

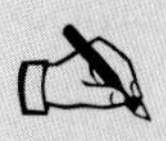

Health-related quality of life in patients with testicular cancer: a comparative analysis according to therapeutic modalities

Miyake H, Muramaki M, Eto H, Kamidono S, Hara I. *Oncol Rep* 2004; **12**: 867–70

BACKGROUND. Primary testicular cancer is the most common solid cancer in men aged 20–45. It is also considered the most curable. However, the malignancy affects men in their prime of life and has the potential to affect work, social life, masculinity and, consequently, HRQoL. Orchidectomy is the primary treatment followed by an array of therapeutic strategies, depending on tumour histology and stage. In their study, Miyake *et al.* aimed to assess HRQoL according to treatment modality post orchidectomy. One hundred and thirty patients, who had been treated for advanced testicular cancer and had been in remission for at least 6 months, were asked to complete the SF-36 questionnaire. Of these, 40 had undergone surveillance monitoring (group A), 64 had been treated with cisplatin-based combination chemotherapy (group B), and 26 had undergone infradiaphragmatic radiotherapy (group C). Of the 64 patients who had chemotherapy, 40 had received standard-dose chemotherapy alone, and 24 had received standard-dose chemotherapy followed by high-dose chemotherapy with peripheral blood stem cell transplantation (PBSCT). Twenty-five of the 64 group B patients had also undergone retroperitoneal lymph node dissection (RPLND) after chemotherapy. When this research was undertaken, no data were available for SF-36 scores for the general population in Japan. SF-36 scores for the general population in the United States were therefore used as a control.

INTERPRETATION. No significant differences were observed in any of the scales of the SF-36 score between patients in the different treatment groups. More importantly, there was no significant difference in SF-36 scores between all three treatment groups and the control population, except in the domains of social functioning, which were found to be lower in the treatment groups, and vitality, which was significantly higher in the treatment groups compared with the control population. Subanalysis of group B revealed no significant difference in SF-36 score between patients who underwent RPLND and those who did not. Results did, however, reveal that high-dose chemotherapy and PBSCT after standard chemotherapy were significantly detrimental to mental health compared with standard chemotherapy alone. Interestingly, there were no significant differences between these two subgroups as measured by the other seven domains of the SF-36 questionnaire.

Comment

With recent advances in multimodal therapy, there are now an increasing number of young survivors of testicular cancer. As such, it is extremely important to investigate the HRQoL of these survivors, not only to assess their outcomes, but also to aid decision-making in those newly diagnosed with testicular cancer. This study aimed to address these issues; however, the results must be interpreted in light of its methodological flaws. The timing of questionnaire completion was significantly different between groups, with group B completing the questionnaire at an earlier follow-up period than either group A or group C. Also, patients in group A almost certainly had lower stage disease than those in group B, and this may have affected the HRQoL scores. The lack of an age- and sex-matched control group is also particularly important. For example, vitality was greater in the testicular cancer survivors than in the control group. This may reflect an appreciation of good fortune in those surviving treatment; however, it may simply reflect cultural differences between the American and Japanese populations. Validated scores for the SF-36 questionnaire are now available in Japanese, and it would be interesting to reanalyse these results using these data. Erectile, ejaculatory and bladder dysfunction are not well detected by the SF-36 questionnaire. It is therefore difficult to determine whether there really were no differences between treatment modality or whether the questionnaire was not specific enough to detect these differences. The inclusion of a questionnaire such as the EORTC QLQ-C30 may have increased the power of this study. Despite these flaws, this study is clinically important as it provides encouraging data for patients recently diagnosed with testicular cancer. It highlights the fact that HRQoL after treatment is generally favourable. Previously published studies support this, reporting that, in the long term (i.e. after the end of treatment), survivors of testicular cancer had a QoL equal to that of the normal age-matched population |**17**|. This study also showed that HRQoL was not affected by treatment modality after orchidectomy. Further research using more specific measures and larger numbers would further clarify these results.

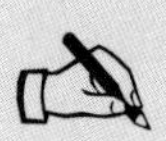

The ED-EQoL: the development of a new quality of life measure for patients with erectile dysfunction

MacDonagh R, Porter T, Pontin D, Ewings P. *Qual Life Res* 2004; **13**: 361–8

BACKGROUND. Erectile dysfunction (ED) is a common problem affecting as many as 10% of healthy men and even greater numbers of men with existing comorbidities such as hypertension (15%) and diabetes (29%). Men with ED may experience a loss of their sense of manhood, humiliation, depression and anxiety. These factors and others can lead to a decrease in overall QoL, which may be long-standing, relating to the chronicity of the condition. As such, accurate analysis of the effect of ED on QoL is essential for planning treatment options for the individual. Several questionnaires have been created to assess ED; however, these often focus on the functional ability alone and not on the resultant effect on QoL, e.g. the International Index of Erectile Function (IIEF). Other questionnaires used to assess ED lack the sensitivity required to detect QoL changes. In this study, the authors aimed to identify issues that have an impact on the QoL of men suffering from ED, and to generate a new ED-specific QoL questionnaire. In-depth qualitative interviews were performed on 29 men with ED from three UK centres. The purpose of the interviews was to explore how ED specifically affected QoL. Further information was gained from discussion with international experts and review of the literature.

INTERPRETATION. The in-depth interviews revealed two main themes: the sense of 'loss with regard to manhood' and the sense of 'being alone with the problem'. Examples of specific issues included feelings of letting the partner down, stigmatization, guilt and embarrassment. Few men acknowledged the multifactorial nature of their problems or had an understanding of the range of available treatment options. A 40-item questionnaire was generated from analysis of the information gained from the interviews, and piloted on 40 men with ED. The results were analysed to find questions that were repetitive or non-discriminative. These questions were removed. This resulted in a 15-item questionnaire which underwent full psychometric testing. The questionnaire had good face and content validity and also the potential to discriminate between men with varying degrees of affected QoL. The questionnaire also demonstrated good internal consistency.

Comment

The incidence of ED is likely to increase as the population ages and men become more able to talk about their health problems. Prior to the development of this questionnaire, there was no measure available in the UK to assess the affect of ED on QoL. The ED-EQoL is fully validated psychometrically, and has been further validated in large multicentre studies, demonstrating excellent responsiveness to change [18]. It is now important to implement this questionnaire into clinical and research practice. The questionnaire can be used not only to assess the degree of impact of ED on QoL, but also to monitor changes in ED with treatment. In the context of clinical practice and research, the use of a validated ED-specific QoL questionnaire in combination with a functional measure such as the IIEF will allow a more holistic assessment of both the physical and the psychological affects of ED in patients and their partners, and help clinicians to target treatment more appropriately.

Conclusion

The recurrent theme of this diverse group of papers is the necessity to assess QoL as well as conventional outcome measures in order to best target treatment to the individual and achieve a holistic approach to healthcare. In an age in which the cost of healthcare is rising and resources are limited, the use of QoL data is imperative to promote the development of national strategies for appropriate resource allocation. Many well-validated questionnaires are now available, and their implementation should be encouraged, not only in research, but also in clinical practice. This will facilitate the collection of data for medical audit and national databases as well as allowing clinicians to standardize patient assessment and care.

In clinical research, the importance of choosing a suitable questionnaire for a particular study cannot be overstated. Validated questionnaires have been psychometrically tested to determine that they are reliable and responsive and that they test the appropriate underlying theories under investigation. There has been an enormous expansion in QoL research in the last 10 years. However, much of the currently published literature describes retrospective studies of QoL with absence of baseline data or control subjects. Further randomized prospective control studies are needed in this exciting and growing field.

There is now a general consensus that the use of survival data, complication rates and symptom responses is no longer enough to assess the impact of disease and its treatment, particularly in patients with chronic or life-threatening disease. In the future, the outcome of treatment must be evaluated, as suggested by the WHO in 1947 |**19**|, on the basis of whether it would result in a life worth living in social and psychological as well as physical terms.

References

1. MacDonagh RP. Quality of life and its assessment in urology. *Br J Urol* 1996; **78**(4): 485–96.
2. Shumaker SA, Anderson RT, Czaijkowski SM. Psychology tests and scales. In: Spilker B (ed). *Quality of life assessments in clinical trials.* New York: Raven Press, 1990; pp 95–113.
3. Jacobsen SJ, Lieber MM. Natural history of prostatism: risk factors for acute urinary retention. *J Urol* 1997; **158**: 481–7.
4. McConnell JD, Roehrborn CG, Bautista OM, Andriole GL Jr, Dixon CM, Kusek JW, Lepor H, McVary KT, Nyberg LM Jr, Clarke HS, Crawford ED, Diokno A, Foley JP, Foster HE, Jacobs SC, Kaplan SA, Kreder KJ, Lieber MM, Lucia MS, Miller GJ, Menon M, Milam DF, Ramsdell JW, Schenkman NS, Slawin KM, Smith JA; Medical Therapy of Prostatic Symptoms (MTOPS) Research Group. The long-term effect of doxazosin, finasteride and combination therapy on the clinical progression of benign prostatic hyperplasia. *N Engl J Med* 2003; **349**: 2387–98.
5. Miyakawa M, Yoshida O. The quality of life in patients with bladder cancer after radical cystectomy with ileal conduit: results of questionnaire surveys to compare the impact of treatments (in Japanese). *J Jpn Soc Cancer Ther* 1987; **22**: 1296–303.
6. Rees J, MacDonagh RP, Waldron D, O'Boyle C. Measuring quality of life in patients with advanced cancer. *Eur J Palliative Care* 2004; **11**(3): 104–6.
7. Woodhouse CR, Christofides M. Modified ureterosigmoidostomy (Mainz II): technique and early results. *Br J Urol* 1998; **81**: 247–52.
8. Mansson A, Davidsson T, Hunt S, Mansson W. The quality of life in men after radical cystectomy with a continent cutaneous diversion or orthotopic bladder substitution: is there a difference? *BJU Int* 2002; **90**: 386–90.
9. Althof SE. Quality of life and erectile dysfunction. *Urology* 2002; **59**: 803–10.

10. Da Silva FC, Fossa SD, Aaronson NK, Robinson MR. The quality of life of patients with newly diagnosed M1 prostate cancer: experience with the EORTC clinical trial 30853. *Eur J Cancer* 1996; **32A**: 72–7.

11. Herr HW, O'Sullivan M. Quality of life of asymptomatic men with non-metastatic prostate cancer on androgen deprivation therapy. *J Urol* 2000; **163**: 1743–6.

12. Newton C, Slota D, Yuzpe AA, Tummon IS. Memory complaints associated with the use of gonadotropin-releasing hormone agonists: a preliminary study. *Fertil Steril* 1996; **65**: 1253–5.

13. Schroder FH, Collette L, de Reijke TM, Whelan P. Prostate cancer treated by anti-androgens: is sexual function preserved? EORTC Genitourinary Group. European Organization for Research and Treatment of Cancer. *Br J Cancer* 2000; **82**: 283–90.

14. Nair B, Wilt T, MacDonald R, Rutks I. Early versus deferred androgen suppression in the treatment of advanced prostate cancer. *Cochrane Database Syst Rev* 2002; (**1**): CD003506.

15. Lubeck DP, Litwin MS, Henning JM, Stoddard ML, Flanders SC, Carroll PR. Changes in health-related quality of life in the first year after treatment for prostate cancer: results from CaPSURE. *Urology* 1999; **53**: 180–6.

16. Litwin MS, Lubeck DP, Spitalny GM, Henning JM, Carroll PR. Mental health in men treated for early stage prostate carcinoma: a post-treatment, longitudinal quality of life analysis from the Cancer of the Prostate Strategic Urologic Research Endeavor. *Cancer* 2002; **95**: 54–60.

17. Dahl AA, Mykletun A, Fossa SD. Quality of life in survivors of testicular cancer. *Urol Oncol* 2005; **23**(3): 193–200.

18. MacDonagh R, Ewings P, Porter T. The effect of erectile dysfunction on quality of life: psychometric testing of a new quality of life measure for patients with erectile dysfunction. *J Urol* 2002; **167**(1): 212–17.

19. World Health Organization. The constitution of the WHO. *WHO Chronicle* 1947; **1**: 29.

4

Trends in diagnostic uropathology

JON OXLEY

Introduction

This chapter discusses recent original articles in the pathology journals that have an impact on diagnostic uropathology. There have been several review articles discussing important issues over the last 12 months, not least is a consensus on Gleason scoring [1]. Previous volumes of this book have discussed discrepancies in Gleason scoring over time, and this consensus article reports our current usage of the Gleason grading system. Alpha-methylacyl CoA racemase (AMACR) immunohistochemistry was experimental 4 years ago but is now widely used, and a recent review on all immunohistochemistry in prostate pathology has also been published recently [2]. Other practical reviews include a guide to cut-up of nephrectomy and radical prostatectomy specimens [3,4]. The molecular pathology of prostate cancer is reviewed by Hughes *et al.* [5].

The original articles in this chapter discuss issues such as margin status in radical prostatectomies, whether vanishing cancer syndrome is in fact switched specimens and how this can be detected using polymerase chain reaction (PCR)-based techniques. Papers on bladder cancer cover a series of small cell carcinomas and whether extracapsular extension of bladder carcinoma in lymph nodes is prognostically important. The incidence and significance of prostate cancer in cystoprostatectomies is also examined. As more localized treatment of renal tumours is being undertaken, so the number of renal tumour biopsies is increasing, and one group's experiences is detailed in another paper. The final paper discusses c-*kit* expression in renal tumours and the possibility of using an anti-tyrosine kinase receptor agent.

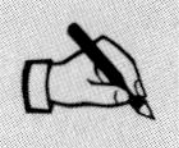

The presence of benign prostatic glandular tissue at surgical margins does not predict PSA recurrence

Kernek KM, Koch MO, Daggy JK, Juliar BE, Cheng L. *J Clin Pathol* 2005; **58**(7): 725–8

Background. Increases in serum prostate-specific antigen (PSA) after radical prostatectomy are thought to indicate recurrent disease, although some suggest that they result from benign prostatic epithelial tissue left at surgical margins.

Interpretation. The authors studied 199 patients with prostate cancer and negative surgical margins. The presence, measured length, anatomical location and extent of benign prostatic tissue at the margin were correlated with clinicopathological characteristics and post-operative PSA increases. Fifty-five (28%) cases had benign prostatic glandular tissue at the surgical margin. The most frequent location of benign prostatic tissue was the apex (40 patients). Presence, anatomical location and length of benign prostatic tissue at the margin were not significantly associated with any of the factors examined, including PSA recurrence. They concluded that the presence of benign prostatic tissue at surgical margins had no prognostic relevance.

Comment

This study addresses the issue of benign prostatic tissue causing biochemical recurrence rather than true cancer recurrence. Biochemical recurrence was defined as a PSA value of at least 0.1 ng/ml after surgery. Only 17 patients out of the 199 studied had a biochemical recurrence in the follow-up period, which ranged from 1.5 to 48 months with a median of 12 months. The short follow-up period is the only fault with this paper, but the numbers studied and the techniques involved are superior to previous studies. The authors postulate that leaving benign tissue behind does not lead to significant serum PSA, as the amount is small and may be damaged by the surgery, so that the pathologist may see glands at a margin but those remaining in the patient have been devitalized and cannot produce PSA. Following these results, the authors do not advocate reporting the presence of benign glands at surgical margins.

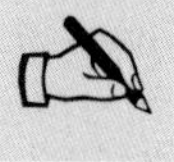

The influence of extent of surgical margin positivity on prostate specific antigen recurrence

Emerson RE, Koch MO, Jones TD, Daggy JK, Juliar BE, Cheng L. *J Clin Pathol* 2005; **58**(10): 1028–32

Background. Positive surgical margins are an adverse prognostic factor in patients undergoing prostatectomy for prostate cancer. The extent of margin positivity varies, and its influence on clinical outcome is uncertain.

Interpretation. The authors examined 86 consecutive margin-positive prostatectomy specimens. The linear extent of margin positivity and the number and location of positive sites were recorded. The linear extent of margin positivity was associated with PSA recurrence in univariate logistic regression ($P = 0.031$). In addition, the extent of margin positivity correlated weakly with pre-operative PSA ($P = 0.017$) and tumour volume ($P = 0.013$), but not with age, prostate weight, Gleason score, pathological stage or perineural invasion. The total number of positive sites was significantly higher in patients with PSA recurrence ($P = 0.037$). The location of the positive margin site was not associated with PSA recurrence. The extent of margin positivity correlated with PSA recurrence in univariate analysis, although it had only marginal predictive value when adjusted for Gleason score ($P = 0.076$). The authors concluded that the extent of margin positivity correlates with PSA recurrence in univariate analysis, although it has no predictive value independent of Gleason score.

Comment

This paper is by the same group as the first paper reviewed and again examines the linear extent of margins and its relationship to recurrence. Once again, the follow-up period was short (range 1.5–48 months with a median of 12 months). From a series of 369 patients, 86 (23%) had positive margins, but these were not divided into intra- or extraprostatic margins. The numbers in this study are small in comparison with previous studies examining margin status, but the authors were addressing the issue of whether measuring the length of positive margin was useful and, although it was significant on univariate analysis, the Gleason score was the only significant factor on multivariate analysis. They concluded that measuring the extent of margin positivity was not required in reporting radical prostatectomy specimens, although a previous study by Epstein *et al.* |**6**| showed significant differences between negative, focally positive (defined by 'the involved site(s) were limited and present in only one or two areas') and extensive.

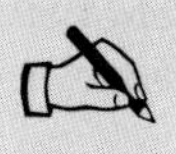

Little or no residual prostate cancer at radical prostatectomy: vanishing cancer or switched specimen? A microsatellite analysis of specimen identity

Cao D, Hafez M, Berg K, Murphy K, Epstein JI. *Am J Surg Pathol* 2005; **29**(4): 467–73

Background. With more vigilant screening for prostate cancer, there has been an associated increase in patients with little or no residual cancer at radical prostatectomy after an initial diagnosis of minute cancer on needle biopsy. This raises a critical question as to whether the biopsy and subsequent radical prostatectomy in these patients are from the same patient.

Interpretation. The authors used PCR-based microsatellite marker analysis to perform identity tests in 46 men (35 with minute cancer and 11 with no residual cancer). Of these, 41 were interpretable; the remaining five cases (four with minute cancer and one with no residual cancer) were considered uninterpretable because of technical problems. All 31 interpretable cases with minute cancer showed a match between the initial biopsy and radical prostatectomy specimens. Nine of the 10 interpretable cases with no residual cancer showed a match and one showed a mismatch. The initial biopsy of the mismatched case had high-grade cancer. Their results confirm that, in most cases of 'vanishing cancer' in radical prostatectomy specimens, it reflects a chance sampling of a minute cancer and not a switch in specimens. However, specimen switch can occur rarely and, if there is high-grade or a lot of cancer on the biopsy with no or very minimal cancer in the radical prostatectomy specimen, one should evaluate for patient identity.

Comment

'Vanishing cancer' is a well-recognized phenomenon in prostate cancer and occurs when the biopsy contains tumour but none can be found in the radical prostatectomy specimen, even when it is completely processed. Bostwick recently reviewed a series of these and found an incidence of 0.2% |**7**|, while this study had an incidence of 0.34%. The authors of this study used microsatellite markers to confirm the identity of the biopsy and the radical prostatectomy. Microsatellite markers are loci or regions within the DNA with short sequences of DNA arranged in tandem arrays (short tandem repeats [STR]). These highly pleomorphic markers are distributed more or less evenly throughout the human genome with a frequency of about one locus per 10 kb. These are stably inherited and unique to an individual, and PCR can enable these regions to be analysed. There were technical difficulties leading to five cases being uninterpretable because of DNA fragmentation, which can occur during formalin fixation and paraffin embedding. The mismatched case had high Gleason score tumour in the cores and the tumour occupied 40% of the tissue, and this in itself would raise concern that a swap had occurred. Specimen swapping does occur in any busy laboratory, and the technology used in this study is now widely available to allow identities to be confirmed. Unfortunately, this is little solace to the patient who has undergone unnecessary surgery, but it may be useful in confirming that a patient really does have vanishing cancer rather than swapped specimens.

Mitochondrial DNA haplotyping revealed the presence of mixed up benign and neoplastic tissue sections from two individuals on the same prostatic biopsy slide

Alonso A, Alves C, Suárez-Mier MP, *et al. J Clin Pathol* 2005; **58**: 83–6

BACKGROUND. DNA typing was used to investigate a presumptive cancer diagnosis error by confirming whether benign and cancerous prostatic tissue in the same presurgical haematoxylin and eosin-stained slide belonged to the same person.

INTERPRETATION. The authors used manual slide dissection to guarantee independent and high-recovery DNA isolation from each tissue section. Nuclear DNA quantification performed by real-time PCR revealed the absence of human DNA for microsatellite analysis. Mitochondrial DNA was only obtained by performing PCR of very short fragments (100 bp), indicating high DNA degradation. Different low-frequency hypervariable region I haplotypes were obtained from each tissue section. Only the normal tissue section haplotype matched that obtained from the patient's blood sample, indicating that the cancer tissue section originated from an unknown patient. These results supported the hypothesis of sample mix-up during block processing or slide preparation by a carryover mechanism. The authors recommended mitochondrial genetic typing when low DNA content and high degradation compromise conventional microsatellite typing.

Comment

Errors in specimen handling do occur, and this paper addresses the problem using a different technique from that of the previous paper reviewed. The authors came across the same problem as in the previous paper insomuch as the DNA had degraded as a result of the processes involved in making the tissue blocks. Mitochondrial DNA haplotyping is a more complex method for microsatellite typing and as such is less available, but this paper highlights its use in instances where there are technical difficulties in recovering DNA.

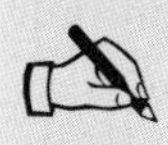

High-grade prostatic intraepithelial neoplasia and atypical small acinar proliferation: predictive value for cancer in current practice

Schlesinger C, Bostwick DG, Iczkowski KA. *Am J Surg Pathol* 2005; **29**(9): 1201–7

BACKGROUND. Prostate cancer (CaP) has been reported to appear in 21–48% of subsequent biopsies for isolated high-grade prostatic intraepithelial neoplasia (PIN) and in 34–60% for isolated atypical small acinar proliferation (ASAP) suspicious for, but not diagnostic of, malignancy.

INTERPRETATION. The authors report the results of follow-up biopsies in a recent cohort of community practice patients who underwent biopsy for PSA abnormalities. The study group consisted of 336 men with initial diagnoses of PIN ($n = 204$), ASAP ($n = 78$) or both lesions ($n = 54$), who underwent at least one repeat biopsy. Mean follow-up intervals in months were 6.0 for PIN, 3.8 for ASAP and 4.9 for PIN/ASAP. Follow-up CaP detection rates were 23%, 37% and 33% respectively. The predictive value of ASAP was significantly higher than that for PIN ($P = 0.0188$). In 23 PIN studies with chronologic midpoints in the early 1990s, follow-up CaP was detected in a mean of 36% of cases, whereas this value was 21% after the year 2000. In 13 ASAP studies, mean CaP detection on follow-up was 45% until 1996 and 39% from 1997 to the present. PIN/ASAP predicted CaP in 33% of cases in our study, similar to ASAP alone ($P = 0.65$), and had a mean predictive value of 44% in the literature. The authors suggest that the decline in PIN predictive values may be due to extended biopsy techniques that yield higher rates of initial cancer detection, lower detection rates for the remaining small cancers that may accompany PIN, and remaining PIN cases may lack concomitant cancer.

Comment

This study looks at current practice and compares it with previous studies over the last 15 years. The diagnosis of ASAP is based on several factors (Table 4.1), and the predictive value of this appears to have decreased slightly from 45% in the studies from 1989 to 1996 to 37% in this study—the authors attribute this to extended biopsy techniques and immunostains such as AMACR. PIN, on the other hand, has shown a more significant fall in its predictive value in the series from before and after 2000, and the authors suggest reasons for this but have not raised the possibility that the diagnosis of PIN is subjective and that trends in our interpretation of certain features may also have a role, in the same way that Gleason grading has changed in the last 15 years. This apart, the most important message is that both PIN and ASAP are more predictive of cancer than a control population, and repeat biopsy should be performed following their diagnosis.

Table 4.1 Factors resulting in ASAP diagnosis

Size
Small number of acini in the focus
Small focus size, average 0.4 mm in diameter
Lesion fracture at core tip (new)
Histology
Lack of clear histological detail, for a variety of reasons
Distortion of acini
Lack of convincing malignant features, e.g. small number of cells with nucleomegaly
Clustered growth pattern
Loss of the focus of concern in deeper levels obtained for high-molecular-weight cytokeratin immunostain
Negative high-molecular-weight cytokeratin immunostain in focus
Presence of associated PIN
Atrophic glands lacking basal cell layer
Inflammation
Prominent inflammation in which the adjacent benign acini show distortion
Inflammatory cellular reactive atypia with nuclear and nucleolar enlargement

Source: Schlesinger *et al.* (2005).

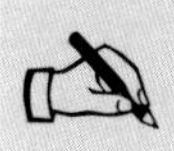

Prognostic implications of extracapsular extension of pelvic lymph node metastases in urothelial carcinoma of the bladder

Fleischmann A, Thalmann GN, Markwalder R, Studer UE. *Am J Surg Pathol* 2005; **29**(1): 89–95

BACKGROUND. The aim of this study was to determine whether extracapsular extension of pelvic lymph node metastases from urothelial carcinoma of the bladder is of prognostic significance.

INTERPRETATION. The authors examined 101 patients with lymph node metastasis from a consecutive series of 507 patients who had undergone radical cystectomy between 1985 and 2000 with standardized extended bilateral pelvic lymphadenectomy in curative intent. These patients were followed prospectively for recurrence-free (RFS) and overall (OS) survival. The median number of nodes examined per patient was 22 (range 10–43). The median number of positive nodes was 2 (range 1–24). Median RFS and OS were 17 and 21 months (range for both 1–191 months) respectively. The 5-year RFS and OS rates were 32% and 30% respectively. There were 59 patients (58%) with extracapsular extension of lymph node metastases. They had a significantly decreased RFS (median 12 vs 60 months; $P = 0.0003$) and OS (median 16 vs 60 months; $P < 0.0001$) compared with those with intranodal metastases (Fig. 4.1). There were no significant differences in survival between pN1 and pN2 categories with extracapsular extension of the lymph node metastases (RFS, $P = 0.70$; OS, $P = 0.65$) or those without extension (RFS, $P = 0.47$; OS, $P = 0.34$). On a multivariate analysis, extracapsular extension of lymph node metastases was the strongest negative predictor for RFS. The authors conclude that meticulous lymph node resection and subsequent thorough histological examination in patients undergoing radical cystectomy for bladder cancer reveal a high incidence of lymph node-positive disease (24%) despite negative pre-operative staging. Lymph node metastases with extracapsular extension in pN1 and pN2 stages carry a very poor prognosis (Fig. 4.2). Therefore, this feature should be used to designate a separate pN category in the staging system. The UICC 2002 classification makes a discrimination between pN1/pN2, which seems arbitrary in the light of these results and of no significant prognostic relevance.

Comment

The extension of tumour outside the lymph node capsule has been shown to be prognostically important in several cancers including prostate and penis, but this has not been thoroughly investigated in bladder cancer until now. Extended lymphadenectomies for bladder cancer are only now becoming standard practice in the UK, so there is a lack of the series that other European countries have. The authors recovered at least ten nodes per patient, and this was partly down to the surgeon submitting tissue from the various regions separately and partly due to meticulous examination by the pathologist. The authors make no reference to using other techniques for lymph node recovery, such as acetone or xylene, which can be

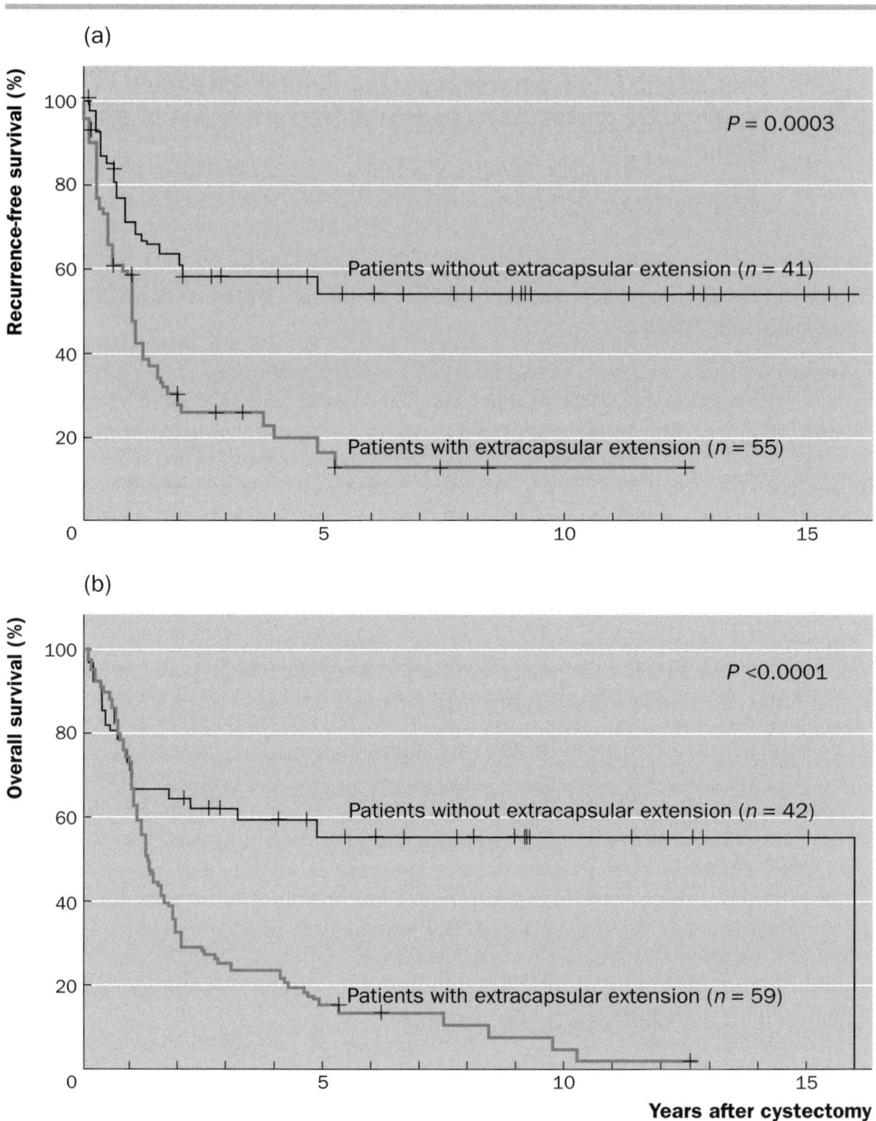

Fig. 4.1 Recurrence-free (a) and overall (b) survival stratified according to the presence or absence of extracapsular extension of lymph node metastasis. Source: Fleischmann *et al.* (2005).

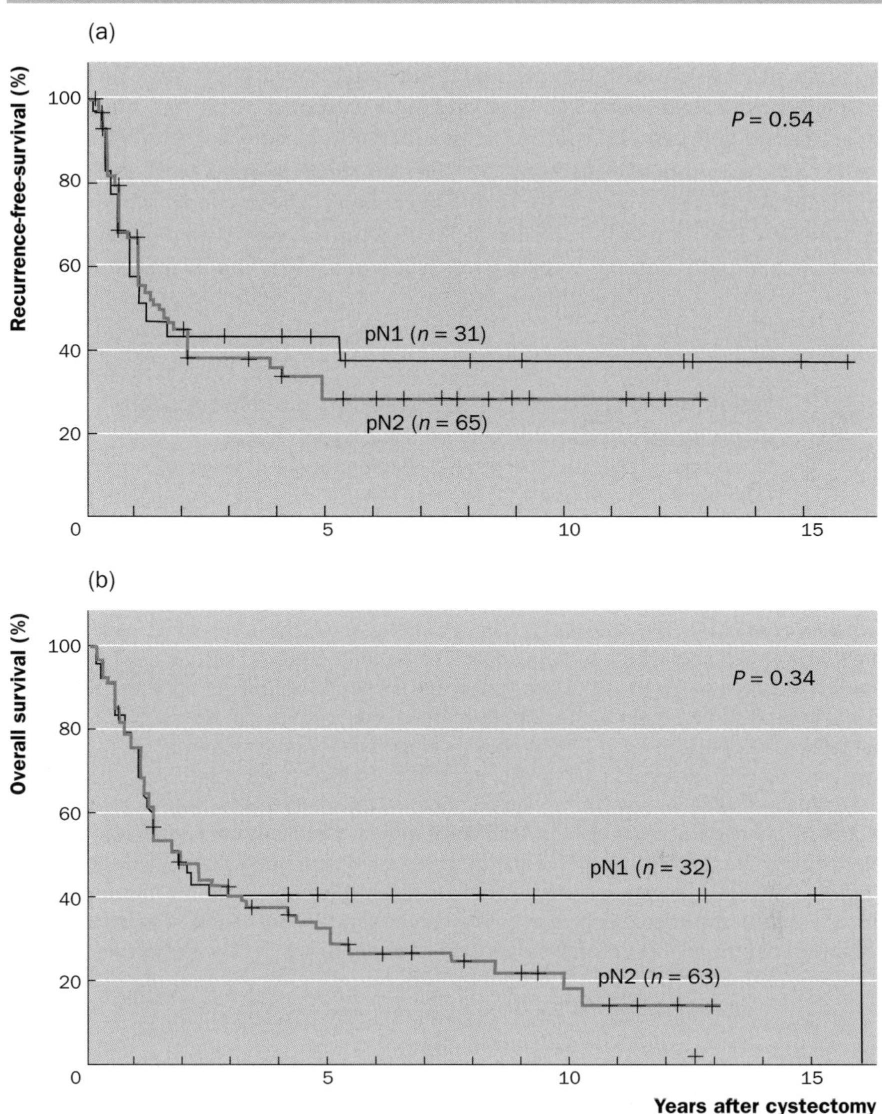

Fig. 4.2 Recurrence-free (a) and overall (b) survival stratified according to nodal status. Source: Fleischmann *et al.* (2005).

used to dissolve the fat. The lymph nodes are often very fatty, and the authors do make reference to the difficulty in determining whether the metastasis was within the node or had invaded the perinodal adipose tissue. They state that, to be considered extranodal, it had to have 'obvious extranodal extension', but this was not accurately defined. The effect of adjuvant chemotherapy was also examined; it did not have a significant effect on the RFS, but those patients receiving it had a significant advantage in overall survival. This may have been selection bias, as only the younger, fitter patients received it. In conclusion, this paper highlights the importance of reporting extracapsular extension in bladder cancer metastasis.

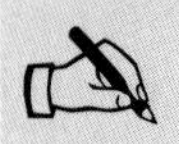

Small cell carcinoma of the bladder: a contemporary clinicopathological study of 51 cases

Abrahams NA, Moran C, Reyes AO, Siefker-Radtke A, Ayala AG.
Histopathology 2005; **46**(1): 57–63

BACKGROUND. Small cell carcinoma is a rare primary malignancy of the urinary bladder with an incidence of less than 2% and a 5-year survival of less than 50%.

INTERPRETATION. The authors present a clinicopathological study of 51 cases of primary small cell carcinoma of the bladder. The patients were 40 men and 11 women between the ages of 39 and 87 years (mean age 67 years). Of the 41 patients with clinical data, 63% had haematuria. Biopsy material was obtained in all the patients. Cystectomy was performed in 20 patients. At diagnosis, clinical stage was as follows: stage I in two (5%), stage II in 18 (44%), stage III in 10 (24%) and stage IV in 11 (27%). Histologically, urothelial carcinoma was present in 70% of the cases, adenocarcinoma in 8% and squamous cell carcinoma in 10% of the cases. Small cell carcinoma was the only histology present in only 12% of the cases studied. Immunohistochemical studies using chromogranin, synaptophysin and neuron-specific enolase were positive in 30%, 70% and 25% of the cases respectively. The patients received a variety of treatment modalities, but the median overall survival for all patients with follow-up data was 23 months with 40% survival at 5 years (Fig. 4.3).

Comment

This study describes the clinicopathological features of a series of small cell carcinoma of the bladder. The authors highlight the fact that it is more often combined with urothelial carcinoma than as a pure tumour. The various treatment modalities and the relatively small numbers make interpretation of the best treatment impossible. They do report that one patient, who had metastatic disease at presentation, responded to chemotherapy and then had a subsequent cystectomy and was still alive 8 years later, which suggests that some are acutely chemosensitive. Unfortunately, the histological characteristics are not specified in this case. The authors found that several of the tumours lacked immunohistochemical expression for chromogranin, synaptophysin and neuron-specific enolase, but they did not

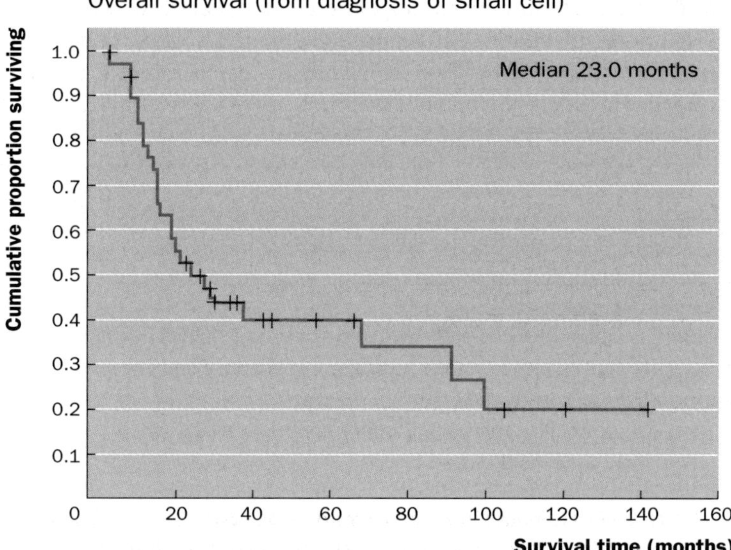

Fig. 4.3 Survival curve for patients with clinical follow-up. Median survival is 23 months with a 5-year cumulative survival of 40%. Source: Abrahams *et al.* (2005).

perform these markers on the whole series. Although they mention that some of the tumours were positive for c-*kit* and epidermal growth factor receptor (EGFR), this was not performed on the whole series. As a pathological series, this paper is useful as it highlights the fact that the light microscopic features are the gold standard in making the diagnosis but, from a treatment point of view, it does not broaden our knowledge.

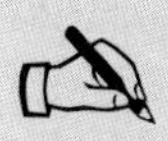

Incidentally detected prostate cancer in cystoprostatectomies: pathological and morphometric comparison with clinically detected cancer in totally embedded specimens

Montironi R, Mazzucchelli R, Santinelli A, Scarpelli M, Lòpez Beltran A, Bostwick DG. *Hum Pathol* 2005; **36**(6): 646–54

BACKGROUND. There are limited data regarding the pathological features of incidentally detected prostate cancer. Examination of cystoprostatectomy specimens obtained during bladder cancer treatment affords a unique opportunity to examine incidentally detected prostate cancer and determine its relationship with clinically detected prostate cancer obtained during radical prostatectomy.

INTERPRETATION. The authors compared the pathological findings of incidentally detected prostate cancer in 132 consecutive cystoprostatectomy specimens from patients treated for bladder cancer with a consecutive series of 228 radical prostatectomy specimens from patients treated for prostate cancer. Incidentally detected cancer was found in 42% of cystoprostatectomy specimens, and the cancers were of lower Gleason score and lower pathological stage with fewer positive surgical margins than in clinically detected cancers in age-matched radical prostatectomies. High-grade PIN was present in 82% of radical prostatectomy specimens, in 70% of cystoprostatectomies with incidentally detected prostate cancer and in 54% of cystoprostatectomies without prostate cancer. Mean nuclear and nucleolar areas were lower in incidentally detected cancer and PIN compared with clinically detected cancer and PIN, respectively, similar to the results with proliferative indices. The authors concluded that incidentally detected cancer is less aggressive than clinically detected cancer.

Comment

The incidence of incidental prostate cancer in cystoprostatectomies is well documented, varying from 23% to 68%. This paper addresses this form of incidental prostate cancer using various techniques (morphology, morphometry and immunohistochemistry) to assess whether it represents a more aggressive form of prostate cancer than that found in radical prostatectomies. Using karyometry, the authors showed that the PIN and the prostate cancer had smaller nuclei and nucleoli in the cystoprostatectomy prostates. The authors make no mention of the tumour volumes or pre-operative serum PSA in the patients undergoing cystectomy. The PSA may not be accurate as these patients may have prostatitis secondary to therapy (e.g. bacillus Calmette-Guérin [BCG] or resection of the bladder tumour). Ward *et al.* looked at incidental prostate cancer and found that, in a series of 1600, 129 (23%) had prostate cancer with PSA values below 2 ng/ml and, of these, 60% had clinically significant tumours (defined as ≥0.5 ml volume, Gleason 4 or 5 architecture, pT3, positive surgical margin, multifocality >3, non-diploid DNA content or proliferation index >5%) |**8**|. Ward *et al.* concluded that the PSA was not useful in predicting clinical significance |**8**|. In this paper by Montironi *et al.*, they use complex karyometry and conclude that it is less aggressive than clinically detected cancer, but their data also suggest that there is a subgroup that is clinically significant, as 12% of the patients had pT3 or pT4 disease (Table 4.2).

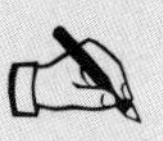

Image-guided biopsy in the evaluation of renal mass lesions in contemporary urological practice: indications, adequacy, clinical impact, and limitations of the pathological diagnosis

Shah RB, Bakshi N, Hafez KS, Wood DP Jr, Kunju LP. *Hum Pathol* 2005; **36**(12): 1309–15

BACKGROUND. With increasing sophistication of imaging modalities, many small indeterminate renal masses are detected, posing therapeutic dilemmas. Minimally

Table 4.2 Stage and margin status of prostate cancer cases (TNM 1997 revision)

	No. of cases with prostate cancer	**pT2a**	**pT2b**	**pT3a**	**pT3b**	**pT4**	**Positive margins**
Cystoprostatectomy specimens (*n* = 132)	55 (42)	33 (60)	15 (28)	4 (8)	2 (3)	1 (1)	4 (7)
Radical prostatectomy specimens (*n* = 228)	228 (100)	24 (10)	73 (32)	79 (35)	38 (17)	14 (6)	119 (52)

The 1997 revision of the TNM was used rather than the 2002 revision to make the data comparable with those already published. Values given in parentheses are percentages.
Source: Montironi *et al.* (2005).

invasive techniques such as radiofrequency ablation (RFA) and cryotherapy are increasingly used in such settings, making it essential to classify renal masses on biopsies.

Interpretation. The authors evaluated indications, adequacy, spectrum and limitations of pathological diagnoses in 52 adequate biopsies that affected management by having conservative therapy (less than total nephrectomy). Indication for biopsies in this group was exclusively for indeterminate mass. Biopsies were categorized as 52% clear cell renal cell carcinoma (RCC); 11% papillary RCC; 23% oncocytic neoplasms, subdivided as oncocytoma (10), chromophobe RCC (1) and cannot rule out RCC (1); 8% spindle cell neoplasms; 2% round blue cell tumours; and 4% inflammatory. After biopsy, 29% underwent nephron-sparing surgery, 36% underwent RFA, and 35% were followed up with observation only. One (2%) unresolved oncocytic neoplasm proved to be a chromophobe RCC in the total nephrectomy. Fifteen of the 19 patients, who underwent RFA after diagnostic biopsy, subsequently underwent post-RFA biopsy to assess therapy response. Complete ablation at first attempt was achieved in 12 out of 15 patients.

Comment

The authors report a series of renal biopsies performed in the setting of incidental tumours and report an adequacy rate of 79%. Biopsies are increasingly performed for incidentally detected renal mass to influence the clinical management, as well as in the scenario of classification of unresectable/metastatic tumours prior to immunotherapy. The efficacy of immunotherapy has been shown to be partially dependent on accurate histological assessment, as response to interleukin (IL)-2-based therapy is largely limited to patients with clear cell rather than papillary morphology. As the authors point out, there may be sampling error and, as a result, they do not Fuhrman grade the clear cell tumours and are cautious with regard to eosinophilic tumours. The immunohistochemical panels for differentiating oncocytomas from chromophobe renal cell carcinoma are not totally specific. Focal areas of oncocytic change can also be seen in conventional RCC, leading to another source of false negatives. In conclusion, the authors found that most biopsies could be classified into clinically relevant categories; however, caution was advised while interpreting oncocytic neoplasms because sampling and tumour heterogeneity may adversely affect interpretation.

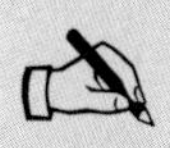

C-*kit* expression in renal oncocytomas and chromophobe renal cell carcinomas

Huo L, Sugimura J, Tretiakova MS, *et al. Hum Pathol* 2005; **36**(3): 262–8

Background. C-*kit* encodes the membrane-bound tyrosine kinase KIT, whose expression has been identified in several types of human neoplasms. Recently, KIT has been reported to be a marker for chromophobe RCC and renal angiomyolipoma. However, expression of this molecule has not been adequately studied in other renal tumours, particularly oncocytoma, which may morphologically resemble chromophobe RCC.

Interpretation. The authors analysed c-*kit* messenger RNA (mRNA) levels in 17 chromophobe RCCs and 20 renal oncocytomas obtained from complementary DNA (cDNA) microarrays. Furthermore, comprehensive immunohistochemical analysis of KIT protein using a monoclonal antibody was performed in 226 renal tumours including chromophobe RCC ($n = 40$), oncocytoma ($n = 41$), clear cell RCC ($n = 40$), renal angiomyolipoma ($n = 29$) and papillary RCC ($n = 21$) on tissue microarrays (TMAs), and was compared with immunostaining results from 25 chromophobe RCCs and 30 oncocytomas using standard sections. The staining intensity was graded semi-quantitatively on a three-tier scoring system. All chromophobe RCCs and oncocytomas showed significant overexpression of c-*kit* mRNA. The average increase in mRNA compared with normal kidney tissue was 7.4-fold for chromophobe RCCs and 7.4-fold for oncocytomas. Immunohistochemical expression of KIT was found in most chromophobe RCCs (95% in TMAs and 96% in conventional sections) and oncocytomas (88% in TMAs and 100% in conventional sections), but was infrequently observed in renal angiomyolipomas (17%), papillary RCCs (5%) and clear cell RCCs (3%). Furthermore, the average KIT immunoreactivity in TMAs was stronger in chromophobe RCC (1.93) and oncocytoma (2.07) than in other subtypes of renal tumours tested, including angiomyolipomas (0.17), papillary RCCs (0.05) and clear cell RCCs (0.03).

Comment

The enthusiastic results of the anti-tyrosine kinase receptor agent imanitib mesylate (Gleevec) in the treatment of gastrointestinal stromal tumours (GISTs) as well as chronic myeloid leukaemia has led to many tumours being examined for expression of KIT. Early results in renal tumours have shown that a proportion of chromophobe renal cell carcinomas and oncocytomas are positive for KIT on immunohistochemistry, but the other subtypes were negative |**9**|. The authors of this earlier study suggested a role for Gleevec in patients with extensive disease, but subsequent authors have shown that, although the tumours express KIT, there is no associated mutation in exons 9 and 11, which are responsible for gain-of-function mutations, and so Gleevec would not be of use |**10,11**|. The paper reviewed here looked at both immunohistochemistry and mRNA levels and found that both were increased in chromophobe renal cell carcinoma and oncocytomas, as opposed to other subtypes of renal cell carcinoma. These results have two implications: one is that KIT expression may be useful in distinguishing chromophobe renal cell carcinoma from other subtypes but, in reality, the main problem is distinguishing oncocytomas from chromophobe carcinomas and, as a result, KIT will not help. The other implication is that these results would suggest that there is overexpression unrelated to the mutations seen in GISTs, and Gleevec may have a role but, as chromophobe renal cell carcinoma has a good prognosis, few patients will have metastatic disease warranting treatment.

Conclusion

The histopathologist can record vast amounts of data when reporting a radical prostatectomy specimen, but it is never very clear what is actually clinically important. The two papers reviewed in this chapter looked at length of margin and found that the length of neither benign nor malignant margin affected the PSA recurrence rate. This comes as a great relief to a pathologist as the prospect of recording these data is daunting. PCR-based technology is having more and more impact in histopathology, and its role in establishing patient identity following specimen mix-up is essential. Microsatellite analysis is now widely available, and this department has used it when specimen identity is unclear with great success. PIN is an ever popular subject in the pathology journals, and the paper reviewed here looked back and compared current with previous rates of both PIN and ASAP. There appears to be a decreased rate of cancer in subsequent biopsies in patients with PIN in their first biopsies when series from the 1990s are compared with those of today. Having said that, it is higher than in a control population, and clinicians should be advising patients to have repeat biopsies following a diagnosis of PIN.

The paper reviewed here shows no prognostic significance of separating pN1 from pN2 in bladder cancer, but extracapsular extension is important. Hopefully, this will be changed in any update of the UICC staging system. Identifying small cell carcinoma as a component of bladder tumours is important, as these can be chemosensitive but, more often, it indicates a poor prognosis. The prognostic importance of incidental prostate cancer in cystoprostatectomies has always been debatable and often not relevant in high-stage bladder cancer. Using karyometry, the authors in the paper reviewed here showed that the tumours showed a less aggressive phenotype in comparison with clinically detected tumours, but the paper does not detail other indicators used by previous authors to define their series better.

The increasing use of minimally invasive therapies for renal tumours has meant that biopsies of tumours are increasing. Learning from other departments' experiences is important, and the paper reviewed here certainly draws attention to the difficult area of oncocytomas, which cannot be reliably diagnosed on core biopsies because of sampling errors. c-*kit* is an evolving area in tumour pathology, and the increased expression of KIT in chromophobe renal cell carcinomas may herald a new treatment modality, but it is early days, and a study looking at patients with recurrent/metastatic chromophobe renal cell carcinomas would take many years to recruit enough patients.

References

1. Epstein JI, Allsbrook WC, Amin MB, Egevad LL; the ISUP Grading Committee. The 2005 International Society of Urological Pathology (ISUP) Consensus Conference on Gleason Grading of Prostatic Carcinoma. *Am J Surg Pathol* 2005; **29**(9): 1228–42.
2. Varma M, Jasani B. Diagnostic utility of immunohistochemistry in morphologically difficult prostate cancer: review of current literature. *Histopathology* 2005; **47**: 1–16.
3. Fleming S, Griffiths DFR. Best Practice No. 180. Nephrectomy for renal tumour; dissection guide and dataset. *J Clin Pathol* 2005; **58**: 7–14.
4. Jhavar SG, Fisher C, Jackson A, Reinsberg SA, Dennis N, Falconer A, Dearnaley D, Edwards SE, Edwards SM, Leach MO, Cummings C, Christmas T, Thompson A, Woodhouse C, Sandhu S, Cooper CS, Eeles RA. Processing of radical prostatectomy specimens for correlation of data from histopathological, molecular biological, and radiological studies: a new whole organ technique. *J Clin Pathol* 2005; **58**: 504–8.
5. Hughes C, Murphy A, Martin C, Sheils O, O'Leary J. Molecular pathology of prostate cancer. *J Clin Pathol* 2005; **58**: 673–84.
6. Epstein JI, Pizov G, Walsh PC. Correlation of pathologic findings with progression after radical retropubic prostatectomy. *Cancer* 1993; **71**(11): 3582–93.
7. Bostwick DG, Bostwick KC. 'Vanishing' prostate cancer in radical prostatectomy specimens: incidence and long-term follow-up in 38 cases. *BJU Int* 2004; **94**(1): 57–8.
8. Ward JF, Bartsch G, Sebo TJ, Pinggera GM, Blute ML, Zincke H. Pathologic characterization of prostate cancers with a very low serum prostate specific antigen (0–2 ng/ml) incidental to cystoprostatectomy: is PSA a useful indicator of clinical significance? *Urol Oncol* 2004; **22**(1): 40–7.
9. Petit A, Castillo M, Santos M, Mellado B, Alcover JB, Mallofre C. KIT expression in chromophobe renal cell carcinoma: comparative immunohistochemical analysis of KIT expression in different renal cell neoplasms. *Am J Surg Pathol* 2004; **28**(5): 676–8.

10. Haitel A, Susani M, Wick N, Mazal PR, Wrba F. c-*kit* overexpression in chromophobe renal cell carcinoma is not associated with c-*kit* mutation of exons 9 and 11. *Am J Surg Pathol* 2005; **29**(6): 842.

11. Petit A, Castillo M, Mellado B, Mallofre C. c-*kit* overexpression in chromophobe renal cell carcinoma is not associated with c-*kit* mutation of exons 9 and 11. *Am J Surg Pathol* 2005; **29**(11): 1544–5.

Part II

Urological oncology

5

Renal cell carcinoma

SIVAPRAKASAM SIVALINGAM, HARTWIG SCHWAIBOLD

Introduction

For many years, renal cell cancer seemed to be the one urological tumour where 'not much happens' in terms of new therapies or diagnostic procedures. However, a closer look reveals the ever-growing impact of modern imaging techniques, which has enabled the detection of early stage tumours. This has created a larger role for surgical intervention, with more elaborate techniques enabling us to perform organ-sparing and minimal invasive procedures.

Prognostic factors too have been evaluated in order to help clinicians to predict the prognosis of tumours and decide which tumour needs treatment and if and when advanced tumours should undergo systemic therapy.

Experimental studies in the field of immunology, gene therapy and dendritic cells are about to reach the clinical trial stage. Promising results have been shown in many of the pre-clinical trials so far.

In this chapter, we reviewed articles on open and laparoscopic surgical techniques, modern imaging tools, prognostic scales for advanced disease, the relevance of microscopic haematuria and the question of whether adrenalectomy makes any sense at all in renal cell cancer.

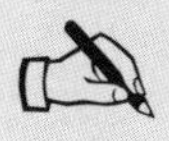

Optical spectroscopy characteristics can differentiate benign and malignant renal tissues: a potentially useful modality

Parekh DP, Lin WC, Herrell SD. *J Urol* 2005; **174**: 1754–8

Background. This study was aimed at assessing the feasibility of using fluorescence and diffuse reflectance spectroscopy to differentiate between cancer and non-cancerous tissue. It was an *ex vivo* study that utilized cancerous and benign tissue obtained from nephrectomy specimens. Ten specimens were obtained; six clear cell renal cell carcinoma (RCC), three papillary RCC and one cystic nephroma. A spectrofluorometer was used to determine the intrinsic fluorescence of the various renal tissues. The tissues were studied within 1 h of resection by preparing them into 5-mm by 20-nm slabs. The optical characteristics of the tissues were further interrogated using a portable fibreoptic spectroscopic kit as shown in Fig. 5.1.

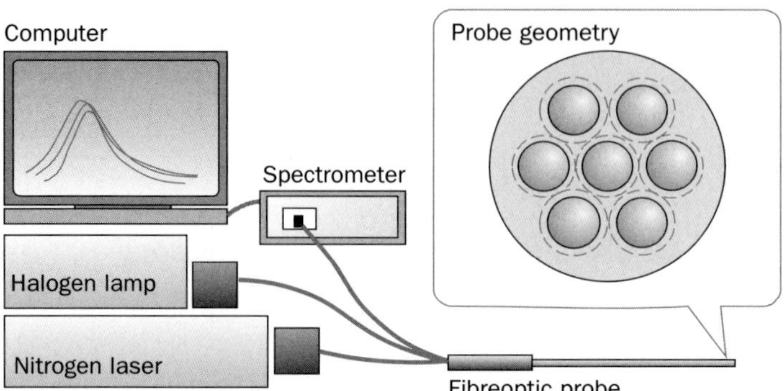

Fig 5.1 Schematic of fibreoptic spectroscopic system. Source: Parekh *et al.* (2005).

Interpretation. The analysis of the emission–excitation matrix of both cancerous and non-cancerous tissues revealed two emission peaks:

Strong Peak A: at 285 nm excitation and 340 nm emission
Weak Peak B: at 340 nm excitation and 460 nm emission

The Peak A of benign tissue locates at the shorter excitation wavelength when compared with cancerous tissue. The intensity of Peak B from benign tissue was greater than that from cancerous tissue. Diffuse reflectance intensity was greater in cancerous tissue compared with benign tissue at the 600- to 800-nm wavelength (Figs 5.2, 5.3 and 5.4).

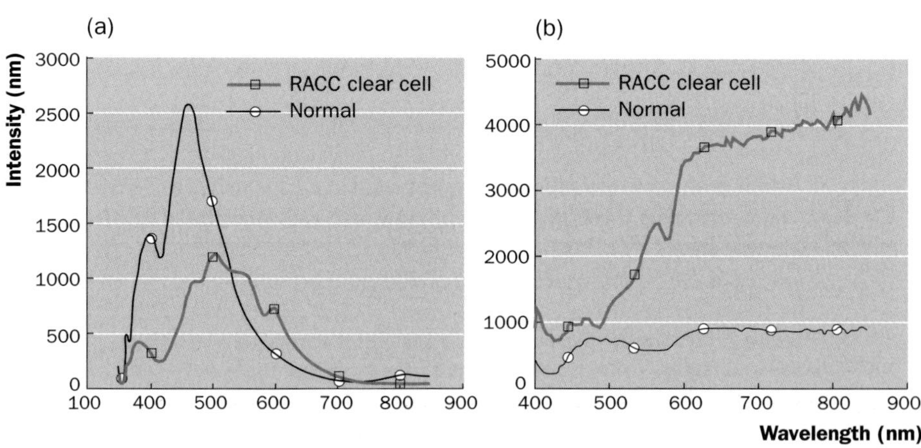

Fig. 5.2 Representative fluorescence (a) and diffuse reflectance spectra (b) from renal cancer carcinoma (clear cell type). Source: Parekh *et al.* (2005).

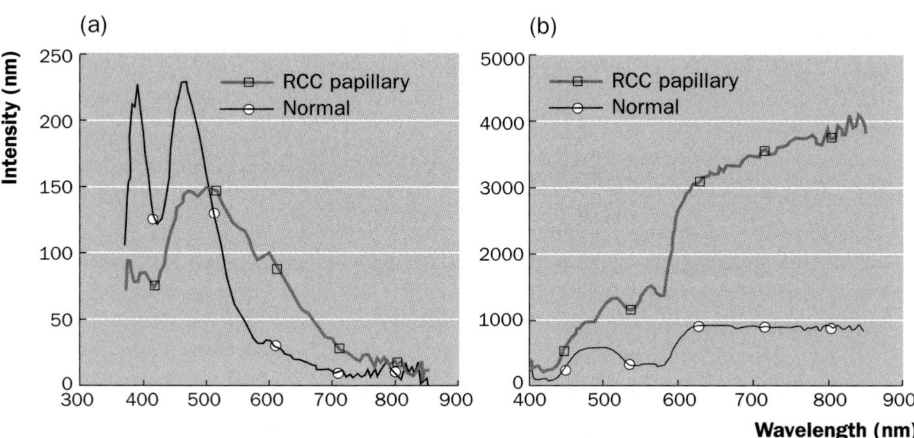

Fig. 5.3 Representative fluorescence (a) and diffuse reflectance spectra (b) from renal cancer carcinoma (papillary type). Source: Parekh *et al.* (2005).

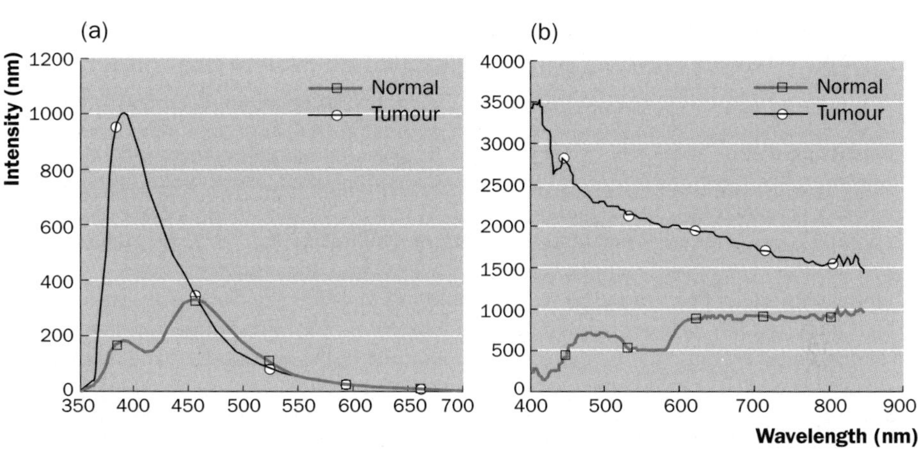

Fig. 5.4 Representative fluorescence (a) and diffuse reflectance spectra (b) from renal cystic nephroma. Source: Parekh *et al.* (2005).

Comment

Although optical characteristics have been studied in other cancers such as oesophageal, cervical, skin and bladder cancer, this is a first of its kind in renal cell cancer. This study is important in the era of nephron-sparing surgery where obtaining clearance of the surgical margin is of immense value to oncological efficacy. The study has demonstrated a significant difference in the optical characteristics of both cancerous and benign tissue during optical interrogation.

Before too much is read into the results, there are limitations to this study that need further elucidation. This was an *ex vivo* study that did not have any significant blood flow during optical interrogation. Chromophores such as haemoglobin absorb much of the light energy in tissue, and the effect of blood flow on the spectral measurements is unknown at this point. The impact of RCC tissue characteristics, such as neovascularity, collagen content, high nuclear density, high lipid and glycogen cytoplasmic content, on spectral analysis also needs further investigation.

The initial findings of this study also suggest that it might be possible to distinguish between the various subtypes of RCC (clear cell and papillary) based on spectral analysis. However, sample sizes in this study are too small to make any definitive statement at present.

This study is a good 'proof of concept', which should now trigger further studies. The ultimate goal for the future should be to develop a tool that would enable intra-operative surgical margin monitoring during resection and the monitoring of tumour response to minimally invasive ablative surgery in renal cell cancers.

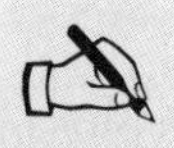

Prospective randomised comparison of transperitoneal versus retroperitoneal laparoscopic radical nephrectomy

Desai MM, Strzempkowski B, Matin SF, *et al. J Urol* 2005; **173**: 38–41

Background. There are two techniques for performing laparoscopic radical nephrectomy: the transperitoneal and the retroperitoneal approach. Each technique has its own advocate. The question of whether one is superior to the other in terms of operative, post-operative and histopathological parameters has yet to be studied in a prospective randomized manner. One hundred and two consecutive patients undergoing radical nephrectomy were randomized to either the transperitoneal approach (*n* = 50) or the retroperitoneal approach (*n* = 52). Randomization was computer generated, and the surgeon was informed of the approach on the morning of surgery. Baseline demographics and tumour characteristics were identical in both patient groups. The exclusion criteria in this study were a body mass index (BMI) >35 and/or previous surgery in the quadrant of concern.

Interpretation. All 102 patients underwent the procedure without the need for open conversion. Continuous variables between the two groups were analysed with the Wilcoxon rank sum test, and categorical variables were compared using the chi-square test. The retroperitoneal approach resulted in a quicker vascular pedicle mobilization and ligation. The total operative time was reduced in the retroperitoneal group (150 min vs 207 min; $P<0.0001$). This parameter was the only statistically significant difference. Factors such as intra-operative and post-operative complications, length of hospital stay, analgesic requirements, resumption of ambulation and oral intake, duration of hospitalization and convalescence were not statistically different between the retroperitoneal and transperitoneal groups. In all cases, the specimen was delivered intact, and no surgical margin involvement was recorded in either patient group.

Comment

This is a unique prospective randomized study comparing the two laparoscopic approaches to radical nephrectomy. Several factors influence the choice of technique used by the operating surgeon. The transperitoneal approach is said to be easier in terms of orientation, as anatomical landmarks are readily identifiable and there is a wider working space. The retroperitoneal technique was believed to result in quicker post-operative recovery, as the risk of ileus in patients was reduced by not entering the peritoneum. In terms of surgical exposure, the retroperitoneal approach provides a limited working space and anatomical orientation. However, there is less interference from bowel loops during dissection and mobilization of the kidney.

This study looked into the purported advantages and disadvantages of both techniques. The only statistically significant difference that the study was able to demonstrate was the reduction in total operating time in the retroperitoneal group. This shortened operating time could be converted into cost savings from improved utilization of the operating theatre facilities. But the authors do state that their preferred technique for routine radical nephrectomy in their centre was the retroperitoneal approach. Therefore, their familiarity with this approach could have accounted for the reduction in operative time demonstrated. In addition, patient numbers in both arms of the study were small, and it was a single centre experience. What this study does demonstrate, however, is that there is no superior approach for laparoscopic radical nephrectomy. Therefore, it should be up to the individual centres to develop their own approach to the procedure.

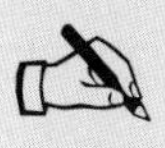

Partial nephrectomy with perfusion cooling for imperative indication: a 24-year experience

Steffens J, Humke U, Ziegler M, Siemer S. *BJU Int* 2005; **96**: 608–11

Background. Nephron-sparing surgery may be indicated for imperative reasons such as solitary kidney, synchronous bilateral tumours or renal failure in the opposite kidney. This may be the only alternative technique to prevent the need for haemodialysis or transplantation in such cases.

In long operative cases, cold ischaemia may be required. This is done either by surface cooling or through the installation of a cold perfusate. In this study, 65 patients undergoing open nephron-sparing surgery between 1980 and 2004 had cold ischaemia through the instillation of Ringer's lactate at 4°C via a clamped and cannulated renal artery. The authors reported on the ischaemia time, complication rate and cancer-specific survival rate in these patients.

Interpretation. All recorded parameters where analysed using the chi-square test, and tumour-specific survival was calculated using the Kaplan–Meier method. The mean operating time was 132 min, mean ischaemia time was 49 min, mean perfusate instilled was 500 ml, and mean operative blood loss was 210 ml. The complications arising from the surgery were post-operative haemorrhage (19%), urinary fistula (8%) and acute renal failure (6%). There were no specific complications arising from the perfusion technique. Although creatinine levels initially increased after surgery, there were no significant rises during the long-term follow-up at up to 111 months.

Comment

Nephron-sparing surgery can be performed by either warm or cold ischaemia techniques. In long cases, where tumours are multiple, intraparenchymal or less accessible, the cold ischaemia technique may be necessary. This can be accomplished by either surface cooling (with ice) or through the instillation of cold perfusate.

Cold perfusion removes blood from the kidney and improves intra-operative visibility, thereby facilitating easy dissection of technically demanding lesions. It also prevents intravascular coagulation and enables the tumour bed to be biopsied more precisely after primary tumour excision. Cold perfusion enables rapid cooling of the renal parenchyma so that anaerobic metabolism of the kidney can be halted more effectively, thereby minimizing ischaemic damage and subsequent renal failure.

To date, there has been no study directly comparing the efficacy of surface cooling and cold perfusion techniques. The authors of this series demonstrated a similar overall complication rate to surface cooling techniques, which is about 30%. The rate of acute renal failure appears to be lower than that published in previous nephron-sparing studies using surface cooling. Surface cooling is technically easier, but the cold perfusion offers better pathophysiological protection during nephron-sparing surgery. A prospective randomized trial comparing the two techniques may be indicated to determine which technique is better in terms of outcomes.

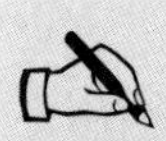

Long-term survival analysis after laparoscopic radical nephrectomy

Permpongkosol S, Chan DY, Link RE, *et al. J Urol* 2005; **174**: 1222–5

BACKGROUND. Intermediate disease-free and cancer-specific survival rates in laparoscopic nephrectomy have been shown to be equal to those in open nephrectomy. However, long-term oncological outcomes comparing open and laparoscopic nephrectomy have been lacking so far. In this retrospective analysis, data from 121 patients who underwent nephrectomy (67 laparoscopic and 54 open) from 1991 to 1999 were analysed. Laparoscopic nephrectomy was performed through the transperitoneal route. Patients were all of clinical stages T1 or T2 N0M0. Patient demographics and tumour characteristics did not differ significantly between the laparoscopic and open nephrectomy groups. The median follow-up for the laparoscopic and open groups was comparable (median of 73 and 80 months respectively).

INTERPRETATION. Kaplan–Meier analysis was used to determine the 5-year and 10-year disease-free, cancer-specific and actuarial survival figures. The results of the

Table 5.1 Kaplan–Meier survival estimates with log-rank comparison for laparoscopic and open radical nephrectomy groups

Stage TxN0M0 (clinical stage)	% Laparoscopic		% Open		P-value (log-rank test)
	5 years	10 years	5 years	10 years	
Disease free					
T1N0M0	98	98	91	91	0.17
T2N0M0	84	84	77	77	0.61
Cancer specific					
T1N0M0	98	98	90	90	0.19
T2N0M0	96	95	84	76	0.21
Actuarial					
T1N0M0	87	76	78	54	0.07
T2N0M0	81	81	77	70	0.63

Source: Permpongkosol *et al.* (2005).

survival estimates for the laparoscopic and open radical nephrectomy groups are shown in Table 5.1. This demonstrates that the disease-free, cancer-specific and actuarial survival rates at 5 and 10 years for the laparoscopic group were comparable to those of the open nephrectomy group.

Comment

Laparoscopic radical nephrectomy was first described in 1991. It has been shown in previous studies to be advantageous to the patient as blood loss, analgesic requirement, time to ambulation, hospital stay and convalescence have all been significantly reduced when compared with open nephrectomy.

Since that time, comparison studies between laparoscopic and open radical nephrectomy have been published demonstrating its oncological efficacy. However, the follow-up interval in these studies has been relatively short; to date, this series has the longest median follow-up of 73 months. On account of the longer follow-up, this is the first series to publish the 5-year and 10-year disease-free, cancer-specific and actuarial survival figures. They showed no incidence of port site metastasis or local recurrence.

Owing to its retrospective nature, this study has biases that need mentioning. Disease selection bias is bound to occur as a result of non-randomization. This usually means that those in the laparoscopic groups would have had smaller and more favourable lesions in terms of resection compared with those in the open group. This could have resulted in artificially better survival outcomes in the laparoscopic group, therefore affecting the overall survival calculations.

Secondly, because of nature of this study, it is also likely that patient selection bias could have been introduced. Patients with a history of obesity and previous intra-abdominal surgery are likely to have undergone an open nephrectomy because of anticipated difficulties with laparoscopy. In these patients, their existing comorbidities could have lowered survival rates, and this could have had a negative impact on the overall survival calculation for the open nephrectomy group.

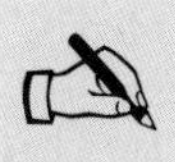

Laparoscopic partial nephrectomy for hilar tumours

Gill IS, Colombo JR, Frank I, Moinzadeh A, Kaouk J, Desai M. *J Urol* 2005; **174**: 850–4

BACKGROUND. Laparoscopic partial nephrectomy had previously been limited to lesions that were small, superficial, exophytic and peripheral tumours. This study is unique as it presents a retrospective series of 25 patients who underwent laparoscopic partial nephrectomy for hilar tumours. The patient demographics are shown in Table 5.2. The authors defined hilar tumours as those that were located in the renal hilum and had demonstrated contact with renal artery and/or vein on a three-dimensional computerized tomographic (CT) reconstruction. All cases were performed by a single operating surgeon. In 22 cases, laparoscopic partial nephrectomy (LPN) was performed through the transperitoneal route and, in the remaining three, retroperitoneally.

INTERPRETATION. All 25 cases had successful laparoscopy without the need for open conversion, although one patient underwent laparoscopic nephrectomy for a thrombus that was found in the renal vein intra-operatively. Mean size of the lesion removed was 3.7 cm. Laparoscopic pelvicaliceal repair was necessary in 22 patients. Mean operating time was 3.6 h, and mean warm ischaemia time was 36.4 min. The mean blood loss was 213 ml, and mean hospital stay for patients was 3.5 days. Seventeen patients had histopathologically confirmed cancer, and 15 were stage pT1a and two pT1b. Fifteen were clear cell carcinoma and two papillary carcinomas. Clear surgical resection margins were achieved in all cases. No kidney was lost for technical reasons. There was no metastasis or recurrence after a mean 21-month follow-up.

Comment

Laparoscopic nephron-sparing surgery had been used for excising small and exophytic peripheral renal tumours. However, its role in the excision of hilar tumours is novel. In laparoscopic surgery of the renal hilum, obtaining a dry surgical field can be technically challenging. This is crucial in order to obtain clear surgical margins during the excision of hilar tumours. The laparoscopic repair of the pelvicaliceal system can be demanding, but it could be facilitated by either retrograde ureteral stenting or dye injection intra-operatively.

Good pre-operative staging is crucial to facilitate operative planning. A three-dimensional CT reconstruction of the hilar lesion and its relationship to the hilar vasculature can facilitate the planning of the surgical approach and the anticipation of probable challenges during excision.

Table 5.2 Demographic data on the 25 patients

No. female (%)	15	(60)
Mean age (range)	61.5	(38–83)
Mean kg/m^2 body mass index (range)	26.3	(20–35)
Mean American Society of Anesthesiologists score (range)	2.5	(2–3)
No. imperative LPN indication (%)	10	(40)
Mean mg/dl pre-op. serum creatinine (range)	0.9	(0.6–2.0)
No. lt kidney (%)	14	(56)
No. laparoscopic approach (%)		
Transperitoneal	23	(92)
Retroperitoneal	2	(8)
No. contralat. kidney status (%)		
Normal	14	(56)
Bilat. tumour	4	(16)
Calculous disease	2	(8)
Solitary kidney	4	(16)
Mean cm tumour size (range)	3.7	(1–10.3)
No. site (%)		
Anterior	23	(92)
Posterior	2	(8)
No. tumours (%)		
Infiltrating	17	(68)
Solid	19	(76)
Cystic	5	(20)
Abutting pelvicaliceal system	19	(76)
No. contact (%)		
Renal artery	7	(28)
Renal vein	10	(40)
Renal artery+vein	8	(32)

Source: Gill *et al.* (2005).

The authors of this study must be lauded for pushing the boundaries of laparoscopic nephron-sparing surgery. The procedure is still new and as yet not well utilized by urological laparoscopists. A note of caution must be added: this procedure should be considered an advanced laparoscopic skill, which must be attempted only by those who have mastered advanced laparoscopic reconstructive skills. For those who wish to embark on this procedure for the first time, a period of laparoscopic mentorship in centres that are currently undertaking this procedure is advised.

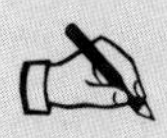

Enhancement of vaccine-mediated antitumour immunity in cancer patients after depletion of regulatory T cells

Dannull J, Su Z, Rizzieri D, *et al. J Clin Invest* 2005; **115**: 3623–33

Background. The authors of this study looked into an innovative strategy for enhancing the immunostimulatory efficacy of tumour RNA transfected dendritic cells

(DC) vaccine therapy in metastatic RCC. This study consisted of *in vitro* and *in vivo* phases involving ten patients with metastatic RCC and one case of metastatic ovarian cancer.

Their strategy was to deplete the $CD25^{high}$-bearing T regulator cells (Tregs) from the peripheral blood mononuclear cells (PBMCs) in patients with RCC. This was accomplished with recombinant interleukin (IL)-2 diphtheria toxin conjugate DAB_{389}IL-2.

INTERPRETATION. The results of the *in vivo* studies on Treg depletion showed significant reduction (26% to 76%) in the CD4/$CD25^{high}$ Tregs population 4 days following infusion of DAB_{389}IL-2 in the six RCC patients who received it. The $CD25^{neg/int}$ Tregs population remain unchanged. Quantitative real time polymerase chain reaction (PCR) showed reduced (30% to 80%) FoxP3 (specific CD4/CD25 Treg marker) mRNA copy numbers in patients receiving the DAB_{389}IL-2. There was only a minor reduction in absolute neutrophil counts.

The specific increases in CD4 and CD8 T cells after vaccination were analysed with the Wilcoxon matched pairs signed rank test to test the null hypothesis that rates of change were equivalent before and after vaccine therapy.

The *in vivo* tumour-specific T-cell response in patients pre-treated with DAB_{389}IL-2 ($n = 6$) prior to vaccine therapy showed a median 7.9-fold increase in the tumour-specific CD8 cell population and a median increase of 7.2-fold in the tumour-specific CD4 cell population. Patients who did not receive DAB_{389}IL-2 ($n = 4$) showed a median 2.7-fold increase in tumour-specific CD8 cells and a 2.0-fold increase in tumour-specific CD4 cells.

Comment

Pre-clinical studies demonstrated that there are three subtypes of CD4 cells based on their CD25 expression; $CD25^{high}$, $CD24^{int}$ and $CD25^{neg}$. The $CD25^{high}$ subtype had been found to be important in immune suppression activity and, physiologically, may be an important mechanism in preventing autoimmunity. However, this can pose a problem as most cancers contain self-antigens, and the presence of the $CD25^{high}$ subtype of CD4 cells could reduce the clinical efficacy of any vaccine-based cancer therapy.

The authors of this study had used a recombinant agent (DAB_{389}IL-2) to eliminate the $CD25^{high}$ subtype of the CD4 population *in vivo*. They have shown that DAB_{389}IL-2 selectively eliminates this CD4 subtype in a dose-dependent manner and leaves other PBMCs, $CD25^{int}$ and $CD25^{neg}$ subtypes, intact.

This study had only a limited number of RCC patients ($n = 10$) and was not randomized. But it has demonstrated that DAB_{389}IL-2 pre-treatment can produce a better tumour-specific immune response in patients receiving vaccine therapy for metastatic RCC. What is uncertain, however, is whether this significant improvement in immune response translates into improved clinical parameters such as symptom control in metastatic disease and prolonged survival. This study should be regarded as a 'proof of concept' study, which should now be taken into the next phase of clinical trials.

This study used our current understanding of immunology to manipulate vaccine response. The outcomes of this study could be beneficial beyond the realms of RCC in other cancer types that have previously been thought to be unresponsive to vaccine therapy.

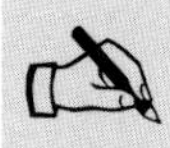

A scoring algorithm to predict survival for patients with metastatic clear cell renal carcinoma: a stratification tool for prospective clinical trials

Leibovich BC, Cheville JC, Lohse CM, *et al.* *J Urol* 2005; **174**: 1759–63

BACKGROUND. The authors of this study designed a clinical tool to predict cancer-specific survival in patients with metastatic clear cell RCC. Between 1970 and 2000, they retrospectively reviewed the records of 727 patients who had metastatic disease at radical nephrectomy ($n = 285$) and patients who developed metastasis subsequently during follow-up ($n = 442$).

INTERPRETATION. The clinical and pathological features of the 727 patients in the series are shown in Table 5.3. Cancer-specific survival was estimated using the Kaplan–Meier method. The association of clinical and pathological features with death from RCC was assessed using Cox proportional hazards regression models. A multivariate model was designed, and the regression coefficients from this model were used to develop a scoring algorithm. The predictive ability of this algorithm was evaluated using a concordance index (c). To develop a scoring system for the algorithm, the authors used the regression coefficients from each feature of multivariate analysis and divided it by the coefficient from liver metastasis, multiplied that by 4 and rounded off the result to the nearest integer. The final scoring algorithm is shown in Table 5.4. After reviewing the median survival figures and performing pairwise comparison between adjacent scores, patients were collapsed into the following score ranges: –5 to –1; 0 to 2; 3 to 6; 7 or 8; and 9 or more, with 5.3, 1.8, 1.3, 0.8 and 0.5 median years of cancer-specific survival respectively. The estimated survival figures for each score range are shown in Table 5.5.

Comment

This algorithm differs from the Survival after Nephrectomy and Immunotherapy score stratified cancer-specific survival and the Mayo Clinic SSIGN (Stage, Size, Grade and Necrosis score) published earlier because it included patients with distant metastases and patients treated for localized cancer in whom metastasis developed subsequently during follow-up. In addition, the features specific to metastasis, such as site of metastasis and treatment of metastasis, were included in this algorithm. The findings from this study indicate that both numbers and specific location of metastasis affect prognosis. It also demonstrates that aggressive treatment of RCC with metastatectomy can improve cancer-specific survival.

This tool could be useful for the selection of metastatic RCC patients into future therapeutic clinical trials. This algorithm has only been validated internally in a

Table 5.3 Clinical and pathological features for 727 patients with metastatic clear cell RCC

Feature	No. (%)
Sex	
Female	239 (32.9)
Male	488 (67.1)
Symptoms at presentation	594 (81.7)
Constitutional symptoms at presentation	322 (44.3)
Pulmonary metastases	389 (53.5)
Bone metastases	186 (25.6)
Liver metastases	73 (10.0)
Metastases in other locations	165 (22.7)
Multiple metastases	97 (13.3)
Years from nephrectomy to metastases	
>2	181 (24.9)
<2	261 (35.9)
0 (metastases at nephrectomy)	285 (39.2)
Complete resection of metastatic RCC	192 (26.4)
Tumour thrombus	270 (37.1)
Tumour thrombus level*	
0	171 (63.3)
I	36 (13.3)
II	40 (14.8)
III	13 (4.8)
IV	10 (3.7)
Primary tumour size (cm)	
<10	431 (59.3)
≥10	296 (40.7)
2002 primary tumour stage	
pT1a	31 (4.3)
pT1b	115 (15.8)
pT2	194 (26.7)
pT3a	109 (15.0)
pT3b	246 (33.8)
pT3c	10 (1.4)
pT4	22 (3.0)
Peripheral perinephric fat invasion	254 (34.9)
Regional lymph node involvement	
pNx+pN0	646 (88.9)
pN1+pN2	81 (11.1)
Nuclear grade of primary tumour	
1	28 (3.9)
2	159 (21.9)
3	398 (54.8)
4	142 (19.5)
Coagulative tumour necrosis	393 (54.1)
Sarcomatoid differentiation	89 (12.2)
Multifocal primary RCC	10 (1.4)

*Percentages reflect only those patients with tumour thrombus.
Source: Leibovich *et al.* (2005).

Table 5.4 Scoring algorithm to predict cancer-specific survival for 727 patients with metastatic clear cell RCC

Feature	Score
Constitutional symptoms at presentation	
No	0
Yes	2
Bone metastases	
No	0
Yes	2
Liver metastases	
No	0
Yes	4
Multiple metastases	
No	0
Yes	2
Years from nephrectomy to metastases	
>2	0
<2	3
0 (metastases at nephrectomy)	1
Complete resection of metastatic RCC	
No	0
Yes	–5
Tumour thrombus	
None or level 0	0
Level I, II, III or IV	3
Nuclear grade of primary tumour	
1, 2 or 3	0
4	3
Coagulative tumour necrosis	
No	0
Yes	2

Source: Leibovich *et al.* (2005).

Table 5.5 Estimated cancer-specific survival by score for 727 patients with metastatic clear cell RCC

		% Estimated cancer-specific survival (no. still at risk)			
Score	**No. (%)**	**Year 0.5**	**Year 1**	**Year 2**	**Year 3**
–5 to –1	96 (13.2)	97.9 (93)	85.1 (79)	70.7 (61)	60.7 (46)
0 to 2	158 (21.7)	83.3 (128)	72.1 (109)	48.5 (69)	35.5 (49)
3 to 6	230 (31.6)	79.7 (179)	58.8 (131)	34.3 (74)	22.1 (44)
7 or 8	119 (16.4)	65.5 (72)	39.0 (41)	18.1 (19)	11.8 (11)
9 or more	124 (17.1)	46.0 (56)	25.1 (29)	8.5 (9)	3.8 (4)

Source: Leibovich *et al.* (2005).

single population, and external validation of the algorithm and its predictive ability is now necessary before it can be implemented in clinical practice. The publication of such validation studies is keenly awaited.

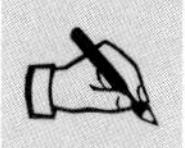

Renal oncocytoma: a clinicopathological analysis of 45 consecutive cases

Gudbjartsson T, Hardarson S, Petursdottir V, Thoroddsen A, Magnusson J, Gudmundur VE. *BJU Int* 2005; **96**: 1275–9

BACKGROUND. Renal oncocytoma is a benign renal tumour that accounts for 3–7% of all renal neoplasms. In an Icelandic population, a retrospective study of patients diagnosed with renal oncocytoma from 1971 to 2000 was undertaken. Forty-five patients were identified in total: 14 cases were post mortem diagnosis and 31 cases were diagnosed when patients were alive. The mean follow-up duration for patients alive at the time of diagnosis was 8.3 years. Thirty patients underwent radical nephrectomy and one had a partial nephrectomy. Histopathological specimens were reviewed by two pathologists and classified according to the 1997 TNM (tumour, node and metastasis) classification. Features such as size, stage, multifocality and concomitant RCC were recorded.

INTERPRETATION. The age-standardized incidence rate was 0.3 per 100 000 per year. Of the 31 patients diagnosed when alive, seven were incidental diagnoses. The mean tumour size was 5.7 cm, and there were three cases of stage 3 cancers. Renal vein invasion, lymph node or distant metastasis were not present in these cohorts. Four patients had coexisting cancers. At follow-up, no metastasis occurred, and there were no deaths from renal oncocytoma. Student *t* test and the Mann–Whitney U test were used to compare groups. Overall survival and disease-specific survival were calculated using the Kaplan–Meier method. Overall survival at 1, 5 and 10 years was 90%, 63% and 51, respectively. Of the 14 diagnosed post mortem, mean tumour size was 3.8 cm, and none was stage 3 disease. Coexisting tumours were also found in four cases.

Comment

This is a unique population-based study on renal oncocytoma. It reaffirms the benign clinical nature of this disease, as there were no cases of lymph node or distant metastasis. No recurrence or deaths were reported in the living diagnosed cohorts during their follow-up after surgical excision.

Renal oncocytoma can be histopathologically difficult to distinguish from chromophobe and granular-type clear cell RCC. CT radiological features of the cancer are also not specific enough for a definitive diagnosis. Needle biopsies of suspected lesions have been shown to be unreliable. Therefore, in most cases, diagnosis is made after histopathological analysis of excised tissue.

Oncocytomas are suitable for nephron-sparing surgery, as most cases appear to be of T1 or T2 stage (42% in the present series). What is uncertain at present, however, is whether, when there is perirenal fat invasion (three cases in the present series), nephron-sparing surgery is sufficient. Non-operative treatment such as radiofrequency ablation and cryotherapy for oncocytoma also needs to be explored in future studies.

The benign nature of this disease makes an argument for conservative management quite compelling. Early data on non-operative management suggest that watchful waiting may be an acceptable management strategy. A single patient with bilateral oncocytoma was left with disease *in situ* in one kidney and remains alive 5 years after the initial surgery to the contralateral kidney. The difficulty in obtaining a firm diagnosis of oncocytoma in the first instance for the reasons stated earlier will continue to remain as an impediment to this strategy.

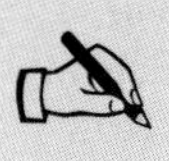

The therapeutic value of adrenalectomy in case of solitary metastatic spread originating from primary renal cell cancer

Kuczyk M, Wegener G, Jonas U. *Eur Urol* 2005; **48**: 252–7

BACKGROUND. Solitary adrenal metastasis occurs in 1.2–10% of RCC patients. The prognostic impact of performing routine adrenalectomy during renal cancer surgery remains uncertain. The authors retrospectively examined the records of 648 patients who underwent adrenalectomy during nephrectomy for RCC between 1981 and 2000. The median age of male patients was 59 years and of females 60 years. The tumour stages were as follows: T1 (37%), T2 (11%), T3 (46%) and T4 (6%). Only 13 cases of solitary adrenal metastasis were identified in this series.

INTERPRETATION. Patient and tumour characteristics were correlated with overall survival by univariate and multivariate statistical analysis. The overall median survival of these cohorts was 4.8 years. The median long-term survival in patients with solitary adrenal metastasis and organ-confined RCC was 11 years and 13.8 years respectively. The long-term survival rates in patients with organ-confined disease and isolated adrenal metastasis at 5 years and 10 years were 66%/50% and 51%/51% respectively. The comparison of long-term survival rates in these two groups did not reveal statistical significance. A multivariate analysis also showed that isolated adrenal metastasis did not predict clinical prognosis in these cohorts (Table 5.6). This supports the claim that isolated adrenal metastasis should be classified separately in the TNM classification system.

Comment

The routine practice of adrenalectomy during nephrectomy for RCC has been questioned recently, first because improvements to current imaging modalities have enabled the detection of early renal cell cancers that have a higher likelihood of being organ confined and, secondly, the results of nephron-sparing surgery have not demonstrated any worsening of the prognosis when adrenal glands have been left untouched. Finally, the low frequencies of adrenal metastasis reported in the published literature mean that routine removal of the ipsilateral adrenal gland during nephrectomy would constitute overtreatment in a majority of patients.

Table 5.6 Prognostic significance of different patient characteristics and metastatic lesions at different organ sites for the long-term survival as determined by multivariate statistical analysis

Variable investigated	*P*-value	RR	95% confidence interval
Age (</≥60years)	0.14		
T-stage (T1/T2 vs T3/T4)	<0.01	2.09	1.52–2.87
Liver metastases	<0.01	2.60	1.76–3.80
Lung metastases	<0.01	2.48	1.87–3.29
Bone metastases	<0.01	1.58	1.14–2.17
Isolated intra-adrenal metastases	0.12	1.31	0.93–1.85
Lymph node metastases	<0.01	1.95	1.45–2.62
Metastases at other sites	<0.01	1.77	1.21–2.58

RR, relative risk for tumour-dependent death.
Source: Kuczyk *et al.* (2005).

Various authors have tried to identify subgroups of patients who would benefit from adrenalectomy based on primary renal tumour stage and size.

The issue of whether adrenalectomy affects clinical prognosis in the setting of isolated metastasis to adrenal glands is controversial. Some series have published no improvement in outcome when adrenalectomy is performed for isolated adrenal metastasis, while others, such as this series, have shown a survival advantage in those undergoing adrenalectomy for the same indication. This variation in findings could be due to the presence of occult metastasis outside the adrenal gland that was not detected during staging procedures. The alternative explanation could be related to the renal cell tumour biology. Histopathological staging and grading may not be sensitive enough to predict the aggressive behaviour of individual renal cancers in terms of tumour progression from isolated adrenal gland metastasis. Molecular tumour markers may be a better alternative but, at present, no such marker exists for clinical use.

Should the upper tracts be imaged for microscopic haematuria?

Feldstein MS, Hentz JG, Gillett MD, Novicke DE. *BJU Int* 2005; **96**: 612–17

Background. This was a quantitative evaluation of the association between renal neoplasms and the different definitions of microscopic haematuria. The aim of the study was to determine whether patients with a positive urine analysis should routinely undergo imaging of the upper tracts to exclude the presence of renal neoplasm. A retrospective case–control study involving 278 patients with previously untreated renal neoplasm was undertaken. Medical records between 1998 and 2003 were examined to select cases and control subjects. Control subjects were matched with cases for age, sex and geographical sites. Both cases and control subjects underwent renal imaging either before or after urine analysis within a 6-month interval.

Gross haematuria and other conditions of microscopic haematuria but not relevant to upper tract imaging were excluded from the study.

INTERPRETATION. Conditional logistic regression was used to compute odds ratios for various definitions of microscopic haematuria. Analysis was stratified to match pairs and adjusted for smoking history, medications and indications for urine analysis. The statistical significance of the comparisons was calculated using the Pearson chi-square test. Sensitivity and specificity were determined by the crude prevalence of microscopic haematuria in matched pairs. The only significant finding was in single urine analysis with a microscopic haematuria value of ≥4 or 5 red blood cells (RBCs)/high power field (HPF). In these cases, there was a statistically significant odds ratio of 2.0 and 2.22, respectively, for renal neoplasm. In a subgroup analysis, symptomatic patients with a urine analysis of 5 RBCs/HPF had a significant odds ratio of 13.68. A subgroup of matched pairs who underwent urine analysis as part of a routine medical examination demonstrated no significant odds ratio for renal neoplasms in any of the microscopic haematuria definitions examined. The sensitivity, specificity and positive predictive values for the different definitions of microscopic haematuria are shown in Table 5.7. The authors also estimated the outcome from analysing urine samples from 10 000 patients from similar demographics to those in this study. The anticipated number of cancers and the number of negative imaging studies are shown in Table 5.8.

Table 5.7 Odds ratio, sensitivity, specificity and positive predictive value for the various microscopic haematuria (MH) definitions

Definition of MH	OR	Sensitivity	Specificity	PPV*
RBC/HPF				
≥3	1.45	24.8	81.3	0.33
≥4	2.00	12.9	92.8	0.45
≥5	2.22	12.6	93.5	0.48
≥20	2.98	5.0	97.8	0.58

*At an assumed prevalence of 0.25%.
Source: Feldstein *et al.* (2005).

Table 5.8 Hypothetical results of 10 000 people undergoing urine analysis

Definition of MH	Number of neoplasms detected by MH*	Number of negative upper tract studies
RBC/HPF		
≥3	6	1866
≥4	3	718
≥5	3	646
≥20	1	215

*Rounded off to the closest whole number. The total number of neoplasms of a possible 25 (prevalence 0.25%) that will be detected by an abnormal urine analysis and the likely number of negative upper tract studies using four different definitions of MH.
Source: Feldstein *et al.* (2005).

Comment

This study attempts to address an important issue of whether upper tract imaging should be performed routinely in patients with unexplained microscopic haematuria to exclude the presence of renal neoplasm. In this retrospective study, cases of previously untreated renal cancer and appropriately matched control subjects were compared for the incidence of microscopic haematuria in their respective groups. The authors stratified the definition of microscopic haematuria into various degrees of severity in terms of RBCs/HPF to see whether there were any safe cut-off levels for the discrimination between the case and control groups.

Urine analysis with ≥4 or 5 RBCs/HPF appears to result in a statistically significant odds ratio for the presence of renal neoplasm. However, the sensitivity of the urine analysis at the aforementioned criteria is low, around 12–13%. At these levels, a negative urine analysis does not reliably rule out the presence of renal neoplasm.

From the data obtained in this study, one can infer that routine renal imaging in asymptomatic microscopic haematuria patients is equivalent to performing a screening test on a normal population, as urine analysis is a poor discriminator for renal cancer in this patient population.

Although renal imaging in unexplained microscopic haematuria is inefficient at picking up renal cancers, it could still help to exclude other pathologies for the microscopic haematuria such as renal calculus or hydronephrosis.

It is difficult to deny a diagnostic test to a patient even if it is on the grounds of providing reassurance that there is no significant underlying pathology such as cancer. But, in the era of health economics and evidence-based medicine, this rationale may not 'hold water' with healthcare managers.

Conclusion

Many papers have been published recently regarding the various developments in RCC. Parekh *et al.* showed a fascinating approach using optical spectroscopy in order to differentiate benign and malignant renal tissue. If this technology could be translated into the operating theatre, then nephron-sparing surgery might reach new levels of accuracy and aggressiveness.

Desai *et al.* attempted to answer the question of whether laparoscopic nephrectomy should be performed retro- or transperitoneally. According to his unique prospective, randomized study, there is no difference in outcome between the two techniques, but the retroperitoneal approach is clearly much faster. Steffens' group proposed perfusion cooling with Ringer's lactate for open nephron-sparing surgery. Their results were impressive, especially with regard to the low renal failure rate of 6%. Permpongkosol *et al.* analysed the outcomes after laparoscopic and open radical nephrectomy and demonstrated equal outcomes regarding cancer-specific and actuarial survival rates. A fascinating paper from the Cleveland clinic demonstrated the feasibility of laparoscopic partial nephrectomy for hilar tumours, an entity that many surgeons would not dare to operate on with an open nephron-sparing technique. The mean tumour size was 4 cm. The post-operative results were impressive with no conversion and positive margins.

Another group presented an innovative strategy for enhancing the efficacy of dendritic cell vaccine therapy, therefore increasing the susceptibility of patients with RCC who undergo vaccination. Leibovich *et al.* from the Mayo clinic developed a scoring algorithm to predict the survival of patients with metastatic RCC. It included site of metastasis and metastatic treatment. They were able to show that aggressive treatment with metastatectomy can improve cancer-specific survival in these patients. A group from Iceland reviewed 45 cases of renal oncocytoma and was able to prove the benign nature of this disease and the advantages of organ-sparing surgery if possible. Kuczyk *et al.* from Hannover analysed more than 700 patients undergoing adrenalectomy during radical nephrectomy. They were able to show that isolated adrenal metastases did not have a negative impact on the prognosis of these patients, and therefore claim that isolated adrenal metastasis should be classified separately in the TNM classification.

Finally, Feldstein *et al.* showed that upper urinary tract screening in patients with microscopic haematuria has a low sensitivity and that routine renal imaging in asymptomatic microscopic haematuria is equivalent to performing a screening test in a normal population.

6

Prostate cancer

JONATHAN OSBORN, KIERAN JEFFERSON

Introduction

Adenocarcinoma of the prostate is a growing health problem, and it is now the most common solid tumour in adult men in the United States. Unlike most malignancies, there is a wide disparity between the prevalence and the mortality of this disease; prostate cancer is present in approximately 30% of 50-year-old men and over 50% of 80-year-old men |**1**|, yet only a small percentage of men actually die from the disease |**2,3**|.

We present papers in the field of prostate cancer ranging from diagnosis and staging strategies to therapeutic techniques, including hormonal therapy. Of particular interest are several papers in the contentious area of watchful waiting (WW) versus radical prostatectomy (RP) in early prostate cancer.

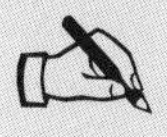

Radical prostatectomy versus watchful waiting in early prostate cancer

Bill-Axelson A, Holmberg L, Ruutu M, et al.; Scandinavian Prostate Cancer Group Study No. 4. *N Engl J Med* 2005; **352**(19): 1977–84

BACKGROUND. In 2002, the Scandinavian Prostate Cancer Group (SPCG) reported the initial results of a trial comparing radical prostatectomy with watchful waiting in the management of early prostate cancer |4|. After a further 3 years of follow-up, the 10-year results were published. Between October 1989 and February 1999, 695 men with early prostate cancer (mean age 64.7 years) were randomly assigned to radical prostatectomy (RP 347 men) or watchful waiting (WW 348 men). The follow-up was complete to 2003, with blinded evaluation of the causes of death. The primary end-point was death due to prostate cancer; the secondary end-points were death from any cause, metastasis and local progression. During a median of 8.2 years of follow-up, 83 men in the surgery group and 106 men in the WW group died (*P* = 0.04). In 30 of the 347 men assigned to surgery (8.6%) and 50 of the 348 men assigned to WW (14.4%), death was due to prostate cancer. The difference in the cumulative incidence of death due to prostate cancer increased from 2.0% after 5 years to 5.3% after 10 years, for a relative risk of 0.56 (95% confidence interval [CI] 0.36–0.88; *P* = 0.01 by Gray's test). For distant metastasis, the corresponding increase was from 1.7% to

10.2%, for a relative risk in the surgery group of 0.60 (95% CI 0.42–0.86; *P* = 0.004 by Gray's test), and for local progression, the increase was from 19.1% to 25.1%, for a relative risk of 0.33 (95% CI 0.25–0.44; *P* <0.001 by Gray's test).

INTERPRETATION. Fewer patients in the RP group died from prostate cancer than in the WW group. The absolute risk reduction between groups increased from 2% at 5 years to 5.3% at 10 years. Patients who received RP also had lower rates of distant metastasis, local progression and death from any cause. The benefit of RP in reducing death from prostate cancer was greatest in men aged <65 years. In men with early prostate cancer, radical prostatectomy reduced death from prostate cancer, distant metastasis, local progression and death from any cause in comparison with watchful waiting, over 10 years of follow-up.

Comment

This is the sequel to the original landmark paper in which 700 men were randomized to watchful waiting or radical prostatectomy |4|. In their previous study, the authors demonstrated that, at 8 years, men who underwent surgery experienced a 50% reduction in progression to metastasis and death from prostate cancer. At the time that article was published, it was criticized because there was no evidence of an improvement in overall survival. At 10 years, the authors argue that men younger than 65 years have an improved survival when treated with radical prostatectomy. However, it seems that this advantage is not present for men older than 65 years at the time of treatment (Fig. 6.1). Furthermore, it is intriguing that 70% of the patients in the placebo arm of the study have not demonstrated evidence of metastatic disease after 10 years. When analysed on the basis of 'number needed to treat', around 19 radical prostatectomies will be performed on men under 65 years to save one life.

Should this paper affect our clinical practice? The study was designed nearly 20 years ago and, since then, *ad hoc* screening and stage migration have changed the clinical picture of early prostate cancer. Until 2003, patients in the WW group who developed local progression were not offered any treatment. Therefore, a disparity existed between the two groups, which biases any conclusions in favour of RP. In addition, in the UK, WW has been replaced by active surveillance, whereby patients are followed closely and, at any hint of disease progression, appropriate systemic therapy is started. This study did not include external beam radiotherapy (EBRT) or brachytherapy. Both treatments are effective in early prostate cancer, but no modern randomized trials have compared radiotherapy with either WW or RP.

The ProtecT study in the UK, which is currently recruiting patients, is comparing active monitoring with RP or EBRT. Only 10% of patients with early prostate cancer will die of prostate cancer—event rates are low, and trials have to be large to show significant differences between treatments. Of particular importance to patients are quality of life issues. All patients allocated to radical prostatectomy may have both acute and chronic symptoms related to the intervention. Patients in the WW group may have a higher risk of symptoms related to disease recurrence or

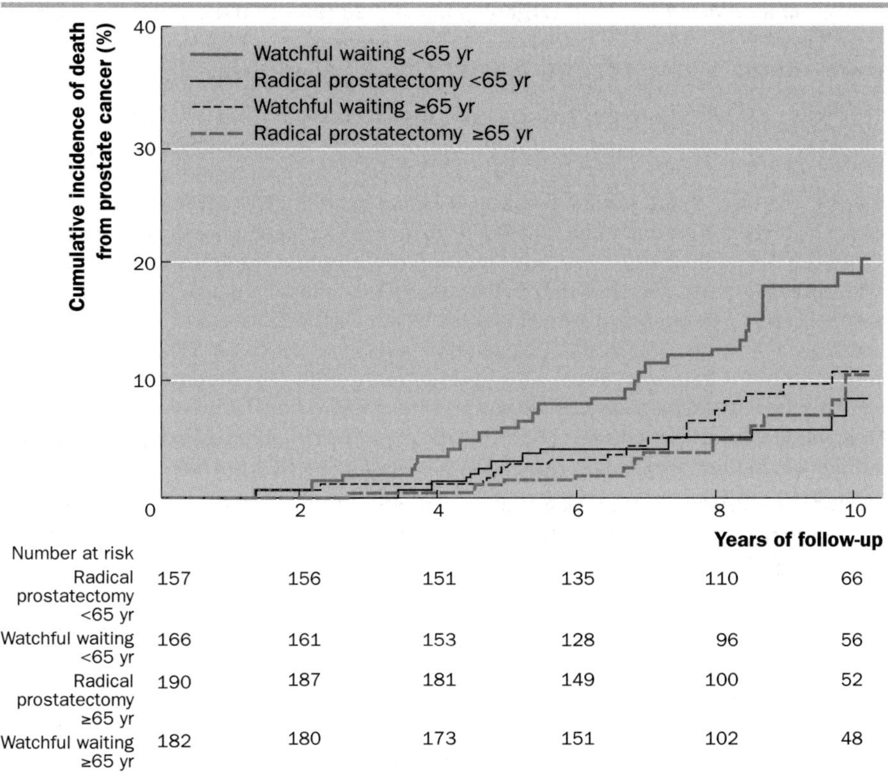

Fig. 6.1 Cumulative incidence of death from prostate cancer in the two study groups according to age. Source: Bill-Axelson *et al.* (2005).

progression, plus any anxieties associated with having untreated cancer. Trade-offs between harms and benefits are complex, particularly when 90% of patients may be at risk of harm without benefit.

Effectively, the authors conclude that healthy men under the age of 65 years with early prostate cancer are more likely to benefit from RP than WW, and this is consistent with the views of most urologists in both the UK and the USA, to some extent dependent on Gleason grade and clinical stage. It is difficult to draw further conclusions from this work in the group of men aged over 65 years.

20-year outcomes following conservative management of clinically localized prostate cancer

Albertsen PC, Hanley JA, Fine J. *JAMA* 2005; **293**(17): 2095–101

BACKGROUND. There is much debate about the appropriate treatment for men with clinically localized prostate cancer. This retrospective population-based cohort study set out to determine the 20-year survival based on a competing risk analysis of men who were diagnosed with clinically localized prostate cancer and treated with observation or androgen withdrawal therapy alone, stratified by age at diagnosis and histological findings. The median observation period was 24 years. The prostate cancer mortality rate was 33 per 1000 person-years during the first 15 years of follow-up and 18 per 1000 person-years after 15 years of follow-up. The mortality rates for these two follow-up periods were not statistically different after adjusting for differences in tumour histology (Fig. 6.2). Men with low-grade prostate cancers have a minimal risk of dying from prostate cancer during 20 years of follow-up. Men with high-grade prostate cancers have a high probability of dying from prostate cancer within 10 years of diagnosis. Men with Gleason scores of 5 or 6 tumours have an intermediate risk of prostate cancer death.

INTERPRETATION. The annual mortality rate from prostate cancer appears to remain stable after 15 years from diagnosis, which does not support aggressive treatment for localized low-grade prostate cancer.

Comment

This paper is an update of the landmark paper by Albertsen *et al.* published in 1998 |**5**|. In their more recent paper, Albertsen *et al.* report that the prostate cancer mortality rate did not increase after 15 years, unlike another large, recently reported cohort study of men with prostate cancer who were managed conservatively |**6**|. As few patients in either cohort lived 15 years, this difference is less important than the substantial difference in prostate cancer mortality over the first 15 years (33 vs 15 per 1000 person-years in the Albertsen and Johansson studies, respectively). This difference is probably due to the higher proportion of men with poorly differentiated tumours in the study by Albertsen *et al.* Indeed, the authors concede that their cohort may include men with extracapsular disease because of the lack of staging and prostate-specific antigen (PSA) data. This hypothesis is supported by the prostate cancer mortality rate of 16 per 1000 person-years in the conservatively managed group in the SPCG-4 trial comparing radical prostatectomy with watchful waiting, which excluded men with high-grade tumours (see Bill-Axelson *et al.* 2005 reviewed above). The outcomes of watchful waiting in these three studies represent 'worst case scenarios' for contemporary men with prostate cancers of similar grades diagnosed in the PSA era. The effects of lead time and overdiagnosis attributable to PSA screening will improve the apparent prognosis regardless of treatment. However, it is hard to estimate the effect of

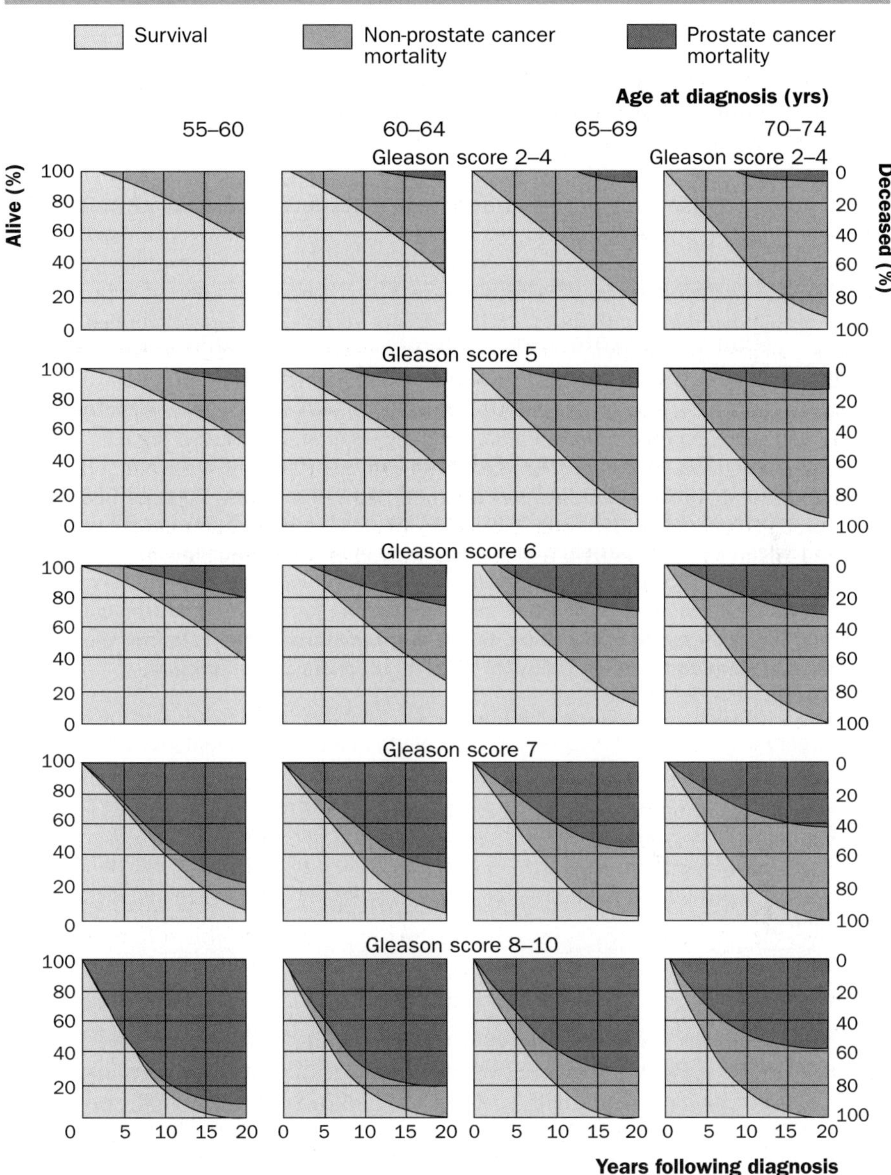

Fig. 6.2 Survival and cumulative mortality from prostate cancer and other causes up to 20 years after diagnosis, stratified by age at diagnosis and Gleason score.
Source: Albertsen *et al.* (2005).

screening on the number needed to treat (NNT) observed in the trial, in which approximately 19 operations were required to prevent a prostate cancer death at 10 years. Most importantly, we do not know the effect of early detection on the subset of poorly differentiated cancers that contribute most to mortality. The Prostate Cancer Intervention versus Observation Trial (PIVOT) of radical prostatectomy versus watchful waiting enrolled men largely discovered by screening, including those with poorly differentiated cancers; it should provide some answers.

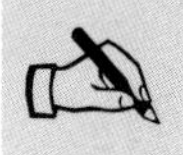

Risk of prostate cancer-specific mortality following biochemical recurrence after radical prostatectomy

Freedland SJ, Humphreys EB, Mangold LA, *et al. JAMA* 2005; **294**(4): 433–9

BACKGROUND. The natural history of biochemical recurrence after radical prostatectomy is variable. This well-designed retrospective cohort study (379 men post-RP) sought to define risk factors for prostate cancer death following RP and to develop tables to stratify patients based on risk of prostate cancer-specific survival. PSA doubling time (PSADT), pathological Gleason score and time from surgery to biochemical recurrence were all significant risk factors for time to prostate-specific mortality. Using these three variables, tables were constructed to estimate the risk of prostate cancer-specific survival at year 15 after biochemical recurrence.

INTERPRETATION. Clinical parameters (PSADT, pathological Gleason score and time from surgery to biochemical recurrence) can help to risk stratify patients for prostate cancer-specific mortality following biochemical recurrence after RP. These preliminary findings may serve as useful guides to patients and their physicians in identifying patients at high risk of prostate cancer-specific mortality following biochemical recurrence after RP to enrol them in early aggressive treatment trials. In addition, these preliminary findings highlight the fact that survival in low-risk patients can be quite prolonged.

Comment

This paper updates the original publication by Pound *et al.* |**7**|, which identifies parameters that predict time to the development of distant metastasis and death from prostate cancer in men with a rising PSA following an RP. With more men followed for longer intervals, the basic findings are the same PSA doubling time (based on the PSA levels during the first 2 years after the first elevation), Gleason score (more or less than 8), and time from surgery to biochemical failure (more or less than 3 years) can be used to stratify patients into risk groups (Fig. 6.3). This will allow clinicians to risk stratify their patients and aggressively treat those at highest risk of early recurrence.

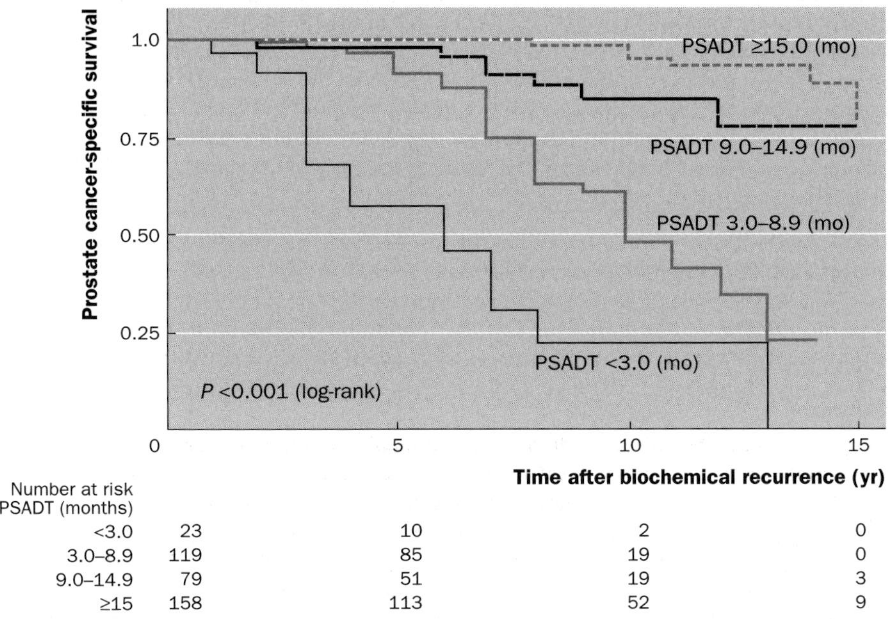

Fig. 6.3 Fifteen-year actuarial Kaplan-Meier prostate cancer-specific survival curves by PSADT. Biochemical recurrence segregated by prostate-specific antigen doubling time among patients who experienced a biochemical recurrence. PSADT, prostate-specific antigen doubling time. Source: Freedland *et al.* (2005).

Maximal tumour diameter and the risk of PSA failure in men with specimen-confined prostate cancer

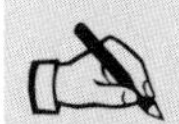

Dvorak T, Chen MH, Renshaw AA, Loffredo M, Richie JP, D'Amico AV. *Urology* 2005; **66**(5): 1024–8

BACKGROUND. The prognostic significance of tumour volume has been debated for many years. Percentage of prostate volume containing tumour and largest tumour volume have been shown to have independent prognostic significance. However, both these techniques require sectioning of the entire prostate, which is both labour intensive and expensive. This paper evaluates the time to PSA failure of maximal tumour diameter (MTD), which is obtained by measuring the maximum dimension of the largest focus of cancer from all 3 mm step sections. Between 1986 and 2002, 781 men with clinical stage T1c–T2 prostate cancer underwent radical prostatectomy. The median follow-up was 5.4 years (range 0.1–14.9 years); 242 men (31%) experienced PSA failure. A Cox regression analysis was used to determine the predictors of time to post-operative PSA failure. Kaplan–Meier estimates of PSA failure-free survival were made, divided about the median MTD value, and compared using a two-sided log-rank test. The value of the MTD was significantly associated

with the time to PSA failure, controlling for pre-operative PSA level (P <0.0001), prostatectomy Gleason score (P <0.0001) and T stage (P <0.0001). When margin status was added (P = 0.0004), the MTD approached statistical significance (P = 0.07). For patients with a pre-operative PSA level of less than 10 ng/ml, prostatectomy Gleason score of 3 + 4 = 7 or less, stage pT2–T3a and negative margins, the value of the MTD significantly (P = 0.05) stratified the time to PSA failure, when divided about the median value (13 mm), with 7-year PSA failure estimates of 17% versus 8%.

Interpretation. The authors conclude that MTD can be used as a proxy for surgical margin status in men treated by radical prostatectomy. However, they do not conclude that MTD should replace percentage of prostate containing tumour until further studies have taken place.

Comment

MTD is a promising prognostic indicator, which may change histological practice. As the authors suggest, most pathologists do not process the whole prostate, and MTD is likely to supersede 'percentage of prostate involved' and 'largest single focus', pending further studies.

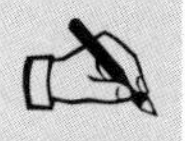

Prostate-specific antigen response duration and risk of death for patients with hormone-refractory metastatic prostate cancer

D'Amico AV, Chen MH, Cox MC, Dahut W, Figg WD. *Urology* 2005; **66**(3): 571–6

Background. A total of 494 men with hormone-resistant prostate cancer were included in four prospective phase 2 clinical trials for thalidomide, ketoconazole, Atrasentan, Taxotere and alendronate (213 in the study group and 281 in the control group). The authors investigated whether the time to return to the baseline PSA level (PSA response duration) is significantly associated with the time to death after randomization for men with hormone-refractory metastatic prostate cancer. Cox regression analysis was used to evaluate whether a significant association existed between the PSA response duration and the time to death after randomization, controlling for treatment and known prognostic factors. A decreasing PSA response duration was significantly associated with a shorter survival after randomization in the study (P = 0.001) and validation (P = 0.02) cohorts, controlling for treatment and known prognostic factors, which included serum PSA, lactate dehydrogenase, alkaline phosphatase and haemoglobin levels and the Eastern Cooperative Oncology Group performance status. The adjusted hazard ratio for death was 1.9 (95% CI 1.4–2.6; P = 0.0002) and 2.1 (95% CI 1.2–3.5; P = 0.01) for men in the study and validation cohorts, respectively, whose PSA response duration was shorter than the median value of 3 months.

Interpretation. The duration of the PSA response to treatment is significantly associated with length of survival for men with hormone-refractory metastatic prostate cancer.

Comment

The PSA response duration may be useful, together with a PSA reduction of >50%, in identifying further agents for use in patients with hormone-resistant prostate cancer. It will also assist doctors in providing more accurate information regarding prognosis to their patients.

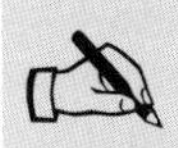

Impact of multiple biopsy cores on predicting final tumour volume in prostate cancer detected by a single microscopic focus of cancer on biopsy

Guzzo TJ, Vira M, Hwang WT, *et al. Urology* 2005; **66**(2): 361–5

Background. It is difficult to estimate tumour volume prior to radical prostatectomy with confidence. With an increasing number of biopsies being taken, the authors questioned whether this practice increases the accuracy of prediction of minimal clinical disease (<5% final tumour volume). This retrospective study identified 102 patients who had undergone radical retropubic prostatectomy for a single microscopic focus of adenocarcinoma. Patients were divided into two groups: those with six biopsies or less and those with seven or more. The Gleason score, margin status, presence of extracapsular extension and percentage of tumour volume were compared. Of these patients, 65 underwent six or fewer biopsies (Group 1) and 37 underwent seven or more (Group 2) at transrectal ultrasonography. Of the 37 patients in Group 2, 27 (73%) had a final tumour volume of less than 5% compared with 24 (37%) out of 65 patients in Group 1 ($P = 0.002$). Of the Group 2 patients, 15 (75%) with stage T1c had an estimated tumour volume of less than 5% compared with only 11 (34%) in Group 1 ($P = 0.01$). No statistically significant difference was noted between the two groups for margin status, presence of extracapsular extension or Gleason score.

Interpretation. The authors conclude that the finding of minimal disease at biopsy cannot be used as an absolute criterion for minimal clinical disease, but may be an aid to decision-making. It is interesting to note that, in the group with fewer than six cores, 37% had a final tumour volume of <5%. In addition, 9% of all men with minimal disease on biopsy had a final tumour volume of >25%.

Comment

Although minimal disease at biopsy may not alter decision-making for most men, specific groups of men may find this information valuable in coming to a decision regarding treatment. Those men with significant comorbidities might be more reassured by minimal disease in multiple biopsies, and therefore more likely to select active surveillance. However, it should be noted that multiple operators performed the biopsies, and also that minimal disease on biopsy does not preclude a >25% cancer volume.

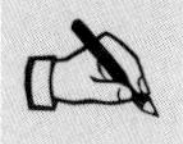

Identifying patients at risk for significant versus clinically insignificant post-operative prostate-specific antigen failure

D'Amico AV, Chen MH, Roehl KA, Catalona WJ. *J Clin Oncol* 2005; **23**(22): 4975–9

BACKGROUND. The authors evaluated whether men at risk of significant versus clinically insignificant PSA failure after RP could be identified using information available at diagnosis. A total of 1011 men treated with RP for localized prostate cancer were included. A pre-operative PSA velocity more than 2.0 ng/ml/year (*P* = 0.001) and biopsy Gleason score of 7 (*P* = 0.006) or 8–10 (*P* = 0.003) were significantly associated with having a post-operative PSADT of less than 3 months. A PSA level less than 10 ng/ml (*P* = 0.005), a non-palpable cancer (*P* = 0.001) with a Gleason score 6 (*P* = 0.0002) and a pre-operative PSA increase that did not exceed 0.5 ng/ml/year (*P* = 0.03) were significantly associated with a post-operative PSADT of at least 12 months or no PSA failure. Most men with these pre-operative characteristics and a post-operative PSADT of 12 months or more had a persistent post-operative PSA level of at least 0.2 ng/ml that did not exceed 0.25 ng/ml after a median follow-up of 3.6 years.

INTERPRETATION. A post-operative PSADT of less than 3 months is associated with a pre-operative PSA velocity of more than 2.0 ng/ml/year and high-grade disease. Selected men with a post-operative PSADT of more than 12 months may not require salvage radiation therapy.

Comment

This paper was designed to identify those men at risk of requiring further treatment, based on information available at the time of diagnosis. It is already known that a significant proportion of men with PSA failure post-RP will develop metastases and will subsequently die of prostate cancer. Post-operative PSADT is acknowledged to detect the majority of these men. Further studies to examine whether adjuvant or neo-adjuvant therapies might improve the prognosis and quality of life of those men at highest risk are required.

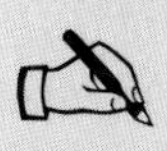

Pre-treatment PSA velocity and risk of death from prostate cancer following external beam radiation therapy

D'Amico AV, Renshaw AA, Sussman B, Chen MH. *JAMA* 2005; **294**(4): 440–7

BACKGROUND. Of men undergoing radical prostatectomy for localized prostate cancer, those who had a pre-operative PSA velocity >2.0 ng/ml/year experience a 10-fold increase in prostate cancer-specific mortality. This study planned to investigate whether a PSA velocity of >2 ng/ml/year in the year prior to treatment is a poor prognostic factor for those men undergoing radiotherapy for localized prostate cancer. A Cox regression multivariate analysis was used to evaluate whether a PSA velocity >2.0 ng/ml per year was significantly associated with prostate cancer-specific mortality and all-cause mortality after controlling for prognostic factors available at diagnosis. A PSA velocity >2.0 ng/ml per year was significantly associated with a shorter time to prostate cancer-specific mortality and all-cause mortality when compared with men whose PSA velocity was 2.0 ng/ml/year or less. Men presenting with low-risk disease and a PSA velocity >2.0 ng/ml per year had a 7-year estimate of prostate cancer-specific mortality of 19% compared with 0% for men whose PSA velocity was 2.0 ng/ml/year or less. The corresponding values for men with higher-risk disease were 24% and 4%, respectively.

INTERPRETATION. A greater than 2.0 ng/ml increase in PSA level during the year prior to diagnosis is associated with a significantly higher risk of death due to prostate cancer following radiotherapy (RT) despite having low-risk disease. Furthermore, the authors recommend that healthy men undergoing RT could be considered for RT combined with androgen suppression therapy because this approach improves survival in men with higher-risk disease (see Trans-Tasman Oncology Group trial reviewed in this chapter; Denham *et al.* 2005).

Comment

Previously, D'Amico and colleagues have shown that men with a PSA velocity of >2 ng/ml/year in the year prior to RP had a markedly increased risk of dying of prostate cancer. In this paper, they show that the same risk applies to patients treated with external beam radiotherapy.

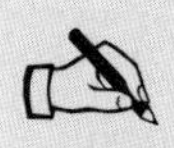

Surrogate end-point for prostate cancer specific mortality in patients with non-metastatic hormone refractory prostate cancer

D'Amico AV, Moul J, Carroll PR, Sun L, Lubeck D, Chen MH. *J Urol* 2005; **173**(5): 1572–6

BACKGROUND. In this paper, D'Amico and colleagues investigated whether PSA velocity can serve as a surrogate end-point for prostate cancer-specific mortality

(PCSM) in patients with non-metastatic, hormone-refractory prostate cancer. Nine hundred and nineteen patients had previously undergone surgery (560) or radiation therapy (359) for clinical stages T1c–4NxMo prostate cancer, followed by salvage hormonal therapy for PSA failure. All patients experienced PSA-defined recurrence while on hormonal therapy. PSA velocity >1.5 ng/ml/year was statistically significantly associated with time to PCSM and all-cause mortality following PSA-defined recurrence while undergoing hormonal therapy.

Interpretation. These data provide evidence to support PSA velocity >1.5 ng/ml/year as a surrogate end-point for PCSM in patients with non-metastatic, hormone-refractory prostate cancer. Enrolling these men onto clinical trials evaluating the impact of chemotherapy on time to bone metastases and PCSM is warranted.

Comment

Changes in PSA with time, including PSA velocity and PSADT, are becoming prognostically important measurements. This paper shows that, in men with non-metastatic, hormone-resistant prostate cancer, the risk of prostate cancer-specific mortality is 200 times higher for men with a PSA velocity of >1.5 ng/ml compared with those with a PSA velocity of <1.5 ng/ml. Smith *et al.* (2005; reviewed later in this chapter) describe the natural history of rising PSA in men with castrate non-metastatic prostate cancer as 'indolent'. Therefore, the early identification of high-risk patients and enrolment into trials (and hence treatments) may significantly improve the quality of life and prognosis of these men.

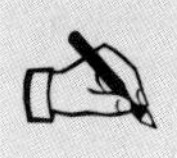

Predictors of short post-operative prostate-specific antigen doubling time for patients diagnosed during PSA era

Lin DD, Schultz D, Renshaw AA, Rubin MA, Richie JP, D'Amico AV. *Urology* 2005; **65**(3): 528–32

Background. This trial was designed to determine the pre-operative and post-operative predictors of a short PSADT after RP for patients diagnosed during the PSA era. A total of 1785 men underwent RP for stage T1c or T2 prostate cancer (as defined by the American Joint Committee on Cancer [AJCC] in 2002). Of these men, 205 had documented PSA failure. Patients with a greater biopsy Gleason score ($P = 0.006$), greater pre-operative risk group ($P = 0.002$), greater prostatectomy Gleason score ($P = 0.0006$), greater 2002 AJCC pathologic stage ($P = 0.01$) or shorter time to post-operative PSA failure ($P = 0.04$) were more likely to have a shorter PSADT.

Interpretation. High-risk disease pre-operatively and a prostatectomy Gleason score of 8–10, seminal vesicle invasion or a time to PSA failure of less than 2 years post-operatively were significant independent indicators of developing a post-operative PSADT of less than 6 months. For these men, trials studying systemic therapy in addition to RP are needed.

Comment

This paper is unusual because it only includes men diagnosed in the PSA era with stage T1c or T2 prostate cancer. These poor prognostic factors (high-risk disease pre-operatively, seminal vesicle invasion, time to PSA failure of <2 years) will help urologists to define those men most in need of adjuvant and neo-adjuvant treatment.

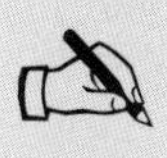

Natural history of rising serum prostate-specific antigen in men with castrate non-metastatic prostate cancer

Smith MR, Kabbinavar F, Saad F, *et al. J Clin Oncol* 2005; **23**(13): 2918–25

BACKGROUND. Smith *et al.* present the results of the placebo group of an aborted randomized controlled trial to evaluate the effects of zolendronic acid in men receiving androgen deprivation therapy. This placebo group provides an insight into the natural history of non-metastatic prostate cancer and rising PSA despite androgen deprivation therapy. At 2 years, 33% of patients had developed bone metastases. Median bone metastasis-free survival was 30 months. Baseline PSA level >10 ng/ml and PSA velocity independently predicted shorter time to first bone metastasis. Baseline PSA and PSA velocity also independently predicted overall survival and metastasis-free survival.

INTERPRETATION. Men with non-metastatic prostate cancer and rising PSA despite androgen deprivation therapy have a relatively indolent natural history. Baseline PSA and PSA velocity independently predict time to first bone metastasis and survival.

Comment

This is a well-designed study that prospectively evaluates the natural history of non-metastatic prostate cancer and rising PSA despite androgen deprivation therapy. As the authors note, laudable features include confirmation of castrate testosterone levels at study entry, documentation of PSA progression with three serial rises and radiographic screening to exclude men with bony metastases at time of study entry. They also performed bone scans every 4 months. The indolent nature of this disease is confirmed by the median metastasis-free survival of approximately 30 months.

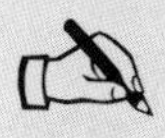

Risk of fracture after androgen deprivation for prostate cancer

Shahinian VB, Kuo YF, Freeman JL, Goodwin JS. *N Engl J Med* 2005; **352**(2): 154–64

BACKGROUND. The use of androgen deprivation therapy (ADT) for prostate cancer has increased substantially over the past 15 years. This treatment is associated with

a loss of bone mineral density, but the risk of fracture after ADT has not been well studied. The records of 50 613 men with prostate cancer were studied. The primary outcomes were the occurrence of any fracture and the occurrence of a fracture resulting in hospitalization. Cox proportional hazards analyses were adjusted for the characteristics of the patients and the cancer, other cancer treatment received and the occurrence of a fracture or the diagnosis of osteoporosis during the 12 months preceding the diagnosis of cancer. Of men surviving at least 5 years after diagnosis, 19.4% of those who received ADT had a fracture, compared with 12.6% of those not receiving ADT (*P* <0.001). In the Cox proportional hazards analyses, adjusted for the characteristics of the patient and the tumour, there was a statistically significant relation between the number of doses of gonadotrophin-releasing hormone received during the 12 months after diagnosis and the subsequent risk of fracture.

Interpretation. Androgen deprivation therapy for prostate cancer increases the risk of fracture.

Comment

This landmark study, which evaluated the records of 50 613 men with prostate cancer, looked at the probability of fracture 5 years after diagnosis. In those patients who received ADT, 19% had a fracture compared with only 12.6% of those not receiving ADT. In this study, only one-third of the patients who received hormonal therapy had distant spread. In their concluding comments, the authors emphasize the need for caution in the use of ADT in settings without clear evidence of benefit. The role of intermittent androgen suppression has yet to be fully evaluated. However, in early studies, intermittent androgen suppression (IAS) seems to reduce the risk of osteoporosis (see Malone *et al.* 2005 reviewed below) with no decrease in oncological control.

Short-term androgen deprivation and radiotherapy for locally advanced prostate cancer: results from the Trans-Tasman Radiation Oncology Group 96.01 randomised controlled trial

Denham JW, Steigler A, Lamb DS, *et al.*; Trans-Tasman Radiation Oncology Group. *Lancet Oncol* 2005; **6**(11): 841–50

Background. Androgen deprivation therapy is an established treatment regimen for disseminated prostate cancer; however, its role in patients with localized cancer is less clear. Several small randomized controlled studies have suggested that short-term ADT improves outcome when given before and during radiotherapy. However, none of these trials gave convincing evidence of the optimum duration of androgen deprivation. This is a large randomized controlled trial designed to determine whether 3 months or 6 months of androgen deprivation given before and during radiotherapy improves outcomes in 818 men with locally advanced prostate cancer. Median follow-up was 5.9 years (range 0.1–8.5 years). Compared with patients assigned no androgen deprivation, those assigned 3 months' treatment had significantly improved local failure, biochemical failure-free survival, disease-free survival and freedom from

salvage treatment. Six months' androgen deprivation significantly improved local failure, biochemical failure-free survival, disease-free survival, freedom from salvage treatment, distant failure and prostate cancer-specific survival compared with no androgen deprivation.

INTERPRETATION. Six months' androgen deprivation given before and during radiotherapy improves the outcomes of patients with locally advanced prostate cancer. Further follow-up is needed to estimate precisely the size of the survival benefits. Increased radiation doses and additional periods of androgen deprivation might lead to further benefit.

Comment

This is a well-designed large randomized trial. The evidence of the benefit of giving ADT is convincing. However, the authors suggest that further trials are needed to examine longer periods of ADT prior to radiotherapy and increasing dosages of radiation. It is also important to note that long-term ADT is associated with significant side effects including osteoporosis (see the paper by Shahinian *et al.* 2005 reviewed above).

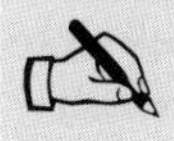

Efficacy of tamoxifen and radiotherapy for prevention and treatment of gynaecomastia and breast pain caused by bicalutamide in prostate cancer: a randomised controlled trial

Perdona S, Autorino R, De Placido S, *et al. Lancet Oncol* 2005; **6**(5): 295–300

BACKGROUND. Gynaecomastia and breast pain are frequent adverse events with bicalutamide monotherapy that might cause some patients to withdraw from treatment. This study aimed to compare tamoxifen with breast radiotherapy for the prevention and treatment of gynaecomastia, breast pain or both during bicalutamide monotherapy for prostate cancer. All treatments were well tolerated. Groups did not differ in disease-free survival rates. Men taking tamoxifen in addition to bicalutamide had significantly fewer reports of gynaecomastia and breast pain than those taking bicalutamide with or without radiotherapy.

INTERPRETATION. Anti-oestrogen treatment with tamoxifen could help patients with prostate cancer to tolerate the hypergonadotrophic effects of bicalutamide monotherapy.

Comment

This paper addresses the important question of breast pain in patients taking bicalutamide for prostate cancer. The bicalutamide Early Prostate Cancer study is currently looking at the benefits of adding bicalutamide to the standard care of patients with early prostate cancer. Breast pain can be a significant quality of life issue in men taking bicalutamide. It is significantly reduced by the addition of tamoxifen, without an increase in other side effects or a decrease in oncological control.

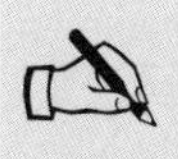

Definitions of biochemical failure that best predict clinical failure in patients with prostate cancer treated with external beam radiation alone: a multi-institutional pooled analysis

Horwitz EM, Thames HD, Kuban DA, *et al. J Urol* 2005; **173**(3): 797–802

Background. PSA failure after radical radiotherapy is usually defined using the 1997 American Society for Therapeutic Radiology and Oncology (ASTRO) definition. Biochemical failure is defined as three consecutive rises in post-treatment PSA after the nadir, with the time of biochemical failure backdated to the time midway between the post-treatment nadir and the first rise. However, some clinicians are keen to tighten up this definition. In this study, the records of 4839 patients with T1–2 prostate cancer treated with EBRT alone were examined. The sensitivity and specificity of several markers of biochemical failure were obtained. In comparison with the 1997 ASTRO definition, three definitions had higher sensitivity and specificity, namely PSA greater than current nadir (lowest PSA prior to current measurement) plus 3 ng/ml (sensitivity 76% and specificity 72%), PSA greater than absolute nadir plus 2 ng/ml (sensitivity 72% and specificity 70%) or two consecutive increases of at least 0.5 ng/ml, (sensitivity 69% and specificity 73%). The sensitivity and specificity of the ASTRO definition in predicting clinical failure were 60% and 72%, respectively.

Interpretation. The authors suggest that the three definitions outlined above might help to improve the 1997 ASTRO definition.

Comment

The 1997 ASTRO definition is a widely accepted benchmark for biochemical failure after radiotherapy in both clinical and research arenas. However, recently, some oncologists have been keen to improve upon the sensitivity and specificity of this definition, particularly to allow closer correlation with surgical series recording any PSA recurrence. This paper gives valuable information to further inform this debate.

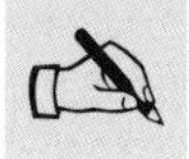

Prostate cancer in patients with screening serum prostate specific antigen values less than 4.0 ng/dl: results from the cooperative prostate cancer tissue resource

Datta MW, Dhir R, Dobbin K, *et al. J Urol* 2005; **173**(5): 1546–51

Background. Since 1990, a PSA level of 4.0 ng/ml or less in men has been widely considered to be indicative that prostate cancer is unlikely to be present. However, prostate cancer can occur in patients with low screening serum PSA values

(<4.0 ng/ml). This paper sought to define whether these tumours are different from prostate cancer in patients with high PSA levels (>4.0 ng/ml). A total of 3416 patients with screening PSA <16.0 ng/ml diagnosed with prostate cancer between 1993 and 2004 were stratified in groups based on screening serum PSA. Of these 468 (14%) patients with screening PSA <4.0 ng/ml, 142 (4.2%) had a PSA of <2.0 ng/ml. This group included 40 black and 376 white patients. Men with low screening PSA treated with RP had smaller cancers, lower Gleason scores, lower pathological tumour (T) stage and lower PSA recurrence rates than men with high PSA levels (4 ng/ml or greater). These differences held true for men who were younger than 62 years or were white, whereas older or black men had tumour characteristics and outcomes similar to those with higher PSA levels.

INTERPRETATION. Young (<62 years) or white patients with screening serum PSA <4.0 ng/ml had smaller, lower grade tumours and lower recurrence rates than patients with PSA 4.0 ng/ml or greater. This was not true for those older than 62 years and for black men.

Comment

The question that remains unanswered by this paper is whether we need to treat men with the relatively low-risk tumours that predominate in patients with low PSA. In this study, approximately 37% of men with 'low' PSA had a Gleason 7–10 prostate cancer. However, the authors admit that the figures are small and should be viewed as preliminary. We await further studies to show the true incidence of high-grade cancers presenting with a PSA <4.0 ng/ml.

The efficacy of sildenafil citrate following radiation therapy for prostate cancer: temporal considerations

Ohebshalom M, Parker M, Guhring P, Mulhall JP. *J Urol* 2005; **174**(1): 258–62; discussion 262

BACKGROUND. Erectile dysfunction is a recognized complication of radiation therapy (EBRT and brachytherapy) for prostate cancer. Sildenafil citrate is a well-known management strategy for erectile dysfunction that has been found to be efficacious across a wide spectrum of comorbidities, including post-radiation erectile dysfunction. This study was designed to discover the efficacy of sildenafil citrate in patients with erectile dysfunction following radiation therapy for prostate cancer and to assess the impact of the interval after radiation on the success of this therapy. Validated questionnaires (International Index of Erectile Function; IIEF) were used post-radiotherapy. All patients were considered to have erectile dysfunction after radiotherapy, and they were prescribed sildenafil citrate. Mean time ± SD between the completion of radiation therapy and the initiation of sildenafil was 8 ± 4 months.

INTERPRETATION. Sildenafil citrate improves erectile function in men in whom erectile dysfunction develops following radiation therapy for prostate cancer. There is clear time dependence for the response to this therapy with a stepwise decrease in all end-points examined serially in a 3-year period.

Comment

This paper addresses an area of radiotherapy that has an impact upon patients' quality of life. It is often stated that some men select brachytherapy because of the lower rates of erectile dysfunction than RP. All men in this trial were impotent after the radiotherapy. Sildenafil has been shown to be effective in improving erectile function in men with post-radiotherapy erectile dysfunction. The response to sildenafil was inversely proportional to the time after radiation therapy. However, there was no control group to show that erectile function would not have resolved without intervention. Another weakness of this paper is the absence of documentation of pre-treatment erectile function scores. Interestingly, response rates were higher in the group that had received brachytherapy rather than EBRT. The authors state that there are ongoing studies to answer these questions.

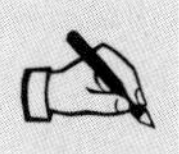

Long-term effects of finasteride on prostate specific antigen levels: results from the prostate cancer prevention trial

Etzioni RD, Howlader N, Shaw PA, *et al. J Urol* 2005; **174**(3): 877–81; Erratum in *J Urol* 2005; **174**(5): 2071

BACKGROUND. Studies have shown that finasteride decreases PSA levels by approximately 50% during the first 12 months of use. This study looked at the long-term effects of finasteride on PSA in men with and without a prostate cancer diagnosis at the end of the study. Serial PSA in participants in the Prostate Cancer Prevention Trial who had an end of study biopsy (928 with cancer and 8620 with negative biopsy) or an interim diagnosis of prostate cancer (671) were analysed.

INTERPRETATION. In men who have been receiving finasteride for more than 1 year, various adjustment factors may be needed to determine whether PSA is in the normal range. In the Prostate Cancer Prevention Trial cohort, the adjustment factor required to preserve median PSA increased from 2 at 24 months to 2.5 at 7 years after the initiation of finasteride.

Comment

This is an elegantly designed study that set out to define the adjustment to the normal range for PSA in men taking finasteride. Of note, the adjustment factor seems to increase with time, from a factor of 2 at 2 years to 2.5 at 7 years. Reassuringly, in men with prostate cancer, the PSA increases equally as rapidly in men taking finasteride as in control subjects.

Intensive lifestyle changes may affect the progression of prostate cancer

Ornish D, Weidner G, Fair WR, *et al. J Urol* 2005; **174**(3): 1065–9; discussion 1069–70

BACKGROUND. Frequently, men with prostate cancer are advised to make changes in diet and lifestyle, although the impact of these changes has not been well documented. This paper was designed to investigate the effects of lifestyle changes on PSA, treatment trends and serum-stimulated LNCaP (a human prostate cancer cell line developed from a lymph node metastasis) cell growth in men with early, biopsy-proven prostate cancer after 1 year. None of the experimental group patients but six control patients underwent treatment for an increase in PSA and/or progression of disease on magnetic resonance imaging. PSA decreased by 4% in the experimental group but increased by 6% in the control group ($P = 0.016$). The growth of LNCaP prostate cancer cells (American Type Culture Collection, Manassas, VA, USA) was inhibited almost eight times more by serum from the experimental than from the control group (70% vs 9%; $P < 0.001$). Changes in serum PSA and also in LNCaP cell growth were significantly associated with the degree of change in diet and lifestyle.

INTERPRETATION. Intensive lifestyle changes may affect the progression of early, low-grade prostate cancer in men. Further studies and longer-term follow-up are warranted.

Comment

It has been suggested that modification of lifestyle factors may be able to restrict both the development and the progression of prostate cancer. Most commonly studied are dietary factors. Of particular interest are lycopene (from tomatoes), vitamins C and E and selenium.

Ornish *et al.* have performed a randomized controlled trial looking at the progression of early low-grade prostate cancer and the effect of diet, exercise and stress reduction. This trial suggests that patients with early low-grade prostate cancer were able to maintain lifestyle changes that significantly reduced serum PSA. It also suggests that serum from patients in the lifestyle modification group inhibited the growth of prostate cancer cells *in vitro*. The accompanying editorial questions the conclusions, based on the inherent variability of the PSA assay, and also points out that a decrease in PSA is not necessarily evidence of any protective effect. Bearing these criticisms in mind, the authors have recommended further studies. Lifestyle and dietary modifications are unlikely to harm the patient, and involving the patient in his active management is likely to improve his psychological well-being, if not his physical health.

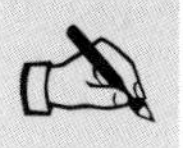

Cross-sectional analysis of sexual function after prostate brachytherapy

Finney G, Haynes AM, Cross P, Brenner P, Boyn A, Stricker P. *Urology* 2005; **66**(2): 377–81

BACKGROUND. Prostate brachytherapy is being used increasingly to treat prostate cancer in the United States, Canada and Australia. It is perceived by some as having a lower side-effect profile than radical prostatectomy, and therefore is selected by some men in whom post-treatment impotence is a major concern. This cross-sectional study consisted of 96 sexually active patients (mean age 64 years) who underwent iodine-125 seed implantation. Validated questionnaires were used. All men were found to have normal sexual function prior to the procedure. No significant relationship was found between sexual function and time since treatment (*P* = 0.9897). Pain on orgasm was reported after brachytherapy by 38 patients (40%) and haemospermia by 16 patients (17%). A negative correlation was observed between pain on orgasm and time since treatment (*P* = 0.021), but no significant relationship was found between haemospermia and time since treatment (*P* = 0.427). A significant difference in sexual function was observed between patients younger than 60 years and patients older than 60 years (66.3 ± 7.0 vs 47.7 ± 7.2; *P* = 0.002).

INTERPRETATION. A large variation in sexual potency is present after brachytherapy with no significant relationship to the time since treatment. Age is an indicator of sexual function after brachytherapy, with younger patients experiencing less sexual dysfunction than older patients. Other aspects of sexual function (pain on orgasm, haemospermia) are also significant side effects of brachytherapy and must be considered in the treatment decision for low-risk prostate cancer.

Comment

This is a cross-sectional study looking at one specific complication of brachytherapy. It shows a mean potency rate of 55%, which is broadly comparable to other studies. Stock *et al.* (2001) **8** reported that 21% of men experienced erectile dysfunction at 3 years post-procedure, whereas Raina *et al.* (2003) **9** reported a 71% rate of impotence at 4 years. Admittedly, these studies all used different measure of impotence, and the current study used different scales to assess pre- and post-treatment potency. The follow-up range (between 3 months and 6.2 years) was large, which makes interpretation difficult. This information will be useful when counselling patients; however, larger studies with longer follow-up are required.

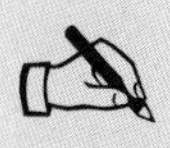

Long-term side effects of intermittent androgen suppression therapy in prostate cancer: results of a phase II study

Malone S, Perry G, Segal R, Dahrouge S, Crook J. *BJU Int* 2005; **96**(4): 514–20

BACKGROUND. Androgen deprivation therapy has been shown to significantly compromise a patient's quality of life. These side effects include decreased bone mineral density, decreased sexual function, muscle mass cognitive function, haemoglobin and energy levels, as well as increased weight and serum cholesterol levels. IAS therapy has been shown to be clinically effective. This paper was designed to show the effect on the quality of life of men with recurrent or metastatic prostate cancer on IAS. In all, 95 patients received 245 cycles; the median duration of rest periods was 8 months, and median time to treatment failure was 47 months. Testosterone recovery during rest periods was documented in 117 (61%) cycles. Anaemia was mild and reported in 33%, 44% and 67% of cycles 1, 2 and 3, respectively. Sexual function recovered during the rest periods in 47% of cycles. There was no significant overall change in body mass index at the end of the treatment period. Osteoporosis was documented in at least one site evaluated in 41 patients (37%).

INTERPRETATION. IAS has the potential to reduce side effects, including recovery of haemoglobin level, return of sexual function and absence of weight gain at the end of the study period.

Comment

ADT is the standard therapy for metastatic prostate cancer. The median survival for men with hormone-resistant disease is approximately 9 months, and IAS has the potential to delay the onset of hormone-resistant disease, while at the same time reducing the side effects compared with ADT. This paper supports the hypothesis that IAS shows an improvement in some quality of life indices. Further validated quality of life studies would confirm this hypothesis.

Conclusion

Recent years have seen a significant shift in our understanding of prostate cancer and its treatment. There is now conclusive evidence from a randomized controlled trial that radical prostatectomy offers a significant but small improvement in overall survival compared with observation. There is also increasing evidence to allow us to identify those patients at high risk of prostate cancer death and disease recurrence. The challenge in the coming years will be to further refine patient selection for the various treatment options and to identify effective treatments for hormone-independent disease.

References

1. Scardino PT. Early detection of prostate cancer. *Urol Clin North Am* 1989; **16**(4): 635–55.
2. Franks LM. Proceedings: etiology, epidemiology, and pathology of prostatic cancer. *Cancer* 1973; **32**(5): 1092–5.
3. Sakr WA, Grignon DJ. Prostate cancer: indicators of aggressiveness. *Eur Urol* 1997; **32**(Suppl 3): 15–23.
4. Holmberg L, Bill-Axelson A, Helgesen F, Salo JO, Folmerz P, Haggman M, Andersson SO, Spangberg A, Busch C, Nordling S, Palmgren J, Adami HO, Johansson JE, Norlen BJ; Scandinavian Prostatic Cancer Group Study Number 4. A randomized trial comparing radical prostatectomy with watchful waiting in early prostate cancer. *N Engl J Med* 2002; **347**(11): 781–9.
5. Albertsen PC, Hanley JA, Gleason DF, Barry MJ. Competing risk analysis of men aged 55 to 74 years at diagnosis managed conservatively for clinically localized prostate cancer. *JAMA* 1998; **280**(11): 975–80.
6. Johansson JE, Andren O, Andersson SO, Dickman PW, Holmberg L, Magnuson A, Adami HO. Natural history of early, localized prostate cancer. *JAMA* 2004; **291**(22): 2713–19.
7. Pound CR, Partin AW, Eisenberger MA, Chan DW, Pearson JD, Walsh PC. Natural history of progression after PSA elevation following radical prostatectomy. *JAMA* 1999; **281**(17): 1591–7.
8. Stock RG, Kao J, Stone NN. Penile erectile function after permanent radioactive seed implantation for treatment of prostate cancer. *J Urol* 2001; **165**(2): 436–9.
9. Raina R, Agarwal A, Goyal KK, Jackson C, Ulchaker J, Angermeier K, Klein E, Ciezki J, Zippe CD. Long-term potency after iodine-125 radiotherapy for prostate cancer and role of sildenafil citrate. *Urology* 2003; **62**(6): 1103–8.

7

Locally advanced and advanced prostate cancer

HEATHER PAYNE, OMAR AL-SALIHI

Introduction

The management of men with all stages of prostate cancer is an increasingly complex process with a variety of available treatments and the involvement of many different disciplines. Locally advanced disease is a common presentation in the UK, accounting for one-third of all new cases. There is no clear consensus on optimal management, and this was highlighted in a recent survey of oncologists and urologists conducted by BUG (British Uro-oncology Group) and the BAUS (British Association of Urological Surgeons) Section of Oncology. Treatment has traditionally included external beam radiotherapy, but more than one-third of patients experience disease progression within 5 years with risk factors including prostate-specific antigen (PSA) ≥10 and any single Gleason score ≥4 on biopsy [1]. There is evidence that increased radiation dose is associated with increased cancer cell kill for men with prostate cancer. The advent of new radiotherapy techniques (three-dimensional conformal [3DCRT], intensity modulated radiotherapy [IMRT], and high dose-rate [HDR] brachytherapy boost) aims to allow increased doses of radiation without unacceptable additional morbidity. The benefits of dose escalation have been demonstrated in a number of clinical trials [2]. A further challenge in treating locally advanced prostate cancer is the concurrent treatment of microscopic metastases at distant sites. This means that, despite improved local treatment, many men will ultimately progress to metastatic disease, which can cause debilitating morbidity including bone pain, fracture, spinal cord compression and urinary dysfunction. There is evidence that the addition of systemic treatment in the form of hormone therapy with androgen suppression is superior to radiotherapy alone in patients with locally advanced disease [3,4]. This combination therapy has been shown to improve survival and increase time to progression. The use of combined modality treatment for locally advanced prostate cancer has been an exciting development, but the optimal duration and timing of the hormone therapy remains uncertain, and the results of further studies are awaited.

Advanced (metastatic) prostate cancer is usually associated with significant morbidity and limited treatment options when the disease becomes hormone refractory (HRPC). Until recently, the standard of care has been mitoxantrone chemotherapy combined with prednisolone |**5**|. This therapy improves bone pain in 30% of men, but has not been associated with increased survival. The results of two independent, international phase 3 studies changed the management approach to HRPC when they reported that taxane-based chemotherapy can lead to a survival benefit for men with HRPC |**6,7**|. Docetaxol was also linked to an increase in times to disease progression, PSA decreases and quality of life. The optimal sequencing of chemotherapy remains uncertain and is again the subject of ongoing clinical trials. There are other drugs showing promise in HRPC, and this remains a challenging therapeutic area.

There have been significant advances in treatment options for men with locally advanced and advanced prostate cancer in the past few years, and it is our pleasure to review some of the important recent papers.

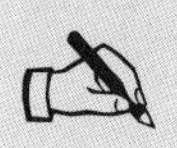

Androgen suppression adjuvant to definitive radiotherapy in carcinomas of the prostate: long-term results of Phase III RTOG 85-31

Pilepich MV, Winter K, Lawton CA, *et al. Int J Radiat Oncol Biol Phys* 2005; **61**: 1285–90

BACKGROUND. This study was designed to evaluate the effectiveness of adding adjuvant androgen suppression, using goserelin, to definitive radiotherapy for men with unfavourable prognosis prostate cancer. A total of 997 men with locally advanced prostate cancer (cT1–2, N+ or T3 any N or after prostatectomy pT3a with tumour at the surgical margin or pT3b) were entered into the study between 1987 and 1992. Stratification was based on histological differentiation, nodal status, acid phosphatase status and prior prostatectomy. Patients were randomized to radiotherapy and adjuvant goserelin starting during the last week of radiation and continuing indefinitely, or radiotherapy alone followed by observation and goserelin at relapse. The minimum radiotherapy target dose to the prostate volume was 65–70 Gy for those men treated definitively and 60–65 Gy in the post-operative setting.

INTERPRETATION. Median follow-up was 7.6 years for all patients and 11 years for living patients. Across the entire study population, there was a significant improvement in estimated 10-year survival with adjuvant goserelin and radiotherapy compared with radiotherapy alone (49% vs 39%; $P = 0.002$). Significant improvements in favour of adjuvant goserelin were also seen for estimated 10-year incidences of local failure (23% vs 38%; $P < 0.0001$), distant metastases (24% vs 39%; $P < 0.0001$) and disease-specific mortality (16% vs 22%). Further analysis of the data was conducted using pre-treatment Gleason grade. This showed that adjuvant goserelin significantly increased estimated 10-year overall survival in patients with Gleason 7 (52% vs 42%; $P = 0.026$) and Gleason 8–10 (39% vs 25%; $P = 0.0046$), but not for those with Gleason grade 2–6.

Comment

RTOG (Radiation Therapy Oncology Group) 85-31 is the largest and longest study of its kind and confirms data from previous trials with shorter duration of follow-up. The results of this highly significant study demonstrate important overall survival benefits. Patients with high Gleason scores have the greatest risk of disease progression and the most significant risk of metastases, and this group (Gleason 8–10) demonstrated the largest benefits from combined modality therapy on subgroup analysis. Earlier analysis of RTOG 85-31 with 5-year estimates of survival showed no significant benefits for any Gleason grade below 8 but, with longer follow-up, this study now demonstrates significant survival benefit for patients with Gleason grade 7. The study is ongoing, and further analyses are awaited to see whether goserelin will provide a long-term survival benefit for patients with lower Gleason grades. Benefits for combined modality treatment for locally advanced (bulky) Gleason grade 2–6 have been demonstrated in RTOG study 86-10 |**8**|, with a significant increase in overall survival and reduction in disease progression seen with the addition of neoadjuvant and concomitant hormone therapy to radiation.

There remain uncertainties regarding the optimal timing and duration of hormone therapy. Timing has varied between different trials. Goserelin was added during the final week of RTOG 85-31, the first week of EORTC 22863 |**3**| and before radiotherapy in RTOG 92-02 |**4**|. There may be an additive or even a synergistic effect of the combination of hormones and radiation, and this could potentially provide further benefits for combination treatments. There were also differences in the duration of adjuvant goserelin therapy between the three studies with hormone

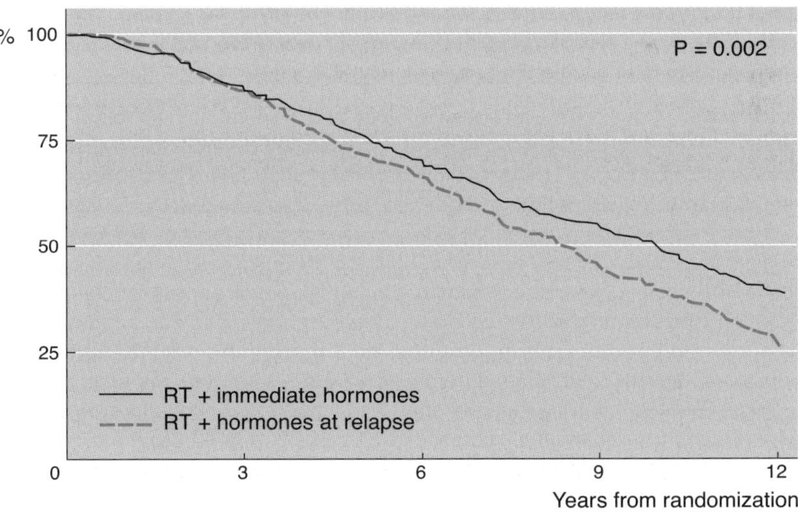

Fig. 7.1 Absolute survival. Source: Pilepich *et al.* (2005).

therapy administered indefinitely (RTOG 85-31), for 3 years (EORTC 22863) or for 2 years plus 2 months neoadjuvant (RTOG 92-02). Patient quality of life is an important issue when deciding on the duration of therapy, and any long-term side effects must also be considered. Further results of these and other studies are awaited to determine the optimal duration of hormone treatment. The introduction of new radiotherapy techniques, as described above, has allowed dose escalation beyond that delivered in RTOG 85-31 and, again, this combination may lead to even greater improvement in outcome. RTOG 85-31 is a very important study demonstrating a durable survival benefit with combined modality treatment, and it is felt that this approach should now be offered to all men with locally advanced prostate cancer.

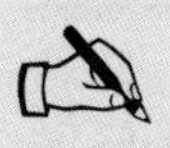

Bicalutamide 150 mg plus standard care versus standard care alone for early prostate cancer

McLeod DG, Iversen P, See WA, Morris T, Armstrong J, Wirth MP; Casodex Early Prostate Cancer Trialists' Group. *BJU Int* 2006; **97**(2): 247–54

Background. The aim of the ongoing Early Prostate Cancer (EPC) study is to evaluate the efficacy and tolerability of adding the non-steroidal anti-androgen bicalutamide 150 mg once daily to standard care (prostatectomy, radiotherapy or watchful waiting) for patients with localized or locally advanced non-metastatic prostate cancer. It comprises three randomized, double-blind, placebo-controlled studies in North America (Trial 23, 3292 men), Europe, South America, Australia, Israel and Mexico (Trial 24, 3603 men) and Scandinavia (Trial 25, 1218 men). The trials were designed and powered for combined analysis. In trial 23, treatment was administered for 2 years but, in studies 24 and 25, it was given for 5 years. The primary end-points were objective progression-free survival (PFS) and overall survival. The median follow-up time at this third analysis was 7.4 years.

Interpretation. Consistent with earlier findings at 5.4 years' median follow-up, the latest analysis at a median of 7.4 years showed no significant difference in overall survival across the programme. However, bicalutamide plus standard care continued significantly to improve objective PFS (hazard ratio [HR] 0.79; 95% confidence interval [CI] 0.73–0.85; *P* <0.001). Exploratory analyses were also conducted to determine the efficacy of bicalutamide in clinically relevant subgroups. In localized disease, there was no significant difference between the treatment groups for overall survival or objective PFS regardless of the standard of care received. Moreover, there was a trend towards decreased survival in patients receiving bicalutamide 150 mg in the watchful waiting subgroup. In locally advanced disease, differences were seen between the standard care subgroups. For men receiving radiotherapy, there was a significant improvement in overall survival with the addition of bicalutamide (HR 0.65; CI 0.44–0.95; *P* = 0.03). There was also a trend towards increased survival for the subgroup treated with bicalutamide who would otherwise have undergone watchful waiting (HR 0.81; CI 0.66–1.01; *P* = 0.06). For radical prostatectomy, no significant benefit in overall survival was seen (HR 1.09; CI 0.85–1.39; *P* = 0.51). A significant improvement in objective PFS in favour of bicalutamide 150 mg for all locally advanced patients was demonstrated irrespective of the standard of care received (HR 0.69; CI 0.58–0.83; *P* <0.001). This benefit was greatest for those receiving radiotherapy (HR 0.56; CI 0.40–0.78; *P* <0.001), but was also seen in the radical prostatectomy (HR 0.75; CI 0.61–0.91; *P* = 0.004) and watchful waiting (HR 0.60; CI 0.49–0.73; *P* <0.0001) groups. Bicalutamide 150 mg was seen to have acceptable tolerability. Mild to moderate gynaecomastia (68.8%) and breast pain (73.6%) were the commonest adverse events described. Other adverse events were infrequent with impotence reported in 9.3%, decreased libido in 3.6%, hot flushes in 9.2% and abnormal liver function tests in 1.7% of men treated with bicalutamide 150 mg.

Comment

The EPC programme is the biggest ever treatment-related study to be conducted in the world with 8113 men randomized between bicalutamide 150 mg and placebo, and it is a goldmine of information. The important findings in this study help to clarify the patients who will most benefit from additional hormone therapy and are also providing invaluable ongoing information on the natural progression of non-metastatic prostate cancer in the 4000 men who received placebo. Most patients were at relatively low risk of progression, with approximately two-thirds of patients having localized disease and a similar number with Gleason grade 6 or below. EPC has shown that this group do not benefit from additional bicalutamide therapy, and these findings are not surprising as no benefits have been shown for castration-based therapy for low-risk patients. It is in the locally advanced group that benefits have been demonstrated. The improvement in overall survival for these men with adjuvant bicalutamide 150 mg and radiotherapy at 7.4 years median follow-up is highly significant. This difference in mortality was driven by a lower risk of prostate cancer-related deaths. These results compare favourably with those discussed for RTOG 85-31 and now allow clinicians and patients a choice of which adjuvant hormone therapy to use without concerns about reducing the efficacy of treatment. This choice is very important with regard to the side effects of treatment. Quality of life advantages have been demonstrated with bicalutamide 150 mg with regard to potency, libido, physical capacity and preservation of bone mineral density at the cost of an increase in breast symptoms. The choice of treatment allows men to tailor side effects of therapy to their own particular needs and lifestyles. A significant benefit for progression-free survival was seen in all locally advanced subgroups. This again is important in delaying the devastating consequences of cancer progression both locally and at distant sites. EPC has demonstrated that bicalutamide is a good alternative treatment choice of hormonal therapy when it is thought to be indicated for locally advanced prostate cancer.

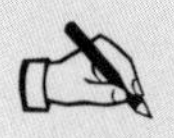

Short-term androgen deprivation and radiotherapy for locally advanced prostate cancer: results from the Trans-Tasman Radiation Oncology Group 96.01 randomised controlled trial

Denham JW, Steigler A, Lamb DS, *et al*; Trans-Tasman Radiation Oncology Group. *Lancet Oncol* 2005; **6**(11): 841–50

BACKGROUND. This large multicentre study was designed to determine whether 3 or 6 months of androgen deprivation (goserelin) given before and during radiotherapy (RT) improves outcome in men with locally advanced prostate cancer. A total of 818 men were treated with 66 Gy in 33 fractions to the prostate and seminal vesicles. They were randomized to no androgen deprivation, 3 months of goserelin (starting 2 months before RT) or 6 months of goserelin (starting 5 months before RT). Patients were stratified by age, stage, tumour differentiation and initial PSA concentration. Primary end-points were time to local failure and prostate cancer-specific survival.

INTERPRETATION. At a median follow-up of 5.9 years, the following results were reported for the 3-month goserelin group and the 6-month goserelin group, both in comparison with the control group. A significant improvement in local failure was seen in both the 3-month group (HR 0.56; 95% CI 0.39–0.79; $P = 0.001$) and the 6-month group (HR 0.42; CI 0.28–0.62; $P < 0.001$) (Fig. 7.2). In terms of prostate cancer-specific survival, patients allocated 3 months of goserelin had no reduction in probability of death from prostate cancer (HR 0.91; CI 0.56–1.48; $P = 0.71$), contrasting with those allocated 6 months of treatment who had a significant reduction (HR 0.56; CI 0.32–0.98; $P = 0.04$) (Fig. 7.3). Secondary end-points including disease-free survival, risk of biochemical failure and freedom from salvage treatment were also evaluated and found to be significant for both groups, but with greater improvements seen in the 6-month group. However, distant failure showed no reduction of risk in the 3-month group, whereas the 6-month group demonstrated a significant reduction.

Comment

This study has investigated the role of short-term androgen deprivation in the management of locally advanced prostate cancer and has provided some interesting results. Three months of goserelin therapy significantly reduced biochemical failure, increased disease-free survival and led to less need for salvage treatment. Six months of goserelin therapy improved these results and also improved prostate cancer-specific survival. The use of shorter duration hormone therapy may have beneficial effects on morbidity when used as part of a combined modality regime. The improvement in local control with the addition of androgen deprivation may have been due in part to the dose of radiotherapy delivered (66 Gy), as the higher doses now used have been shown to improve local tumour control. Therefore, the question is whether the magnitude of observed benefit with added goserelin would be less with higher doses of radiotherapy. Overall, a trend for increasing treatment effect was found with higher Gleason scores and PSA concentration, and this is consistent with other studies of combination therapy.

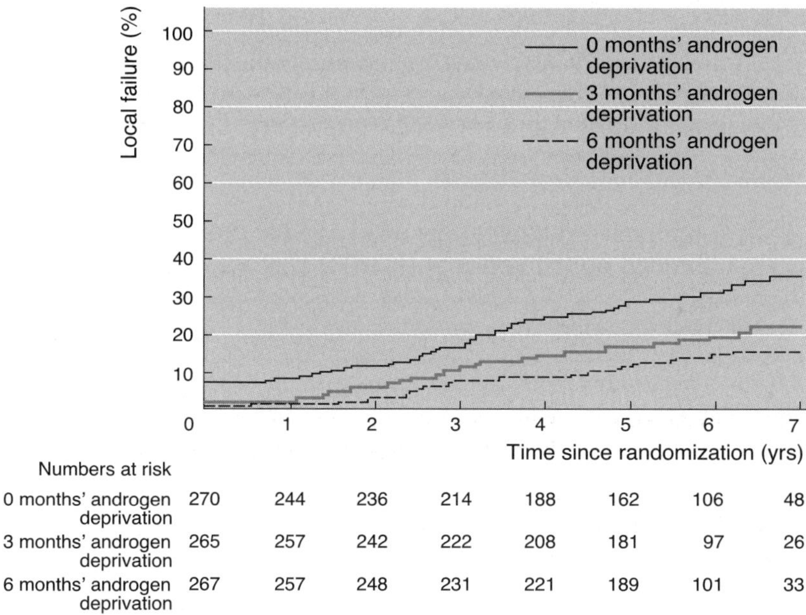

Numbers at risk	0	1	2	3	4	5	6	7
0 months' androgen deprivation	270	244	236	214	188	162	106	48
3 months' androgen deprivation	265	257	242	222	208	181	97	26
6 months' androgen deprivation	267	257	248	231	221	189	101	33

Fig. 7.2 Local failure. Source: Denham *et al.* (2005).

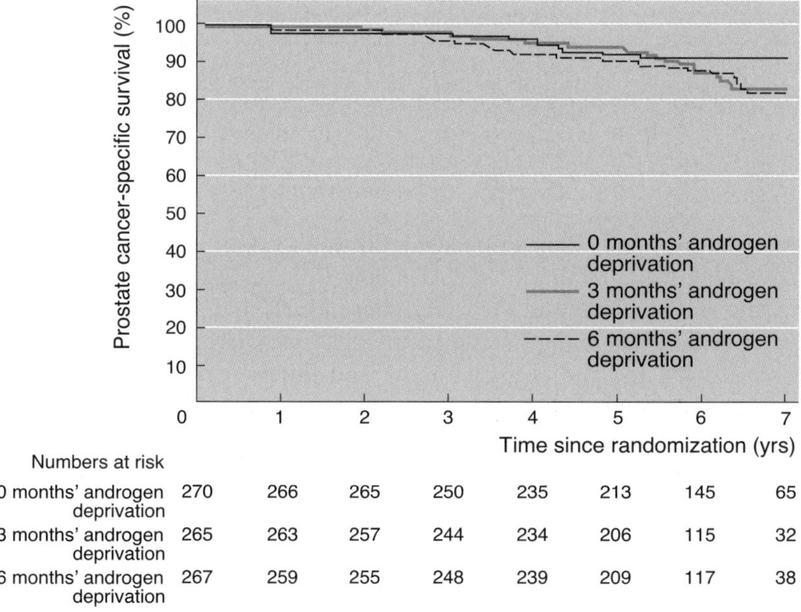

Numbers at risk	0	1	2	3	4	5	6	7
0 months' androgen deprivation	270	266	265	250	235	213	145	65
3 months' androgen deprivation	265	263	257	244	234	206	115	32
6 months' androgen deprivation	267	259	255	248	239	209	117	38

Fig. 7.3 Prostate cancer-specific survival. Source: Denham *et al.* (2005).

The optimal timing and duration of hormone therapy in combination with optimal radiotherapy for locally advanced prostate cancer has yet to be defined, and further studies are needed to answer this important question. The median follow-up in this study was only 5.9 years with a range of 0.1–8.5 years, and the results of longer follow-up are awaited to quantify further the size of the survival benefit.

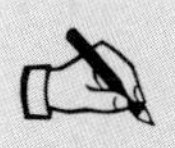

Post-operative radiotherapy after radical prostatectomy: a randomised controlled trial (EORTC trial 22911)

Bolla M, van Poppel H, Collette L, *et al.*; European Organization for Research and Treatment of Cancer. *Lancet* 2005; **366**(9485): 572–8

BACKGROUND. This study was designed to investigate the benefit of immediate post-operative radiotherapy in patients with pT3 disease or positive surgical margins, as opposed to radiotherapy offered for biochemical or clinical relapse. A total of 502 patients were randomized to the immediate treatment arm and received a dose of 60 Gy/30 fractions with non-conformal radiotherapy. Of the 503 patients randomized to the delayed radiotherapy arm, 113 were treated. The primary end-point was biochemical progression-free survival (bPFS) (Fig. 9.4).

INTERPRETATION. After a median follow-up of 5 years, bPFS was significantly improved in the immediate radiotherapy group (74.0% vs 52.6%; $P < 0.0001$). Clinical PFS was also significantly improved ($P = 0.0009$), and the cumulative rate of locoregional failure was significantly lower ($P < 0.0001$), both in favour of the group treated with immediate radiotherapy. There was no significant difference for overall survival (in the region of 92% for both groups at 5 years). In terms of toxicity, at 5 years, the cumulative incidence of events of grade 3 toxicity was 2.6% in the wait-and-see group and 4.2% in the immediate radiotherapy group ($P = 0.0726$) (Fig. 9.5). No grade 4 events were recorded.

Comment

The question of how and when to treat men with pT3 disease after radical prostatectomy remains one of the most challenging for urologists and oncologists. There is a known risk of tumour recurrence both locally and at distant sites. The combination of adjuvant radiotherapy and/or systemic therapies currently with hormone treatment and the optimal timing and duration of these treatments remain unclear. This study is therefore very important, as it addresses the issue of radiotherapy in a large randomized study in an attempt to gain some clarity as to when this treatment should be introduced. Limitations of the trial include the low dose of radiation used (60 Gy) as dose escalation of 64–66 Gy is now the current standard with a three-dimensional conformal approach. There was also variable PSA nadir and variation in the indications and type of therapies used in the wait and see arm. However, the fact that a significant improvement in biochemical PFS and local control with immediate post-operative radiotherapy has been demonstrated is highly significant. The important question of whether immediate

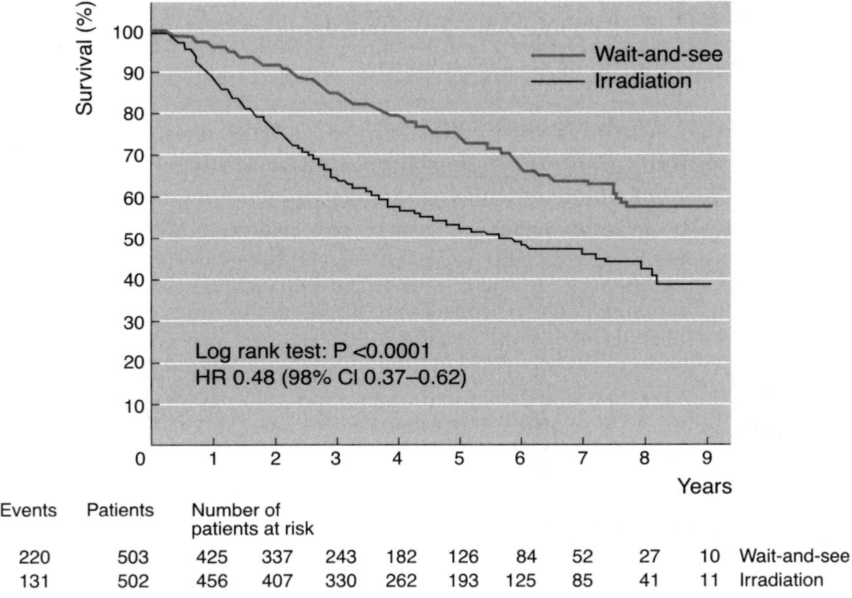

Fig. 7.4 Biochemical progression-free survival. Source: Bolla *et al.* (2005).

radiotherapy will lead to an increase in overall survival and reduction in distant metastases will need longer follow-up, and further results are eagerly awaited.

The treatment of these men may be best achieved with a stratified approach, as risks for local and distant recurrence will vary depending on other prognostic factors and, consequently, the benefits of radiotherapy and hormone therapy will differ. Other ongoing studies (including the proposed Radicals Study) will help to address these complex issues.

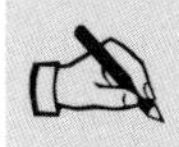

Phase III pilot study of dose escalation using conformal radiotherapy in prostate cancer: PSA control and side effects

Dearnaley DP, Hall E, Lawrence D, *et al. Br J Cancer* 2005; **92**(3): 488–98

BACKGROUND. This pilot study from the Royal Marsden Hospital randomized 126 men with T1b–T3b N0 M0 prostate cancer to 74 Gy vs 64 Gy of conformal radiotherapy. The aims were to test the effects on tumour control and side effects of escalating radiotherapy dose and the appropriate target volume margin (1 cm vs 1.5 cm), using a 2 by 2 factorial trial design. All men had been treated with an initial 3–6 months of androgen deprivation. The primary end-points were comparison of

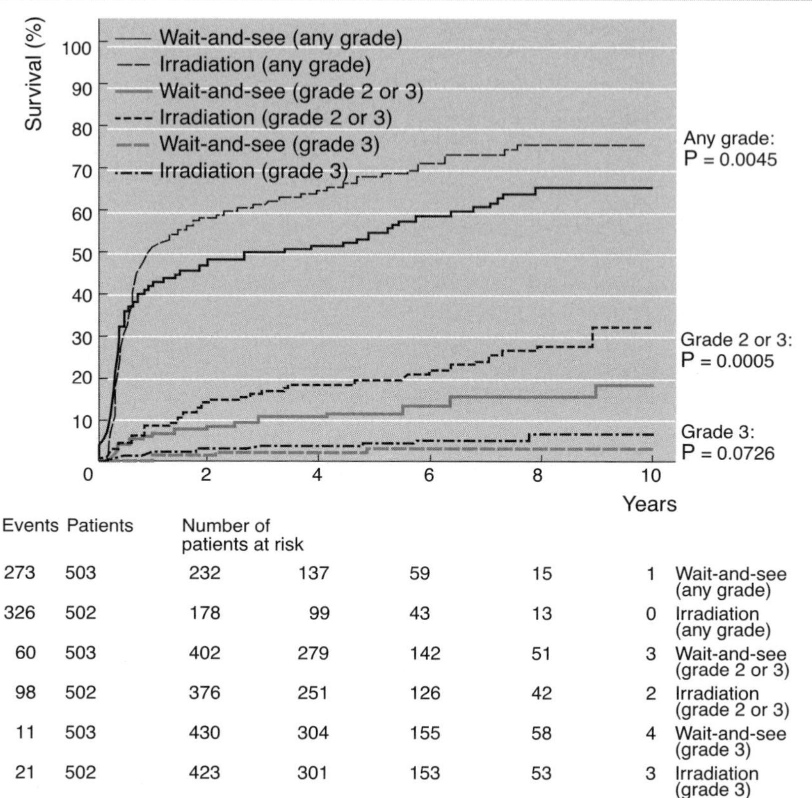

Events	Patients	Number of patients at risk					
273	503	232	137	59	15	1	Wait-and-see (any grade)
326	502	178	99	43	13	0	Irradiation (any grade)
60	503	402	279	142	51	3	Wait-and-see (grade 2 or 3)
98	502	376	251	126	42	2	Irradiation (grade 2 or 3)
11	503	430	304	155	58	4	Wait-and-see (grade 3)
21	502	423	301	153	53	3	Irradiation (grade 3)

Fig. 7.5 Cumulative incidence of late complications. *P*-values indicate comparison of wait-and-see with irradiation groups. Source: Bolla *et al.* (2005).

disease control and treatment-related side effects. Tumour control was monitored by PSA testing and clinical examination.

Interpretation. Patients in the 74-Gy arm had a trend to better biochemical control with 5-year actuarial control of 71% (95% CI 58–81%) in the 74-Gy compared with 59% (CI 45–70%) for the 64-Gy group. For acute side effects, there were statistically significant increases in acute bladder effects in the 74-Gy group and in bowel and bladder effects for the men treated with a 1.5 cm margin (Table 7.1). However, these effects were of short duration. With regard to late side effects, a statistically significant increase in late bowel effects was seen in the 74-Gy group and the 1.5 cm margin group. Sexual function deteriorated after treatment, but no consistent difference was seen between the treatment groups. No difference in tumour control was seen between the 1 cm and 1.5 cm margin groups (5-year actuarial control rates 67%; CI 53–77% vs 63%; CI 50–74%) (HR 0.97; CI 0.50–1.86; $P = 0.94$).

Comment

Radiotherapy techniques for prostate cancer and the doses administered have experienced revolutionary changes in the last few years. This pilot study has demonstrated that dose escalation from 64 Gy to 74 Gy using conformal radiotherapy may improve local tumour control but at the price of an increase in late rectal toxicity. A treatment margin of 1.5 cm did not produce superior results with respect to PSA control and, moreover, was associated with an increase in acute bladder and bowel effects and late rectal toxicity. This carefully executed trial has been vitally important in setting some uniformity in the delivery of radiotherapy treatments in the UK, as it has led directly into the multicentre MRC RT01 conformal radiotherapy study comparing standard dose 64 Gy with 74 Gy. This completed patient accrual in 2001, and the results are expected in 2006.

Table 7.1 Time to prostate-specific antigen (PSA) failure analysis

		% PSA failure free (95% CI)		
Year	**64 Gy dose**	**74 Gy dose**	**1.0 cm margin**	**1.5 cm margin**
2	89 (78–95)	90 (80–95)	87 (76–93)	92 (82–97)
3	78 (65–86)	89 (77–94)	84 (72–91)	82 (70–90)
4	64 (51–75)	78 (65–87)	72 (59–82)	70 (57–80)
5	**59 (45–70)**	**71 (58–81)**	**67 (53–77)**	**63 (50–74)**
6	57 (43–68)	67 (53–78)	60 (53–77)	63 (50–74)

Bold represents 5-year results.
Source: Dearnaley *et al.* (2005).

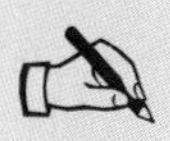

Randomized trial comparing iridium implant plus external-beam radiation therapy with external-beam radiation therapy alone in node-negative locally advanced cancer of the prostate

Sathya JR, Davis IR, Julian JA, *et al.* *J Clin Oncol* 2005; **23**: 1192–9

BACKGROUND. This study investigated the effects of radiotherapy dose escalation using a combination of external beam radiotherapy (EBRT) and temporary brachytherapy iridium implantation into the prostate. A total of 104 patients with T2/T3 prostate cancer were randomized to EBRT alone (66 Gy/33 fractions) or iridium implant (35 Gy delivered to the prostate in 48 h) combined with EBRT (40 Gy/20 fractions). The primary outcomes were biochemical or clinical failure (BCF), which were defined by biochemical failure, clinical failure or death as a result of prostate cancer. Secondary outcomes included 2-year post-radiation biopsy, toxicity and survival.

INTERPRETATION. The results were reported with a median follow-up of 8.2 years. In the combination therapy group, 29% of men had experienced BCF compared with 61% in

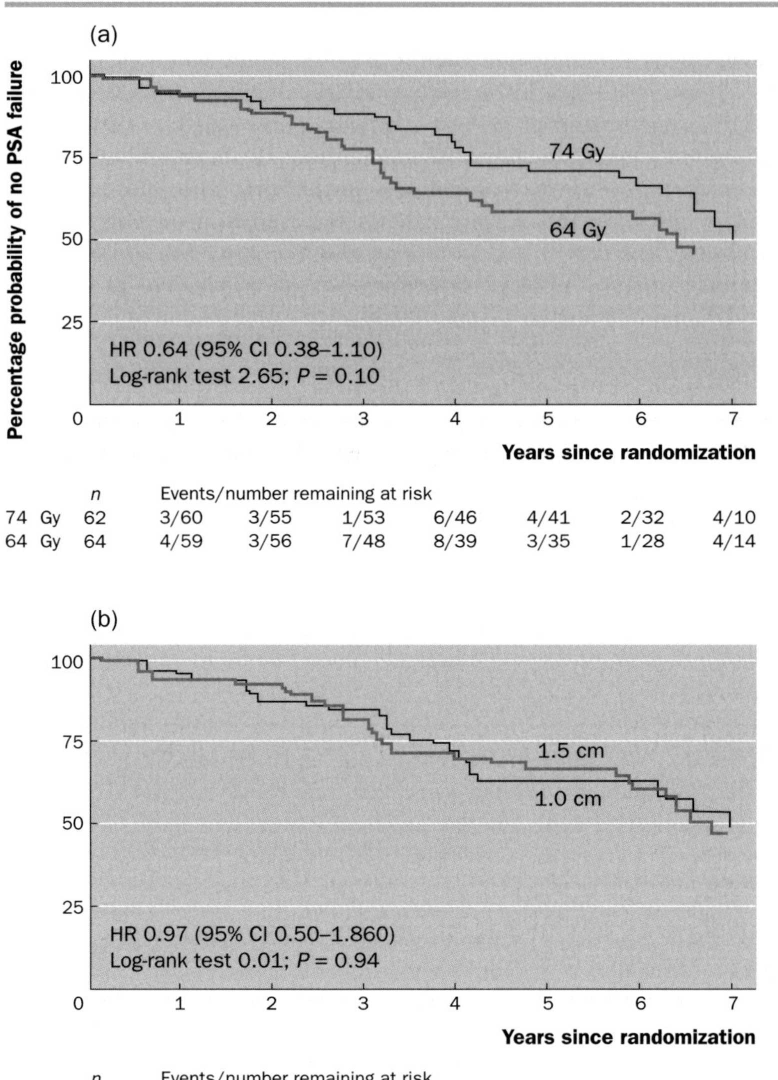

	n	Events/number remaining at risk						
74 Gy	62	3/60	3/55	1/53	6/46	4/41	2/32	4/10
64 Gy	64	4/59	3/56	7/48	8/39	3/35	1/28	4/14

	n	Events/number remaining at risk						
1.0 cm	63	3/60	5/55	2/51	7/43	3/40	3/29	3/12
1.5 cm	63	4/59	1/56	6/50	7/42	4/36	0/31	5/12

Fig. 7.6 (a) Time to PSA failure: 74 vs 64 Gy dose randomization; (b) time to PSA failure: 1.5 vs 1.0 cm margin randomization. Source: Dearnaley *et al.* (2005).

the EBRT-only group ($P = 0.0024$). Two-year post-radiation biopsies were performed on 87 patients, and these were positive in 10/42 (24%) of the implant plus EBRT group and in 23/45 (51%) of the men treated with EBRT alone ($P = 0.015$). Overall survival was 94% in the combination group and 92% in the EBRT-only group.

Comment

This randomized study also shows the benefits of radiotherapy dose escalation with improvement in local and biochemical control. The method of achieving dose escalation with a combination of iridium implantation and EBRT allows higher doses to be delivered within a short duration, and this may be beneficial for prostate cancer, which has recently been reported to have a low alpha/beta ratio. The use of hypofractionated radiotherapy, which may have a radiobiological advantage, is currently under investigation in several large international studies of EBRT. The treatment-related toxicity was similar in both groups. There was no difference in overall survival at the time of reporting.

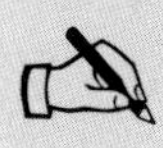

Increased risk of biochemical and local failure in patients with distended rectum on planning CT for prostate cancer radiotherapy

de Crevoisier R, Tucker SL, Dong L, *et al. Int J Radiat Oncol Biol Phys* 2005; **62**(4): 965–73

BACKGROUND. This retrospective study investigated the hypothesis that rectal distension on planning computed tomography (CT) is associated with an increased risk of biochemical and local failure (measured by biopsy) in patients receiving prostate radiotherapy. A total of 127 patients treated between 1993 and 1998 with conformal radiotherapy to 78 Gy were evaluated. Patients were initially treated with a four-field box to 46 Gy followed by a six-field boost. Rectal distension was assessed by calculating the average cross-sectional area (CSA) and measuring three rectal diameters on the planning CT.

INTERPRETATION. The incidence of biochemical failure was significantly higher for patients with distended rectums (CSA >11.2 cm^2) on the planning CT scan ($P = 0.0009$, log-rank test). A multivariate analysis, in which disease risk group (low vs intermediate vs high) and CSA were used, selected high risk and CSA as independent factors having an adverse effect on biochemical control. In fact, patients with intermediate-risk disease and distended rectums achieved inferior biochemical control rates to patients with high-risk disease and non-distended rectums. The probability of having a 2-year biopsy positive for tumour but with no radiation effect increased significantly with rectal distension, as determined by logistic analysis of positive biopsy vs CSA ($P = 0.010$).

Comment

This is an interesting paper that provides for the first time 'proof of principle' that eliminating simple sources of systematic treatment errors (in this case specifically by reducing rectal distension) may produce substantial improvement in outcome. This needs further confirmation. The group suggests that ensuring an empty rectum at the time of planning may optimize results and, in addition, image-guided prostate localization should be used for each fraction during treatment to prevent 'geographical miss' and to improve local control.

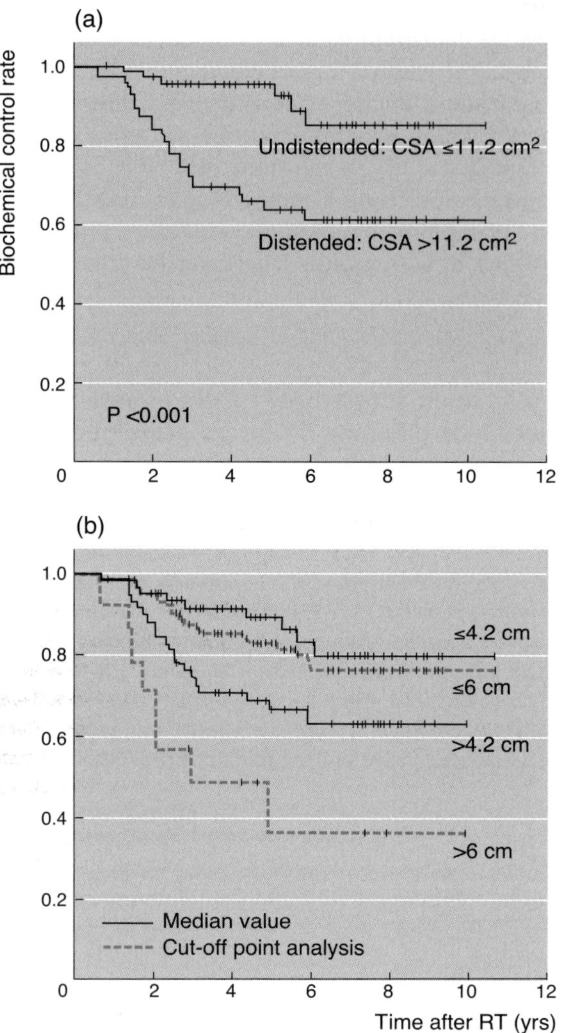

Fig. 7.7 (a) Biochemical control by rectal distension according to cross-sectional rectal area (entire cohort divided in two groups at the median value of CSA). (b) Biochemical control by rectal distension according to rectal diameter at base of prostate (entire cohort divided into subgroups at the median value [*solid curves*] and at 6 cm by optimal cutoff point analysis [*dashed curves*]). CSA, cross-sectional rectal area; RT, radiotherapy Source: de Crevoisier *et al.* (2005).

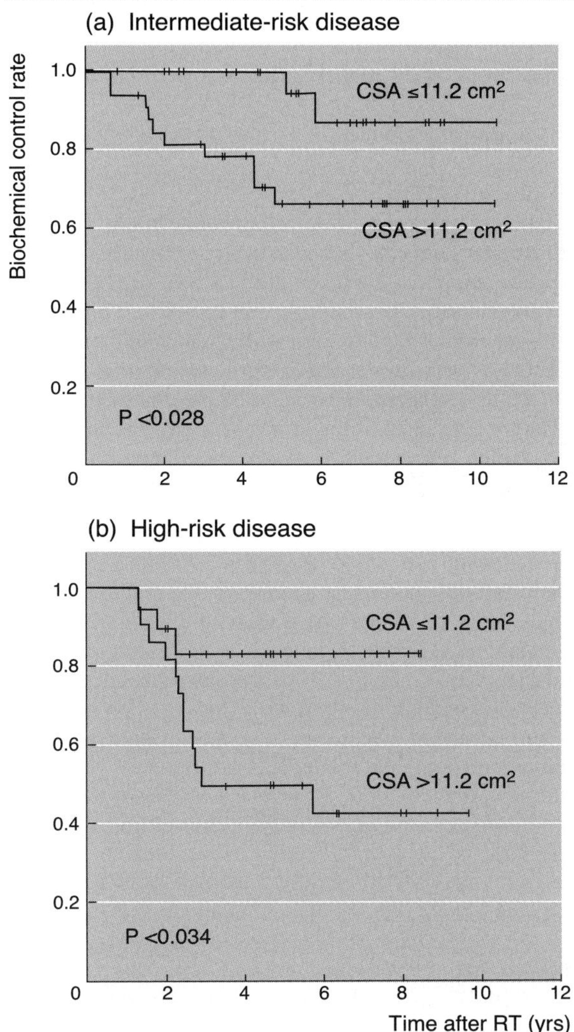

Fig. 7.8 (a) Biochemical control by rectal distension (median cross-sectional rectal area) for intermediate-risk group. (b) Biochemical control by rectal distension (median cross-sectional rectal area) for high-risk group. CSA, cross-sectional rectal area; RT, radiotherapy. Source: de Crevoisier *et al.* (2005).

Risk of fracture after androgen deprivation for prostate cancer

Shahinian VB, Kuo YF, Freeman JL, Goodwin JS. *N Engl J Med* 2005; **352**(2): 154–64

BACKGROUND. Androgen deprivation (AD) therapy is commonly used in the treatment of prostate cancer with excellent effects. One side effect of this therapy is loss of bone mineral density. This study aimed to clarify the associated risk of fracture using information from the linked Surveillance, Epidemiology, and End Result program (SEER) and Medicare database. The records of 50 613 men with diagnosed prostate cancer between 1992 and 1997 and aged 66 years or above were evaluated to assess the risk of fracture associated with AD by orchidectomy or gonadotrophin-releasing hormone agonists (GnRHa). The primary outcomes of the study were any fracture and fracture resulting in hospitalization. Secondary outcomes were a new diagnosis of osteoporosis and fractures at specific sites.

INTERPRETATION. The use of AD was seen to increase during the study period (from 26.5% in 1992 to 40% in 1997). An increased rate of the use of therapy (within 6 months of diagnosis) was demonstrated with increasing age, stage and grade of cancer and the presence of comorbid conditions. There was a significant increase in recorded fractures in the 12- to 60-month period from diagnosis in men treated with AD (19.4%) and those untreated (12.6%) (P <0.001) (Table 7.2). In the same period, 5.2% of those on AD were hospitalized for fractures compared with 2.4% of those not on therapy (P <0.001). The relative risk of fracture increased with number of doses of GnRHa and reached 1.45 for men receiving nine or more doses in the first 12 months after diagnosis and 1.54 for those treated with orchidectomy. If analysis was limited to patients receiving AD as primary or adjuvant treatment, the relative risks of fracture were calculated as 1.44 and 1.53, respectively.

Table 7.2 Estimated number needed to harm for the occurrence of any fracture within 12 to 60 months after diagnosis, according to age and extent of androgen deprivation

Age (years)	Gonadotrophin-releasing hormone agonist			Orchidectomy
	1–4 doses	5–8 doses	≥9 doses	
	No. needed to harm (95% CI)			
66–69	74 (50–146)	42 (29–73)	18 (16–24)	15 (13–18)
70–74	69 (46–146)	39 (27–71)	17 (15–20)	14 (12–17)
75–79	61 (41–125)	34 (24–61)	15 (14–17)	13 (11–15)
≥80	46 (32–91)	26 (19–45)	12 (11–13)	10 (9–11)

Estimates were calculated on the basis of adjusted rates of fracture 5 years after diagnosis from a Cox model with any fracture as the outcome. Doses of a gonadotrophin-releasing hormone agonist were grouped according to the number of doses received within the 12 months after diagnosis. CI, confidence interval.
Source: Shahinian *et al.* (2005).

Comment

This is a large and powerful study, although there are some limitations in that the data are retrospective and fractures related to bone metastases were not excluded. However, the fact that there is known to be a loss of bone mineral density in the first 6–12 months of treatment |**9**| and that the use and indications of AD have increased to include treatment in the neoadjuvant and adjuvant settings for non-metastatic disease need to be recognized. Risk benefits need to be discussed fully with patients and, moreover, interventions to lower the risk of fracture or alternative hormone therapies with anti-androgens (as discussed above), where appropriate, should be considered for men with locally advanced disease.

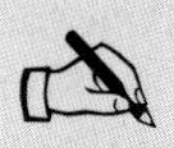

Phase III trial of satraplatin, an oral platinum plus prednisone versus prednisone alone in patients with hormone-refractory prostate cancer

Sternberg CN, Whelan P, Hetherington J, *et al*; Genitourinary Tract Group of the EORTC. *Oncology* 2005; **68**: 2–9

BACKGROUND. Satraplatin is an oral platinum complex that has shown some activity against hormone-refractory prostate cancer (HRCaP) in platinum-resistant tumour models and also in a small clinical phase II trial. It can be administered orally and seems to have a favourable toxicity profile. This planned multicentre study aimed to randomize 380 men with HRCaP to satraplatin 100 mg/m^2 for 5 days every 35 days plus prednisolone 10 mg orally bid (continuously) up to eight cycles or prednisolone alone. After 50 men had been recruited with good compliance and tolerability, the study was closed because of a decision by the sponsoring company. The *ad hoc* analysis of the available data was reported.

INTERPRETATION. At the time of analysis, 48/50 patients had progressed and 42 had died, mostly from prostate cancer. Median overall survival was 14.9 months on the satraplatin combination arm and 11.9 months on the prednisolone arm. A >50% decrease in PSA was seen in 9/27 (33%) treated with satraplatin and prednisolone and 2/23 (8.7%) in the prednisolone-only arm. Progression-free survival was significantly increased in favour of the satraplatin combination (5.2 months vs 2.5 months; $P = 0.023$). Toxicity was generally minimal in both arms.

Comment

The early closure of the study meant that the analysis lacks power because of the small number of patients entered, and no definitive conclusions can be made on the impact of the combination of satraplatin and prednisolone on pain or overall survival. This study has been included because this drug shows considerable promise, from the limited data available, and could potentially be an important future therapy in HRCaP. It also has the considerable advantages of being administered orally and appears to be very well tolerated. The satraplatin and prednisolone combination needs to be evaluated further, and this is currently being tested in a large-scale multicentre, multinational, double-blind, randomized phase III trial. Further results are awaited with great interest.

Conclusion

These reviews highlight some of the new and emerging data published recently and have helped to clarify a number of issues in the management of locally advanced and advanced prostate cancer. There has been ongoing evidence for the significant survival benefits of combined modality treatment with hormones and radiotherapy in locally advanced disease, demonstrated for both goserelin and bicalutamide. This allows clinicians a choice of hormonal agents in this setting, depending on the patient's individual needs and lifestyle. There has also been interesting data for the efficacy of radiotherapy, including new techniques and the benefits of dose escalation. The need to reduce systematic errors in radiotherapy set up in order to achieve superior outcomes has been described. There has also been evidence of emerging data from new systemic therapies and chemotherapy.

References

1. Zagars GK, Pollack A, von Eschenbach AC. Management of unfavourable locoregional prostate carcinoma with radiation and androgen ablation. *Cancer* 1997; **80**: 764–75.
2. Pollack A, Zagars GK, Starkschall G, Antolak JA, Lee JJ, Huang E, von Eschenbach AC, Kuban DA, Rosen I. Prostate cancer radiation dose response: results of the MD Anderson phase III randomized trial. *Int J Radiat Oncol Biol Phys* 2002; **53**(5): 1097–105.
3. Bolla M, Gonzalez D, Warde P, Dubois JB, Mirimanoff RO, Storme G, Bernier J, Kuten A, Sternberg C, Gil T, Collette L, Pierart M. Improved survival in patients with locally advanced prostate cancer treated with radiotherapy and goserelin. *N Engl J Med* 1997; **337**: 295–300.
4. Hanks GE, Pajak TF, Porter A, Grignon D, Brereton H, Venkatesan V, Horwitz EM, Lawton C, Rosenthal SA, Sandler HM, Shipley WU; Radiation Therapy Oncology Group. Phase III trial of long-term adjuvant androgen deprivation after neoadjuvant hormonal cytoreduction and radiotherapy in locally advanced carcinoma of the prostate: the Radiation Therapy Oncology Group Protocol 92-02. *J Clin Oncol* 2003; **21**: 3972–8.
5. Tannock IF, Osoba D, Stockler MR, Ernst DS, Neville AJ, Moore MJ, Armitage GR, Wilson JJ, Venner PM, Coppin CM, Murphy KC. Chemotherapy with mitoxantrone plus prednisone or prednisone alone for symptomatic hormone-resistant prostate

cancer: a Canadian randomized trial with palliative end points. *J Clin Oncol* 1996; **14**(6): 1756–64.

6. Tannock IF, de Wit R, Berry WR, Horti J, Pluzanska A, Chi KN, Oudard S, Theodore C, James ND, Turesson I, Rosenthal MA, Eisenberger MA; TAX 327 Investigators. Docetaxel plus prednisone or mitoxantrone plus prednisone for advanced prostate cancer. *N Engl J Med* 2004; **351**(15): 1502–12.
7. Petrylak DP, Tangen CM, Hussain MH, Lara PN Jr, Jones JA, Taplin ME, Burch PA, Berry D, Moinpour C, Kohli M, Benson MC, Small EJ, Raghavan D, Crawford ED. Docetaxel and estramustine compared with mitoxantrone and prednisone for advanced refractory prostate cancer. *N Engl J Med* 2004; **351**(15): 1513–20.
8. Pilepich MV, Winter K, John MJ, Mesic JB, Sause W, Rubin P, Lawton C, Machtay M, Grignon D. Phase III Radiation Therapy Oncology Group (RTOG) trial 86-10 of androgen deprivation adjuvant to definitive radiotherapy in locally advanced carcinoma of the prostate. *Int J Radiat Oncol Biol Phys* 2001; **50**: 1243–52.
9. Sieber PR, Keiller DL, Kahnoski RJ, Gallo J, McFadden S. Bicalutamide 150 mg maintains bone mineral density during monotherapy for localized or locally advanced prostate cancer. *J Urol* 2004; **171**(6 Pt 1): 2272–6.

8

Phytotherapy in urology

PAUL CROW, MARK STOTT

Introduction

The use of complementary therapies is widespread in many fields of medicine, but particularly so within urology. Natural remedies are often attractive to patients who can see them as preferential to using prescribed medicines. Whereas there is little doubt as to the efficacy of some phytotherapeutic agents, many preparations are regarded with suspicion by medical practitioners. Much of this scepticism is due to the lack of scientific evidence as to their effectiveness. In recent years, the popularity of complementary medicines has demanded that scientific trials are undertaken to ensure the safety and efficacy of these preparations, as well as to understand better potential mechanisms for their actions. In this chapter, a range of recent studies looking at the use of phytotherapies within the field of urology are reviewed. The majority of the work within this area looks at the use of these agents in the prevention or treatment of benign and malignant prostatic pathologies. It is, therefore, not surprising that the majority of papers included within this review pertain to prostatic disease. Also included are papers that give a flavour of how phytotherapies are being investigated within other urological fields.

The use of phytotherapy in the prevention or treatment of prostatic adenocarcinoma

The incidence of prostate cancer (CaP) varies significantly between different geographical regions of the world [1]. In some instances, it has been shown that the risk of a population of men moving from a low CaP incidence region to a high CaP incidence region increases to the background rate of the new region [2,3]. This has been used to hypothesize an environmental aetiology for the disease, in particular a dietary aetiology. Numerous dietary factors have been implicated, often based on their differential consumption by men in high and low CaP incidence regions or on the potential biological activity of the substance. Once a potential environmental factor has been identified, population studies can be used to compare exposure to this factor with CaP incidence or to compare serum/tissue levels of the factor in

Table 8.1 Potential phytotherapeutic agents for use in the chemoprevention of CaP

Agent	Dietary source
Selenium	Bread, cereals, meat, fish
Vitamin A	Vegetables
Vitamin D	Milk, vegetables (sunlight exposure)
Vitamin E	Lettuce, watercress
Phyto-oestrogens	Legumes (soy, beans)
Carotenoids	
Lycopene	Tomatoes (processed)
β-Carotene	Carrots

men with and without CaP. Laboratory-based studies can be used to investigate the effects of the factor on prostate cancer cell proliferation or biochemistry. Table 8.1 details some of the phytotherapeutic agents that show potential utility in the chemoprevention of CaP.

Inevitably, there tends to be a large crossover between the substances investigated to prevent CaP and those studied to treat CaP. Often, evidence that suggests that a substance has utility in one of these areas is also used to propose its potential for use in the other. It is for this reason that papers have been considered on both prevention and treatment of CaP together.

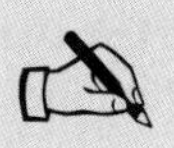

Prostate cancer in native Japanese and Japanese–American men: effects of dietary differences on prostatic tissue

Marks LS, Kojima M, Demarzo A, *et al. Urology* 2004; **64**(4): 765–71

Background. Japanese men have the lowest worldwide incidence of CaP, but this relative protection is lost when they emigrate to the west. This suggests an environmental cause for the disease, with dietary factors as the chief suspects. Most evidence to date relating diet and CaP has been epidemiologic. In contrast, this study examines how differences in diet (with particular emphasis on fat and soy intake) relate to carcinogenic effects in prostatic tissue.

Interpretation. Twenty-five Japanese men (NJ) and 25 American-born Japanese men (J-A) who had undergone radical prostatectomy were identified. Each man was interviewed post-operatively, and a dietary questionnaire was completed together with clinical measurements including assessment of body fat and analysis of urine and serum samples. Benign and malignant areas from the resection specimen were examined retrospectively using tissue microarrays along with histological, immunohistochemical and quantitative grading of nuclei (QNG) techniques |**4**|.

The two groups were well matched, save for the J-A men being 5 years older on average. Surprisingly, the diet questionnaire showed little difference between the two groups, but J-A men had a greater percentage of body fat. Serum studies showed significantly higher oestradiol and lower triglyceride levels in NJ men compared with J-A men, but testosterone and other lipid components showed no significant differences. Urine metabolites of soy were significantly higher in NJ men. The Gleason grade and stage of the tumours in J-A and NJ groups were similar, as was the expression of the majority of biomarkers studied. Lipoxygenase, an enzyme believed to prevent apoptosis and to be stimulated by dietary fat, was increased in the cancer cells of both J-A and NJ men. In contrast to expectation, however, lipoxygenase expression was greater in NJ men than in J-A men. Caspase-3, an androgen-sensitive enzyme that promotes apoptosis, was also found to have greater expression in NJ men than in J-A men, although its expression in benign and malignant tissues was equal. The QNG studies showed that the nuclear chromatin was similar for benign cells in both NJ and J-A men. For cancerous cells, however, the chromatin varied significantly between NJ and J-A men. This raises the possibility of gene–nutrient interaction leading to different patterns of CaP seen in Japan compared with western countries.

Comment

This is a well-conceived and well-executed study, which hoped to link environmental factors to pathological findings in genetically similar men with CaP. By the authors' own admission, the study was limited by its retrospective nature and in terms of its small sample size. The biggest limitation, however, was the surprisingly similar diet of the NJ and J-A men. It would seem that to study the effects of a 'highly protective' diet would require the recruitment of a rural population who rarely undergo collection of CaP tissue. There is no doubt that the NJ men in this study did have a higher phyto-oestrogen content in their diet and lower body fat, but it proved hard to link this to definite pathological findings.

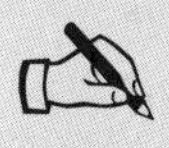

Effects of a diet rich in phytoestrogens on prostate-specific antigen and sex hormones in men diagnosed with prostate cancer

Dalais FS, Meliala A, Wattanapenpaiboon N, *et al.* *Urology* 2004; **64**(3): 510–15

Background. As already discussed, men from regions with high soy intake have a low incidence of CaP. Linseed has also been linked with a reduction in CaP risk |5|, although there have been conflicting data on this |6|. This Australian randomized, double-blind, placebo-controlled study investigates the effect of supplementing dietary soy and linseed on CaP biomarkers in men with CaP.

Interpretation. Twenty-nine men with CaP, awaiting radical prostatectomy, were randomized into three groups: soy (high phyto-oestrogen), soy/linseed (high phyto-oestrogen) and wheat (control group low phyto-oestrogen). The dietary supplementation was given as four slices of bread consumed for between 20 and 30 days before surgery. Serum prostate-specific antigen (PSA), free PSA and sex hormone assays were performed. Compliance was confirmed by measuring urinary soy metabolites.

Statistically significant differences were seen between the soy group and the control group for percentage change in total PSA (–12.7% vs 40%; $P = 0.02$) and free/total PSA ratio (27.4% vs –15.6%; $P < 0.01$). Statistically significant differences were also seen between the soy and soy/linseed groups for percentage change in free androgen index (16.4% vs –15.5%; $P = 0.04$) and percentage change in free/total PSA ratio (27.4% vs –10%; $P = 0.007$). The authors concluded that soy appeared to favourably affect serum markers of CaP, but that this effect was lost when linseed was added to soy.

Comment

The small sample size and short period of study make it difficult to draw definite conclusions from this study. It may be that soy does play a protective role which is negated by linseed, but this would be at odds with the majority of previous work into linseed |6|. If phyto-oestrogen is protective, then this study suggests that it acts by a mechanism independent of sex hormone production, as there was no statistically significant difference in hormone levels between the soy and control groups.

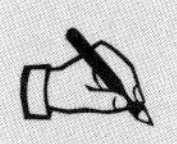

Selenium levels of patients with newly diagnosed prostate cancer compared with control group

Lipsky K, Zigeuner R, Zischka M, *et al.* *Urology* 2004; **63**: 912–16

BACKGROUND. Selenium is an essential trace element that has an antioxidative effect in the cell membrane |7|. Selenium intake varies greatly between geographical regions, largely reflecting soil concentrations. Several epidemiological studies have suggested a protective effect of selenium on the incidence and progression of CaP |8|, although its role within the field remains controversial |9|. This Austrian study aimed to determine whether a link exists between CaP and long-term selenium intake, as demonstrated by toenail selenium levels.

INTERPRETATION. Selenium levels were measured in the toenail clippings of 70 men with CaP and 80 men with benign urological disease presenting over a 2-year period beginning in 2001. In addition, each subject's body mass index (BMI), smoking habits and dietary habits were ascertained. Patients taking selenium supplements, finasteride or lipid-lowering drugs were excluded. No correlation was demonstrated between selenium levels and the diagnosis of CaP, smoking status, age or BMI using the Wilcoxon test.

Comment

An argument against a protective role for selenium is that American men are known to have high selenium levels and yet have among the highest worldwide incidences of CaP. The US Health Professional Follow-Up Study of more than 50 000 men found that those in the highest quintile of selenium levels had a reduced incidence of advanced CaP, but no reduction in early CaP. The cancer group in this Austrian study predominantly comprises men with early CaP (median PSA 8.2) and finds them to have similar selenium levels to men without CaP. Thus, the authors conclude that selenium may have a role in reducing the progression of CaP without reducing its incidence. The Selenium and Vitamin E Cancer Prevention Trial (SELECT) has been designed to evaluate the effect of both selenium and vitamin E on the incidence of CaP in more than 32 000 men. The results are expected in 2013 and will hopefully help to determine whether selenium does offer protection from CaP. For now, the jury remains out.

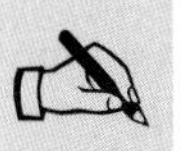

Retinol, carotenoids and the risk of prostate cancer: a case–control study from Italy

Bosetti C, Talamini R, Montella M, *et al. Int J Cancer* 2004; **112**: 689–92

BACKGROUND. Vitamin A or retinol is a fat-soluble vitamin that is either consumed in its true form in animal foods or as the pro-vitamin β-carotene in vegetables. Other carotenoids, such as lycopene, have no pro-vitamin A action. Studies have given contrasting results for the use of retinol and carotenoids in the prevention of CaP, but, most famously, the US Health Professional Follow-Up Study suggested a protective role for lycopene |10|. This Italian case–control study set out to determine the relationship between dietary consumption of these substances and CaP.

INTERPRETATION. A total of 1294 men admitted to hospital with histologically proven CaP were controlled with 1451 patients admitted to the same hospitals with a wide range of non-neoplastic conditions. Personal information, including dietary habits, was collected via an interview-administered validated questionnaire. Odds ratios (OR) were calculated using unconditional multiple logistic regression models. The risk of CaP in the highest quintile of consumption for each substance was compared with that for the lowest quintile of consumption.

Cases were somewhat older and more educated than control subjects, with a greater family history of CaP, lower physical activity but similar BMI. The risk of CaP tended to be reduced with increased intake of retinol (OR 0.79), carotene (OR 0.70), α-carotene (OR 0.85) and β-carotene (OR 0.72), but was only significant for carotene and β-carotene. Lycopene showed no meaningful association with CaP.

Comment

The weak protective role for β-carotene found in this study is in contrast to the findings of the Finnish Alpha-Tocopherol Beta-Carotene Cancer Prevention (ATBC) study, which showed greater incidence and mortality from CaP in men supplemented with β-carotene |**11**|. Lycopene was found to be protective in the US Health Professional Follow-Up Study |**10**|, but not in this Italian study. Interestingly, both studies showed reduced risk for men with high tomato product intake. In the American study, this effect was attributed to lycopene, but the Italian authors point out that tomatoes contain other carotenoids, which may also explain the apparent protective effect. β-carotene is being investigated further in 15 000 subjects as part of the Physicians' Health Study II. It is hoped that, once available, the results will help to throw further light on this controversial subject.

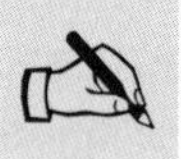

Lycopene: a novel drug in hormone refractory metastatic prostate cancer

Ansari MS, Gupta NP. *Urol Oncol* 2004; **22**(5): 415–20

BACKGROUND. Approximately 80% of men with metastatic CaP become hormone refractory within 12–18 months of starting androgen manipulation therapy. These men are difficult to manage, generally deteriorating rapidly despite treatment. Newer approaches using chemotherapeutic agents such as taxanes or growth factor inhibitors have met with some success, but have not provided a solution to the problem. Lycopene, as discussed in the previous paper, is a carotenoid that has powerful antioxidant properties. A number of studies have shown it to have activity against CaP, although others, such as the previous study, have not confirmed this. This Indian study looks at the use of lycopene in the treatment of hormone refractory CaP (HRCaP).

INTERPRETATION. Twenty consecutive patients with metastatic HRCaP and median PSA of 50.1 ng/ml were treated with lycopene. HRCaP was defined as PSA >8 despite castrate levels of testosterone. Patients had previously been treated with bilateral orchidectomy or flutamide and subsequent androgen withdrawal. Lycopene (10 mg/day) was given for 3 months, and response was assessed using PSA together with measures of bone pain, lower urinary tract symptoms (LUTS) and performance status (Table 8.2). One patient had complete response with PSA falling from 960 ng/ml to 3.6 ng/ml. Six had partial response, ten had stable disease and three had progressive disease. No patients had an adverse reaction to lycopene.

Table 8.2 Criteria for response rate to lycopene in HRCaP

	PSA	Bone pain	Performance status	LUTS
Complete response (CR)	<4 ng/ml	None	No change or improved	No change or improved
Partial response (PR)	>50% decrease	Improved	No change or improved	No change or improved
Stable disease (SD)	<50% decrease or <25% increase	No change or improved	No change or improved	No change or improved
Progressive disease (PD)	>50% increase	No change or deteriorated	No change or deteriorated	No change or deteriorated

Source: Ansari and Gupta (2004).

Comment

This small study, together with others of similar size, seems to suggest that treatment with lycopene can have a favourable effect on CaP. The results of this trial were based on a small number of patients treated without the use of gonadotrophin-releasing hormone (GnRH) analogues, as would be typical in the UK. The results, particularly the single dramatic complete response, are encouraging and warrant further investigation. The authors feel that the innocuous nature of lycopene means that it should be considered before the use of more toxic options when treating HRCaP.

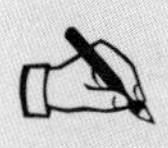

The combined treatment of 1,25-dihydroxyvitamin D_3 and a non-steroid anti-inflammatory drug is highly effective in suppressing prostate cancer cell line (LNCaP) growth

Gavrilov V, Steiner M, Shany S. *Anticancer Res* 2005; **25**(5): 3425–9

BACKGROUND. The incidence of CaP is known to increase with latitude |12|. This led to the hypothesis that low vitamin D levels secondary to reduced sun exposure might predispose to the disease. Population studies have shown that low levels of serum vitamin D are associated with increased risk of developing CaP |13|. Subsequently, *in vitro* studies have shown that vitamin D, acting via specific receptors, can exhibit anti-proliferative effects in CaP cells |14|. Unfortunately, hypocalcaemia limits the doses of vitamin D that can be used clinically. There is extensive *in vitro* and *in vivo* evidence that non-steroidal anti-inflammatory drugs (NSAIDs) are effective against CaP via multiple pathways |15|. The aim of this study was to determine whether the active metabolite of vitamin D_3 ($1,25(OH)_2D_3$) and NSAIDs used in combination might have an improved action against CaP.

INTERPRETATION. The androgen-sensitive CaP cell line LnCaP was cultured in a medium with or without dihydrotestosterone (DHT) and subsequently treated with $1,25(OH)_2D_3$ or ibuprofen or both. The effects of the culture conditions on the LNcaP cells were analysed in terms of proliferation, cell cycle and apoptosis. In cells grown without DHT, treatment with $1,25(OH)_2D_3$ or ibuprofen decreased proliferation by 24% compared with control cells. When used together, an additive effect was seen, with cell proliferation reduced by 42%. When $1,25(OH)_2D_3$ and ibuprofen were used together on cells grown in the presence of DHT, a synergistic effect was seen, with proliferation reduced by 67%. This effect was shown to be mediated by decreasing cell transition from G1 to S phase of the cell cycle and increased apoptosis.

Comment

The study supports previous work suggesting cross-talk between vitamin D and androgens. It also suggests that concomitant use of ibuprofen may allow reduction in the dose of vitamin D that is effective against CaP. This is clinically important as it may allow vitamin D to be employed at levels that will not cause hypocalcaemia. *In vivo* studies will be required to determine whether these promising results translate from the laboratory to the clinic.

The use of phytotherapy in relation to benign prostatic disease

Phytotherapeutic agents have been used extensively to treat LUTS associated with benign prostatic disease. The majority of the work has been in relation to bladder outlet obstruction secondary to benign prostatic hyperplasia (BPH) but, more recently, studies on inflammatory prostatic conditions have been undertaken.

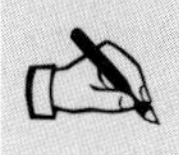

Association between serum concentrations of micronutrients and lower urinary tract symptoms in older men in the Third National Health and Nutrition Examination Survey

Rohrmann S, Smit E, Giovannucci E, Platz EA; Third National Health and Nutrition Examination Survey. *Urology* 2004; **64**: 504–9

BACKGROUND. As discussed in the previous section of this chapter, numerous micronutrients have been investigated with regard to their activity against CaP; however, there are few data as to their relationship to LUTS. This study examines the relationship between LUTS in men aged 60 and over with plasma micronutrient levels measured between 1988 and 1994.

INTERPRETATION. A total of 2497 men who had serum concentrations of vitamin A, vitamin C, vitamin E, carotenoids and selenium measured previously were assessed as to their LUTS. Cases were 298 men with three out of four of the following symptoms: nocturia, hesitancy, incomplete emptying and weak stream. Control subjects were 624 men without any of these symptoms. The two groups were adjusted for age and race, and analysis was undertaken using logistic regression. Vitamin E ($P = 0.03$) and selenium ($P = 0.06$) were significantly lower in men with LUTS compared with control subjects. Vitamin A and other carotenoids showed no relationship to LUTS.

Comment

This study demonstrates that some of the micronutrients that have been associated with reduced risk of CaP in some studies are also associated with a reduced risk of LUTS. Many of these micronutrients have antioxidant properties and may exert their effects by reducing the prostatic inflammation that is associated with BPH. The role of these micronutrients in CaP remains unclear, but it is reassuring that encouraging increased intake would seem to be unlikely to adversely affect LUTS and may actually improve them.

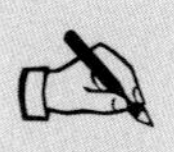

A prospective, 1-year trial using saw palmetto versus finasteride in the treatment of category III prostatitis/chronic pelvic pain syndrome

Kaplan SA, Volpe MA, Te AE. *J Urol* 2004; **171**: 284–8

BACKGROUND. Chronic non-bacterial prostatitis/chronic pelvic pain syndrome (CPPS) is a poorly understood, but relatively common entity, which causes considerable morbidity in its sufferers. Commonly employed pharmaceutical treatment options include antibiotics, anti-inflammatory drugs, α-blockers and 5α-reductase inhibitors. Saw palmetto is a herbal, lipid extract from the berry of the *Sable serrulata* plant (American dwarf palm tree). It is known to be an inhibitor of both type I and type II 5α-reductase and has been studied extensively with respect to the treatment of BPH. Finasteride is a type I 5α-reductase inhibitor with proven efficacy in the treatment of BPH. A recent study comparing finasteride with placebo in patients with inflammatory CPPS showed an advantage for finasteride |16|. This study aimed to compare the efficacy of saw palmetto with that of finasteride in treating men with CPPS who had failed first-line treatment.

INTERPRETATION. A total of 64 men fitting the National Institutes for Health (NIH) criteria for CPPS were randomized to each treatment arm. The NIH Chronic Prostatitis Symptom Index (NIH-CPSI) was measured at 3-month intervals up to 1 year. Both treatment arms show a similar significant symptomatic improvement at 3 months, but thereafter the finasteride group continued to improve to 1 year (NIH-CPSI decrease from 23.9 to 18.1; $P < 0.003$), whereas the saw palmetto group returned to baseline (NIH-CPSI decrease from 24.7 to 24.6; $P = 0.41$). At the end of the study, 41% of the saw palmetto group and 66% of the finasteride group continued treatment.

Comment

Both treatments produced similar symptomatic improvement at 3 months, but this improvement was not durable for saw palmetto. Without a placebo arm, it is not possible to say whether the short-term response to saw palmetto represented anything more than a placebo effect. The results of this study would suggest that finasteride showed a significant advantage over the phytotherapeutic agent in the treatment of CPPS.

The use of phytotherapy in the bladder and upper urinary tract

Whereas the majority of phytotherapy research has concentrated on prostatic disease, there have also been other studies looking at its use within other areas of urological practice. Two papers are reviewed in this section, one looking at the use of mistletoe in the treatment of bladder cancer, and the other looking at the use of green tea in the prevention of urolithiasis.

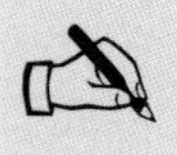

Adjuvant intravesical treatment of superficial bladder cancer with a standardized mistletoe extract

Elsasser-Beile U, Leiber C, Wolf P, Lucht M, Mengs U, Wetterauer U. *J Urol* 2005; **174**: 76–9

BACKGROUND. European mistletoe (*Viscum album* L.) has been used widely to treat a variety of conditions for more than 70 years. More recently, mistletoe lectins have been shown to have immunomodulatory, cytotoxic and pro-apoptotic activity against human cancer cell lines |17|. Intravesical therapy is widely practised as an adjunct to the surgical treatment of superficial bladder transitional cell carcinoma (TCC) and has been shown to reduce recurrence rates. This German study examined the use of intravesical mistletoe in patients with superficial TCC.

INTERPRETATION. Thirty patients with G1/G2 pTa/pT1 TCC were treated intravesically with differing concentrations of mistletoe lectins (between 10 and 5000 ng/ml). Six instillations were given on a weekly basis, starting 1 month after the initial resection. Urine samples were taken for cytokine analysis, and patients were followed up for recurrent TCC for 1 year. The treatment was well tolerated, and the recurrence rate for patients with G2 TCC was 33%, similar to a local control group treated with bacillus Calmette-Guérin (BCG) (28%). No change in urinary cytokine concentration was seen following treatment, and there was no correlation between mistletoe lectin concentration and recurrence rate.

Comment

The results of this small study suggest that intravesical instillation of mistletoe lectin is well tolerated, but it has not given insight into its potential mechanism of action or suggested an optimum preparation concentration. Larger studies will be required to make meaningful comparison with existing intravesical adjuvant treatments for superficial TCC.

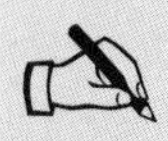

Preventive effects of green tea on renal stone formation and the role of oxidative stress in nephrolithiasis

Itoh Y, Yasui T, Okada A, Tozawa K, Hayashi Y, Kohri K. *J Urol* 2005; **173**: 271–5

BACKGROUND. The formation of calcium-containing renal stones shares a number of similarities with arteriosclerosis. Green tea contains catechins, which have antioxidant effects and have been shown to have anti-arteriosclerotic activity by preventing the degradation of low-density lipoprotein (LDL) |18|. This Japanese animal

study set out to determine whether green tea could be used to prevent the development of renal stones.

Interpretation. One hundred and twenty Wistar rats were divided into four dietary groups: a control group (saline), a stone group (ethyl glycol and vitamin D_3), a fluid green tea group (ethyl glycol, vitamin D_3 and green tea [40 mg of catechins]) and a powder green tea group (ethyl glycol, vitamin D_3 and green tea [169 mg of catechins]). Ethyl glycol and vitamin D_3 stimulate the formation of renal stones. The effects of green tea were determined by measuring serum and urinary metabolites, together with number of calcium oxalate deposits and markers of oxidative stress in harvested kidneys.

The green tea groups showed a significant reduction in urinary oxalate and citrate excretion compared with the stone group ($P < 0.05$). The powder green tea group showed a significant reduction in serum calcium compared with the stone group ($P < 0.05$). Histological examination of the kidneys showed a significant reduction in the number of calcium oxalate deposits found in the green tea groups compared with the stone group. Markers known to indicate degree of oxidative stress varied significantly between the green tea and the stone groups.

Comment

This rat study shows that green tea can reduce factors associated with the formation of renal stones. The biochemical analyses performed suggest that it exerts this effect via antioxidant activity. Clinical studies are required to determine the role of green tea in preventing stone formation in urological practice.

Conclusion

The papers reviewed in this chapter demonstrate the range of research currently being undertaken within the field of phytotherapy in urology. The fact that the ten studies reviewed came from groups working in eight separate countries serves to illustrate the worldwide interest in this area. The range of study types also demonstrates the different approaches being employed to determine the effectiveness or otherwise of the phytotherapeutic agents. Currently, the majority of the work is being undertaken in relation to the chemoprevention of CaP. As with many aspects of CaP research, the slow progression and multifactorial aetiology of the disease make it difficult to investigate. Long periods of follow-up together with large sample sizes are likely to be required to provide the answers that are being sought. At present, there is little concurrence as to the role of any of the phytotherapies in the prevention of CaP. Large, well-designed studies such as SELECT are in progress, and it is hoped that they will provide some definitive answers. Unfortunately, the long follow-up periods mean that the results of these trials remain some way off. The incongruity in the existing data may point to each of these individual substances having a relatively small effect on CaP risk. Once effective preparations are identified, it might be that their combined use, together with other lifestyle modifications, gives the best protection against CaP.

References

1. Parkin MD, Pisani P, Ferlay J. Global cancer statistics. *CA Cancer J Clin* 1999; **49**: 33–64.
2. Shimizu H, Ross RK, Bernstein L, Yatani R, Henderson BE, Mack TM. Cancers of the prostate and breast amongst Japanese and white immigrants in Los Angeles County. *Br J Cancer* 1991; **63**: 963–6.
3. Watanabe M, Nakayama T, Shiraishi T, Stemmermann GN, Yatani R. Comparative studies of prostate cancer in Japan versus the United States. A review. *Urol Oncol* 2000; **5**: 274–83.
4. Veltri RW, Partin AW, Miller MC. Quantitative nuclear grade (QNG): a new image analysis-based biomarker of clinically relevant nuclear structure alterations. *J Cell Biochem* 2000; **35**(Suppl): 151–7.
5. Thompson U. Flaxseed, lignans and cancer. In: Cunane SC, Thompson LU (eds). *Flaxseed in human nutrition.* Chicago: AOCS Press, 1995; pp 219–36.
6. Connor WE. Importance of omega-3 fatty acids in health and disease. *Am J Clin Nutr* 2000; **71**(Suppl): 171–5.
7. Rotruck JT, Pope AL, Ganther HE, Swanson AB, Hafeman DG, Hoekstra WG. Selenium: biochemical role as a component of glutathione peroxidase. *Science* 1973; **179**: 588–90.
8. Brooks JD, Metter EJ, Chan DW, Sokoll LJ, Landis P, Nelson WG, Muller D, Andres R, Carter HB. Plasma selenium level before diagnosis and the risk of prostate cancer development. *J Urol* 2001; **166**: 2034–8.
9. Moyad MA. Selenium and vitamin E supplements for prostate cancer: evidence or embellishment? *Urology* 2002; **59**(4 Suppl 1): 9–19.
10. Gann PH, Ma J, Giovannucci E, Willett W, Sacks FM, Hennekens CH, Stampfer MJ. Lower prostate cancer risk in men with elevated plasma lycopene levels: results of a prospective analysis. *Cancer Res* 1999; **59**(6): 1225–30.
11. Albanes D, Heinonen OP, Huttunen JK, Taylor PR, Virtamo J, Edwards BK, Haapakoski J, Rautalahti M, Hartman AM, Palmgren J, *et al.* Effects of alpha-tocopherol and beta-carotene supplements on cancer incidence in the Alpha-Tocopherol Beta-Carotene Cancer Prevention Study. *Am J Clin Nutr* 1995; **62**(6 Suppl): 1427S–30S.
12. Schwartz GG, Hulka BS. Is vitamin D deficiency a risk factor for prostate cancer? *Anticancer Res* 1990; **10**: 1307–11.
13. Ahonen MH, Tenkanen L, Teppo L, Hakama M, Tuohimaa P. Prostate cancer risk and pre-diagnostic serum 25-hydroxyvitamin D levels. *Cancer Causes Control* 2000; **11**: 847–52.
14. Tokar EJ, Webber MM. Cholecalciferol inhibits growth and invasion by up-regulating nuclear receptors and 25-hydroxylase in human prostate cancer cells. *Clin Exp Metastasis* 2005; **22**: 275–84.
15. Nelson JE, Harris RE. Inverse association of prostate cancer and non-steroidal anti-inflammatory drugs (NSAIDS): results of a case–control study. *Oncol Rep* 2000; **7**: 169–70.

16. Leskinen M, Lukkarinen O, Marttila T. Effects of finasteride in patients with inflammatory chronic pelvic pain syndrome: a double-blind, placebo-controlled, pilot study. *Urology* 1999; **53**(3): 502–5.

17. Mengs U, Gothel D, Leng-Peschlow E. Mistletoe extracts standardized to mistletoe lectins in oncology: review on current status of preclinical research. *Anticancer Res* 2002; **22**(3): 1399–407.

18. Maeda K, Kuzuya M, Cheng XW, Asai T, Kanda S, Tamaya-Mori N, Sasaki T, Shibata T, Iguchi A. Green tea catechins inhibit the cultured smooth muscle cell invasion through the basement barrier. *Atherosclerosis* 2003; **166**(1): 23–30.

9

Bladder cancer

STEVE WILLIAMS, HARTWIG SCHWAIBOLD, JOHN PROBERT

Introduction

The collection of papers presented in this chapter represents a sampling of some of the best recent papers in the world of urology. Various papers on the subject of bladder cancer have been selected and evidence analysed according to principles of evidence-based medicine. The twelve papers reviewed in this chapter represent exciting developments across the clinical spectrum. It is hoped that the reader will find it as stimulating and informative a read as we found it a pleasure to write.

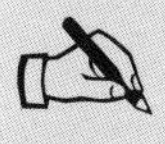

Use of the novel marker BLCA-1 for the detection of bladder cancer

Myers-Irvin JM, Lansittel D, Getzenberg RH. *J Urol* 2005; **174**: 64–8

BACKGROUND. The current methods applied for detection of bladder cancer lack sensitivity for the detection of low-grade tumours. It is important to detect bladder cancer in the early stages because the 5-year survival rate is 94% when this cancer is detected at an early stage. The current standard for bladder cancer detection involves the use of cystoscopy and urine cytology. Cystoscopy is an invasive procedure, and urine cytology, although highly specific, lacks sensitivity for detecting low-grade tumours (approximately 50%). The specific nuclear structural proteins BLCA-1 to -6 are specifically expressed in bladder cancer tissue. The expression pattern of BLCA-4 has been determined previously, and specific antibodies against this protein have been produced. Sequence data from BLCA-1 protein have been elucidated recently and used to produce antibodies. This study looks at the use of these antibodies to examine BLCA-1 expression in bladder urine and tissue via Western blots and enzyme-linked immunosorbent assay (ELISA).

INTERPRETATION. Urine was collected from 25 patients with bladder cancer as well as from 18 with no urological abnormalities. Urine was also collected from eight spinal cord-injured patients, 10 patients with renal cell carcinoma and from 10 with prostate cancer. ELISA and Western blots were used to demonstrate the presence of BLCA-1 in the urine and bladder tissue. Patients with spinal cord injury represent a unique population in which to use this assay because they are at high risk of bladder cancer and other urinary conditions, such as chronic catheterization and cystitis.

Table 9.1 Values in each patient group tested

	Av (odu)	Median ± SD (odu)	*P*-value vs bladder cancer
Normal	0.028	0.015 ± 0.047	0.007
SCI	0.020	0.012 ± 0.021	0.001
Prostate cancer	0.009	0.004 ± 0.008	1.0E-04
Kidney cancer	0.009	0.006 ± 0.007	1.1E-04
Bladder cancer	0.078	0.047 ± 0.079	

odu, optical density units.
Source: Myers-Irvin *et al.* (2005).

BLCA-1 was detectable in tissue from patients with bladder cancer but not adjacent areas of the bladder or in normal donor bladder tissue. BLCA-1 protein in patients with bladder cancer was statistically higher than in normal individuals ($P = 0.007$), those with spinal cord injury ($P = 0.001$), individuals with prostate cancer ($P = 1.0$E–04) or patients with kidney cancer ($P = 1.1$E–04) (Table 9.1). Using a cut-off of 0.025 optical density units (absorbance value), BLCA-1 was detectable in 20 out of 25 urine samples from patients with bladder cancer but in only 6 of 46 normal, high-risk, prostate or renal cancer samples tested, resulting in a test with 80% sensitivity and 87% specificity. Expression of the protein did not appear to correlate with tumour grade.

Comment

This research seems to indicate that an antibody has been successfully produced against the bladder cancer-specific biomarker BLCA-1. This antibody was used in immunoblots to detect BLCA-1 in the tissue and urine of patients with bladder cancer, but not in that of normal donors. A limitation of this study was the small number of low-grade tumours. This assay has a slightly lower specificity for bladder cancer detection than cytology but a higher sensitivity. This assay may therefore be clinically useful in increasing the sensitivity of bladder cancer detection, particularly in conjunction with the already developed BLCA-4 urine-based ELISA.

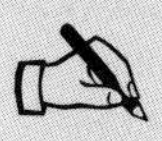

Bacillus Calmette–Guerin versus epirubicin for primary, secondary or concurrent carcinoma *in situ* of the bladder: results of a European Organization for the Research and Treatment of Cancer-Genito-Urinary Group Phase III Trial (30906)

De Reijke TM, Kurth KH, Sylvester RJ, *et al.*; European Organization for the Research and Treatment of Cancer (EORTC) Genito-Urinary Group. *J Urol* 2005; **173**: 405–9

Background. Carcinoma *in situ* (CIS) should be considered pre-invasive bladder cancer, with time to muscle invasive progression reported to be between 18 and

77 months with various primary or adjuvant treatment schemes. Different forms may be discriminated, namely primary: no concurrent or prior urothelial tumour; concurrent: CIS combined with a papillary urothelial tumour; and secondary: CIS detected during follow-up of papillary urothelial cancer. If not treated with intravesical therapy after diagnosis, the chance of progression to muscle invasion or regional or distant metastases has been reported to be between 0% and 83%. Various intravesical regimens have been applied, and they induce a complete response in 50–80% of cases. This randomized European Organisation for Research into the Treatment of Cancer (EORTC) phase III study was performed in patients with CIS of the bladder to compare the efficacy and side effects of bacillus Calmette–Guérin (BCG) and epirubicin.

INTERPRETATION. Between 1993 and April 1999, 168 patients were randomized at 28 institutions. These patients had biopsy-proven primary, secondary or concurrent CIS of the bladder and were randomized to 81 mg of BCG-Connaught (6 weekly instillations, i.e. one a week for 6 weeks) or 50 mg of epirubicin (8 weekly instillations, i.e. one a week for 8 weeks) (Table 9.2). Previous intravesical treatment with cytotoxic drugs other than epirubicin and doxorubicin was permitted as long as the interval between the end of the previous cytotoxic treatment and the initiation of the protocol was more than 1 month. Exclusion criteria were CIS in the prostatic stroma, bladder capacity below 150 ml, chronic urinary tract infection, cured or active tuberculosis, previous pelvic irradiation, concurrent or previous muscle invasive disease, another malignancy (except well-treated basal cell carcinoma), intravesical obstruction with a residual urine more than 100 ml, pregnancy or lactation and a concurrent tumour of the upper urinary tract. Seven patients, including four in the epirubicin group and three in the BCG-Connaught group, were ineligible and were excluded from the analysis.

Follow-up cystoscopy under general anaesthesia was performed at 10 weeks after the start of instillation, when select site biopsies were performed and urine cytology taken. If there was a complete CIS response, maintenance instillation therapy was started at 3 months. If persistent CIS or a papillary tumour was found that had been completely resected, the patient received a second induction course, followed by repeat cystoscopy and biopsies 10 weeks after the start of the second course. Crossover between treatment groups was not part of the study. Treatment was stopped in cases of allergic reactions or severe systemic toxicity.

Overall follow-up was for a median of 5.6 years (maximum 9.7 years). Eighty-two patients were randomized to the epirubicin group and 80 patients to the BCG group. The overall complete response (CR) rate after one or two cycles was 56% for epirubicin and 65% for BCG-Connaught (Table 9.3). The difference in overall CR rates was not statistically significant ($P = 0.21$). The time to the first papillary or CIS recurrence was longer in those treated with BCG-Connaught, with a median of 1.4 years on epirubicin and 5.1 years on BCG (Fig. 9.1). This was statistically significant ($P = 0.0004$). More complete responders in the CIS group than in the CIS group had recurrent CIS (45% vs 16%) (Table 9.4). Cystectomy was due to bladder cancer (persistent CIS and/or the persistence/development of other T1 or greater urothelial tract tumours) (Table 9.5). No significant differences were noted in time to progression within the bladder ($P = 0.17$) or duration of survival ($P = 0.26$). In the epirubicin group, 23 patients progressed and 34 died, including 13 of bladder cancer, while in the BCG group 15 progressed and 26 died, including 9 of bladder cancer. Ten patients (12%) on epirubicin had secondary primary tumours compared with seven (8%) on BCG.

Table 9.2 Characteristics of all randomized patients

	No. epirubicin % **84**	**No. BCG-Connaught** % **84**	**Total no.** % **168**
Age			
<60	19 (23)	22 (26)	41 (24)
60–69	28 (33)	27 (32)	55 (33)
70–79	32 (38)	30 (36)	62 (37)
≥80	4 (5)	4 (5)	8 (5)
Unknown	1 (1)	1 (1)	2 (1)
Sex			
M	75 (89)	79 (94)	154 (92)
F	9 (11)	5 (6)	14 (8)
CIS type			
Primary	19 (23)	20 (24)	39 (23)
Secondary	22 (26)	19 (23)	41 (24)
Concurrent	43 (51)	44 (52)	88 (52)
Biopsies taken			
≤6	7 (8)	8 (10)	15 (9)
7	38 (45)	32 (38)	70 (42)
8	18 (21)	21 (25)	39 (23)
≥9	20 (24)	22 (26)	42 (25)
Unknown	1 (1)	1 (1)	2 (1)
Biopsies with CIS			
0	1 (1)	0	1 (1)
1	26 (31)	23 (27)	49 (29)
2	24 (29)	21 (25)	45 (27)
3–4	13 (15)	22 (26)	35 (21)
≥5	19 (23)	17 (20)	36 (21)
Unknown	1 (1)	1 (1)	2 (1)
Cytology			
Normal	9 (11)	10 (12)	19 (11)
Inflammation	4 (5)	2 (2)	6 (4)
Moderate dysplasia	7 (8)	6 (7)	13 (8)
Severe dysplasia	3 (4)	9 (11)	12 (7)
Malignant cells	45 (54)	43 (51)	88 (52)
Other	2 (2)	3 (4)	5 (3)
Unknown	14 (17)	11 (13)	25 (15)

Source: DeReijke *et al.* (2005).

Of the patients on epirubicin, 82 received one to eleven cycles (median three cycles), while 81 on BCG received one to 13 cycles (median four cycles). Local and systemic side effects were observed in a higher percentage of patients in the BCG treatment group, and these side effects were more frequently the reason for stopping treatment.

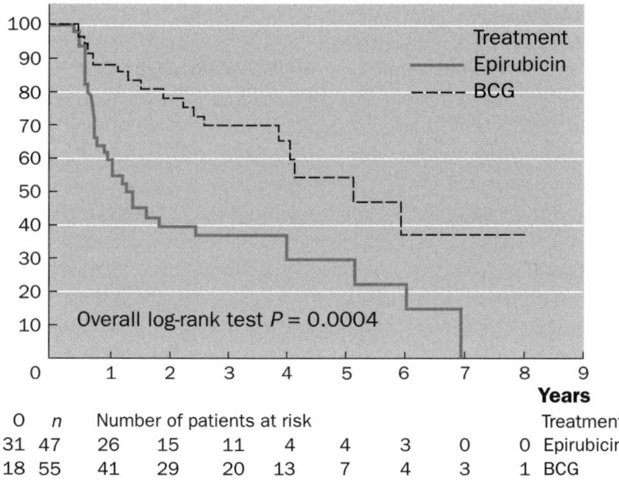

Fig. 9.1 Time to first recurrence after CR. O, observed. *n*, total number. Epi, epirubicin. Source: De Reijke *et al.* (2005).

Comment

This randomized phase III trial shows no statistically significant difference in the completed response rates in patients with CIS treated with BCG or epirubicin. Based on a median follow-up of 5.6 years, time to first recurrence in complete responders was significantly longer in patients on BCG. The study duration is short, so it is difficult to derive any conclusions regarding progression and survival. Nevertheless, this good study seems to suggest that BCG significantly prolonged time to recurrence after complete response, and more CIS recurrences were noted

Table 9.3 Response to treatment

Response	**No. epirubicin** %	**No. BCG-Connaught** %	**Total no.**
CR			
Overall	47 (56)	55 (65)	102
After course 1	35 (42)	48 (57)	83
Partial response	11 (13)	3 (4)	14
No change	5 (6)	6 (7)	11
Progression	4 (5)	4 (5)	8
Unknown	17 (20)	16 (19)	33
Total	84	84	168

Source: De Reijke *et al.* (2005).

Table 9.4 First recurrence type after CR

	No. epirubicin %	No. BCG-Connaught %
No. pts	47	55
Papillary	10	9
CIS	12	7
CIS + papillary	9	2
Totals	31	18

Source: De Reijke *et al.* (2005).

Table 9.5 Reason for cystectomy

Reason	No. epirubicin	No. BCG-Connaught	Total no.
CIS alone	5	5	10
CIS + pT1	3	1	4
CIS + pT2 or greater	8	5	13
pT1 alone	2	0	2
pT2 or greater alone	6	7	13
Prostate cancer	1	0	1
Frequency	0	1	1
Totals	25	19	44

Source: De Reijke *et al.* (2005).

on epirubicin. The incidence of side effects was greater in the BCG group. Longer term data are awaited to compare time to progression and duration of survival.

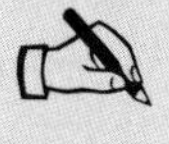

Intraoperative sentinel node detection improves nodal staging in invasive bladder cancer

Leidberg F, Chebil G, Davidsson T, Gudjonsson S, Mansson W. *J Urol* 2006; **175**: 84–9

BACKGROUND. Nodal status remains one of the most important predictors of outcome of radical cystectomy for muscle invasive bladder cancer. Published 5-year survival data for radical cystectomy with node-positive disease ranges from 23% to 35%. Controversy remains regarding the appropriate extent of lymphadenectomy and the number of nodes that should be dissected.

Knowledge of the pathway of the spread of tumour cells is important for complete clearance and is also the basis of the sentinel node concept. The sentinel node concept suggests that tumour metastasizing via the lymphatics enters the sentinel node, which is the first node of the regional lymph node basin, prior to disseminating sequentially to other nodes. It is believed that the sentinel node is specific for each

individual and is detected by radio-guided surgery. This entails injecting γ-emitting substances close to the tumour and the use of a γ-detecting probe to detect the sentinel node. This pilot study looked at sentinel node detection in patients with invasive bladder cancer in conjunction with limited lymphadenectomy. The aim was to determine whether nodal staging in such cancer cases could be improved by sentinel node detection.

Interpretation. The study was performed on 75 patients from May 2001 to December 2004, including 59 men and 16 women at a mean age of 65 years (range 46–81 years) for locally advanced urothelial carcinoma of the bladder. Two patients were clinical stage T4b and received neoadjuvant chemotherapy prior to cystectomy. Immediately prior to cystectomy, cystoscopy was performed, and 2 ml of ^{99m}Tc-nanocolloid (70 MBq/ml) and 1 ml of Patent Blue were injected near the tumour into the detrusor muscle. Extended lymphadenectomy was subsequently performed, and examination of the lymphatic tissue was performed using a handheld γ probe. Radioactivity was measured in counts per second, and nodes that were radioactive were sent in fractions for pathological evaluation as sentinel nodes. Intraoperative blue nodes were identified visually.

An average of 40 nodes (range 8–67) were removed at lymphadenectomy. Of the 75 patients, 32 (43%) were lymph node positive. Sentinel nodes were found in 65 of 75 patients (87%) with the handheld γ probe, and intraoperative dye detection identified sentinel nodes in two patients. In seven patients, sentinel nodes were identified after the completion of extended lymphadenectomy and cystectomy. Sentinel nodes were found outside the obturator fossa in 35 of 65 patients (54%). Of the 32 lymph node-positive cases, 26 (81%) were found to have a positive (metastatic) sentinel node; in 14 of the 32 (44%), the metastatic sentinel node was the only lymph node involved. A false-negative sentinel node was defined as a benign sentinel node despite lymph node metastases in other nodes. The false-negative rate for identified sentinel nodes was 19% (6 of 32 cases). Five of the six patients with false-negative sentinel nodes had macroscopically enlarged hard nodes and/or perivesical metastases. Nine of the 65 patients (14%) had a sentinel node that contained micrometastases (less than 2 mm), which was the only metastatic deposit in five cases. These micrometastases were found by extensive serial sectioning combined with immunohistochemistry techniques, a procedure not done routinely by pathologists.

Comment

A false-negative rate of 19%, as quoted by the authors of this study, is quite high, and it would therefore not be feasible to omit lymphadenectomy in patients with negative sentinel lymph nodes at cystectomy. Two explanations proposed by the authors include obstruction of lymphatic channels by extensive metastasis, thereby altering lymph flow, and difficulty with identification of the sentinel node due to radioactivity interference from the primary injection site (Fig. 9.2). This is, however, a worryingly high number. The authors concluded that nodal staging was improved in nine patients, and that surgery was optimized in a further seven. This study shows the feasibility of detecting small-volume nodal metastases. The question remains whether this finding would alter their prognosis, as most of these

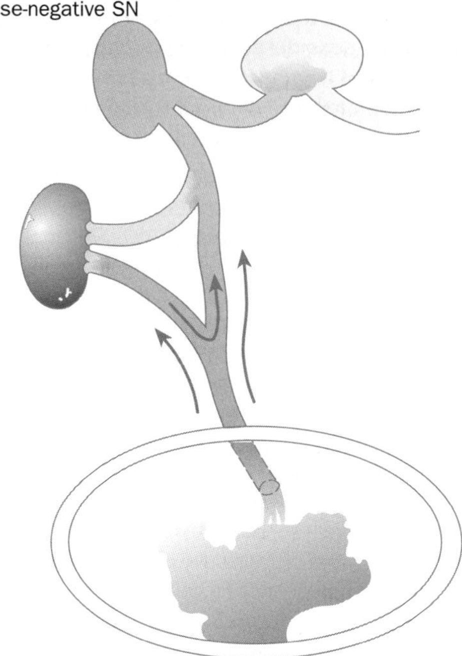

Fig. 9.2 Lymph nodes with extensive metastasis might obstruct lymph vessels, altering lymph flow and generating false-negative sentinel node (SN). Source: Leidberg *et al.* (2006).

patients, by virtue of their tumour stage, would already have been candidates for adjuvant chemotherapy. A long-term prospective randomized trial to investigate the efficacy of sentinel node biopsy in bladder cancer is required.

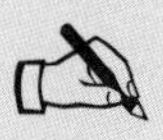

Does the management of bladder perforation during transurethral resection of superficial bladder tumors predispose to extravesical tumor recurrence

Skolarikos A, Chrisofos M, Ferakis N, Papatsoris A, Dellis A, Deliveliotis C. *J Urol* 2005: **173**: 1908–11

Background. Bladder perforation is the second most common complication of transurethral bladder tumour resection (TURBT) with a reported incidence rate of 1.3–5% in various series. Extraperitoneal perforation accounts for the great majority of the cases (83–89%) and is usually managed conservatively. Intraperitoneal perforation is a more serious condition, with the risk of systemic absorption of fluid or bowel injury. Intraperitoneal injuries are traditionally repaired surgically. A major

concern of bladder perforation is the possibility of tumour cell dissemination into the perivesical area, which potentially increases the tumour stage to T3 or higher and may predispose to metastases. This study evaluated the impact of inadvertent bladder perforation during TURBT of superficial transitional cell carcinoma (TCC) on extravesical tumour recurrence and on patient prognosis. The study also evaluated the potential risk factors for extravesical tumour recurrence, prospectively assessing whether open surgical repair vs conservative management of bladder perforations affected extravesical recurrence and overall prognosis.

Interpretation. Between September 1990 and September 2000, 34 patients were identified from patient records as having documented bladder wall perforation at TURBT with a history of superficial tumour. Twenty-six were treated conservatively with an indwelling urethral catheter for 1 week following TURBT. Four patients were managed by a silicone drain in the perivesical space inserted under ultrasound guidance, and four patients required an open surgical procedure. None of the patients received immediate intravesical chemotherapy.

Of the 34 patients, four (11.8%) presented with extravesical tumour recurrence during follow-up. All had an open surgical treatment of their bladder perforation and presented with extravesical tumour recurrence after a mean follow-up of 7.5 months. On univariate analysis, open surgical repair, intraperitoneal perforation and tumour location at the time of perforation were the most important parameters. Multivariate logistic regression analysis revealed that the only important factors associated with extravesical tumour recurrence were the open management of bladder perforation ($P < 0.001$), followed by an intraperitoneal localization of the perforation ($P = 0.0003$) and the size of the tumour ($P = 0.01$). Disease-specific survival was 100% for those who were managed by either conservative drainage or percutaneous drainage after a median follow-up of 60 months, compared with 25% for the patients treated with open surgery after a median follow-up of 15 months ($P < 0.001$).

Comment

This study shows that inadvertent bladder perforation may lead to extravesical recurrence and reduced long-term survival, particularly after intraperitoneal-type perforation. It is unclear whether bladder perforation should be treated with chemotherapy or radiotherapy to reduce extravesical recurrences and progression. Animal studies suggest that intraperitoneal application of a cytostatic agent such as gemcitabine or doxorubucin in combination with a fibrinolytic agent (rt-PA) may prevent the growth of peritoneally injected tumour cells.

This study is hampered by its small size, short duration and retrospective nature and, as a result, it is difficult to draw firm conclusions because of the inherent bias. Nevertheless, this remains the first study in the literature to document the incidence of extravesical tumour recurrence following TURBT, its predisposing risk factors and its influence on patient prognosis.

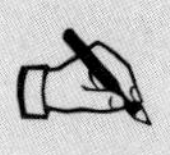

Four years' experience in bladder preserving management for muscle invasive bladder cancer

Lodde M, Palermo S, Comploj E, *et al.* *Eur Urol* 2005; **47**: 773–9

BACKGROUND. Radical cystectomy is the gold standard for muscle invasive TCC of the bladder. In selected cases, bladder-preserving strategies have been used, particularly in patients not fit for surgery. This is because of either reduced general health (ASA score 3 and 4) or advanced age and therefore limited life expectancy. Some authors have reported 5-year cancer-specific survival rates with bladder-preserving strategies similar to those obtained in some radical cystectomy series. The authors report their experience in patients managed conservatively.

INTERPRETATION. From January 2000 to May 2004, a total of 24 patients (mean age 81 years, range 68–92 years) with primary muscle invasive TCC who had refused surgery or were not eligible for cystectomy were followed up for a period of up to 4 years. All underwent complete transurethral resection (TUR) of the lesion. All patients had a negative workup for metastasis (bone scan, liver function tests, abdominopelvic computed tomography [CT] scan, intravenous pyelogram).

Six weeks after the primary TUR, a second look TUR was performed to confirm the complete resection or to remove the residual neoplastic material completely. Thereafter, the patients underwent radiation therapy and/or chemotherapy. The patients were followed up for a mean time of 680 (range 182–1253) days.

During the observation period, two (8.3%) patients remained free of tumour. The mean re-admission rate was 8.0 per patient. All patients complained of frequency, urgency and severe nocturia. The second most frequent complication was bleeding, which required a salvage cystectomy in seven cases and formolization in one patient. Twenty-two patients (92.7%) experienced a local or systemic progression. Other major complications were intestinal occlusion in three cases, an enterovesical fistula, brain metastases requiring neurosurgical intervention, bone metastases in the cervical column and chronic renal failure. The mean time spent in hospital was 109 (range 13–253) days. Twelve patients (50%) died during this time, with 10 cancer-related deaths. Fifteen patients needed chronic pain medication.

Comment

This study seems to show that, in this group of patients, current bladder-preserving strategies failed to improve their quality of life and resulted in insufficient local control. Complications such as bleeding and frequency due to reduced bladder capacity forced a salvage cystectomy to be carried out in nearly half the cases. Long-term survival was also reduced when compared with radical cystectomy. It suggests that, even in elderly patients with muscle invasive disease, a radical surgical approach should help to better retain the patient's quality of life and to avoid complications that result from an insufficient local tumour control.

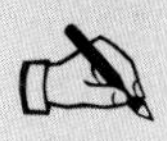

Cyclooxygenase-2 inhibition: A potential mechanism for increasing the efficacy of bacillus Calmette–Guerin immunotherapy for bladder cancer

Dovedi SJ, Kirby JA, Atkins H, Davies BR, Kelly JD. *J Urol* 2005; **174**: 332–7

Background. Immunotherapy with intravesical bacillus (BCG) is now standard therapy for the treatment of superficial urothelial bladder cancer. The precise mechanism by which BCG exerts its immune effect is still unknown, but there is evidence that the induction of a cascade of immunological events is central to engendering an anti-tumour immune response. The presentation of immunogenic BCG peptides by antigen-presenting cells (APC) such as dendritic cells is fundamental to the activation of T cells. The production of T-helper cells (Th1 and Th2) from a precursor stage (Th0) is stimulated by BCG-activated dendritic cells (DCs). Th1 cells predominantly function to coactivate cytotoxic T cells, and they are characterized by their production of the proinflammatory cytokines interleukin (IL)-12 and interferon-γ. The activation and differentiation of Th cells to Th1 cells is fundamental to the activation of CD8+ cytotoxic T cells. The depletion of CD4+ and CD8+ cells has been shown to inhibit BCG-mediated anti-tumour immunity. Th2 cells perpetuate the activation of B cells via the production of IL-10, IL-4 and transforming growth factor-β.

The urinary cytokine profile following BCG treatment indicates that both Th1 and Th2 cytokines are produced. These cytokines are mutually antagonistic, and the presence of Th2 cytokines significantly decreases the immune response. This cytokine response is indicative of the induction of a poorly focused Th1 and Th2 cell containing immune response. The efficacy of BCG therapy may be enhanced when treatment is supplemented with exogenous IL-12. This focused Th1 response is demonstrated further by clinical studies demonstrating high levels of Th2 cytokines IL-10 and IL-6 in the urine of patients who are responsive to BCG therapy. IL-10 is a cytokine with potent anti-inflammatory and immunosuppressive activity, which acts to polarize the immune system to a Th2 response. Prostaglandin E_2 (PGE_2), a product of the arachidonic acid cascade and an immune modulator, significantly downregulates IL-12 expression and is a potent stimulator of IL-10 production. The rate-limiting step in PGE_2 production is the activity of the cyclooxygenase enzyme (COX). Cox-2, one of the two major isoforms of this enzyme, is not normally expressed, but can be induced in response to inflammatory cytokines, such as IL-1 and tumour necrosis factor.

This study aimed to show that augmenting BCG with COX inhibitors would increase the efficacy of BCG therapy for urothelial carcinomas by inhibiting PGE_2 formation, thereby polarizing the response towards a Th1 phenotype. This potential was investigated in the context of a BCG-treated murine model for bladder cancer.

Interpretation. Murine bone marrow-derived DCs were cultured with IL-4 and granulocyte–macrophage colony-stimulating factor. After 7 days, the cells were stimulated with BCG. Cell surface expression of co-stimulatory molecules and phagocytic ability were measured by flow cytometry analysis to verify cell activation. The cultured DCs were treated with PGE_2, IL-10, anti-IL-10 antibody, NS-398 (COX-2 selective blocker) and indomethacin (partially selective COX-2 blocker), and then the presence of IL-12 and IL-10 was measured by ELISA.

PGE_2 increased the DC production of IL-10 but had no effect on IL-12 synthesis. The production of IL-10 by DCs stimulated with BCG in the presence of exogenous PGE_2 for 72 h increased significantly compared with DCs stimulated with BCG alone. This was a dose-dependent phenomenon that was statistically significant ($P < 0.001$). In contrast, the level of IL-12 did not vary significantly following culture of BCG-activated DCs compared with BCG stimulation alone ($P < 0.05$). In the absence of BCG stimulation, PGE_2 had no effect on DC IL-10 and IL-12 production ($P < 0.05$). IL-10 significantly decreased Il-12 production ($P < 0.001$), while IL-10 blockade with antibodies significantly increased IL-12 levels ($P < 0.05$). The COX-2 inhibitor NS-398 caused a dose-dependent increase in the concentration of IL-12 produced by BCG-activated DCs ($P < 0.01$), an effect also noted with indomethacin ($P < 0.05$). Neither inhibitor had an effect on IL-10 or IL-12 levels in the absence of BCG stimulation.

Comment

COX-2 is overexpressed in many solid tumours, including TCC of the bladder. Current evidence suggests that COX-2 inhibitors can decrease tumour cell population, inhibit angiogenesis and promote tumour cell apoptosis. The authors suggest that COX inhibition may exert an immunomodulatory role in combination with BCG. The inhibition of PGE_2 synthesis by COX inhibitors favoured the production of IL-12 by BCG-activated DCs, while at the same time decreasing IL-10 production. The therapeutic potential of the use of COX-2 inhibitors to potentiate the immune-mediated cytotoxicity associated with BCG for TCC is clear. Further investigations in the form of a randomized controlled prospective trial are clearly warranted however.

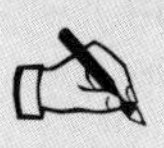

Improved detection and treatment of bladder cancer using hexaminolevulinate imaging: a prospective, phase III multicenter study

Jocham D, Witjes F, Wagner S, *et al. J Urol* 2005; **174**: 862–6

BACKGROUND. At first follow-up, the recurrence rate of bladder cancer is between 3.4% and 20.6% for single tumours and 7.4–45.8% for multiple tumours. The high recurrence rate of bladder cancer is of some concern, as it may be due to poor detection at investigation or regrowth of residual tumour after incomplete transurethral bladder resection (TURB). Diagnosis is usually made using urine cytology and white light cystoscopy. Macroscopic tumours are relatively easy to visualize, but dysplasia and CIS can be overlooked. Random biopsy rarely results in the identification of additional neoplasms, and it may increase tumour seeding. White light cystoscopy is inadequate for detecting many lesions, particularly dysplasia and CIS. A technique that would improve their detection would therefore have an impact on initial treatment and diagnosis and subsequently on prognosis.

Hexaminolaevulinate (HAL) is a lipophilic ester of 5-aminolaevulinic acid (5-ALA), a precursor of photoactive porphyrin that was developed for fluorescence diagnosis of bladder cancer using blue light illumination. A previous study of 52 patients with

primary or recurrent bladder cancer suggested that HAL imaging has 96% sensitivity compared with 73% for white light cystoscopy, and is particularly useful in the detection of CIS. This study was an open, comparative, within-patient, controlled phase III study that investigated whether improved detection of bladder tumours with HAL imaging would lead to improved treatment in patients according to European Association of Urology (EAU) bladder cancer guidelines.

Interpretation. A total of 146 patients with known or suspected bladder cancer diagnosed by cystoscopy or positive urine culture were recruited. Exclusion criteria included gross haematuria and BCG treatment or chemotherapy within 3 months of inclusion. An exception was made if patients had received only a single course of chemotherapy immediately following TURB. Half the patients (73) had newly diagnosed cancer and half had recurrent disease. Of the patients, 18% had previously received BCG immunotherapy, and 18% had received intravesical chemotherapy. Patients received intravesical HAL for 1 h and were assessed with standard white light and blue cystoscopy. Blue light cystoscopy was supplied by placing a band filter over a xenon arc lamp, supplying light at 380–440 nm in patients randomized to continue. All lesions and their type (e.g. flat or papillary) were mapped on a bladder chart, and biopsies were taken from suspicious areas for assessment by an independent pathologist. To avoid bias, an average of two patients per centre were randomized not to undergo blue light cystoscopy after white light cystoscopy. After white light cystoscopy, a sealed envelope was opened to determine whether the patient would continue to blue light cystoscopy. Patients not continuing were given standard treatment and included in the safety population but not in the efficacy calculations.

An independent urologist blinded to the detection method used recommended treatment plans based on biopsy results and medical history according to EAU cancer guidelines. Any differences in recommended treatment plans arising from the two cystoscopy methods were recorded. The primary efficacy end-point was treatment plan comparison, that is the difference in treatment (more or less aggressive) following diagnosis with white or blue light. This was assessed by rating the severity of treatment (none to cystectomy) and comparing the two plans for each patient. The most severe intervention was compared to establish which diagnostic technique would have resulted in the most complete treatment. If the entire treatment plans were the same for the two techniques but more lesions were detected with blue than with white light, resection would be more extensive and, therefore, the patient was deemed to undergo more complete treatment.

Secondary end-points were the detection rate and the false detection rate of white and blue light cystoscopy, as confirmed by biopsy and histology for dysplasia, CIS, Ta and T1 to T4, and the number of patients with a different number of CIS lesions found by white or blue light cystoscopy.

Adverse events and concomitant medications were recorded. A limited physical examination and vital signs were recorded before and after instillation with HAL. Safety assessments were also made 7 days after cystoscopy.

Of the 146 patients, 28 (19%) had no disease. Overall, HAL imaging improved tumour detection. Of all the tumours, 96% were detected with HAL imaging compared with 77% using standard cystoscopy (Table 9.6). This difference was particularly noticeable for dysplasia (93% vs 48%), CIS (95% vs 68%) and superficial papillary tumours (96% vs 85%). The total number of false-positive lesions detected by HAL imaging was 185, and

Table 9.6 Patients in whom lesions were detected

Lesion type	Total no. pts*	No. with more lesions detected %		
		HAL	Neither technique	Cystoscopy
Mild or moderate dysplasia	19	9 (47)	9 (47)	1 (6)
CIS	29	12 (41)	15 (52)	2 (7)
pTa	66	13 (20)	48 (73)	5 (8)
pT1 (pT1a + pT1b)	16	1 (6)	14 (88)	1 (6)
pT2–pT4	22	3 (14)	18 (82)	1 (4)

*>100% due to multiple tumour types in some patients.
Source: Jocham *et al.* (2005).

it was 89 for standard cystoscopy. The false detection rate was the number of suspected lesions per technique that had negative histology divided by the total number of areas biopsied with that technique. The mean false-positive rate of biopsy for HAL was 37% compared with 26% for standard cystoscopy (Table 9.7). There was a large variation in the false-positive rate among centres for HAL imaging and standard cystoscopy (range 4–53% and 16–45% respectively; Table 9.8). As a result of improved detection, additional post-operative procedures were recommended in 15 patients (10%), and more extensive treatment was done intraoperatively in a further 10 patients. Overall, 17% of patients received more appropriate treatment at the time of the study following blue light fluorescence cystoscopy, that is 22% or 1 in 5 patients without tumours were excluded. HAL imaging was well tolerated. Overall, 47 patients (29%) reported 75 adverse events, mainly dysuria, bladder pain and bladder spasm, two of which were considered to be treatment related. One patient died as a result of a cerebrovascular accident considered to be unrelated to the study medication.

Table 9.7 False-positive detection rates

	HAL	Cystoscopy
No. false-positive lesions*	185	89
Total no. lesions examined	499	343
% false-positive (95% CI)	37 (33–41)	26 (21–31)
% false-positive range among centres	4–53	16–45

*Of tumours 66 were falsely identified as positive by each technique.
Source: Jocham *et al.* (2005).

Comment

This well-designed study will most probably lead to changes in the investigation, detection and surveillance of bladder cancer. The greatest benefit of HAL blue light cystoscopy comes from its increased sensitivity in the detection of CIS. The authors

Table 9.8 False-positive rate by patient type

	No. pts %	No. false-positive %		
		HAL	Cystoscopy	2 techniques
Tumour	115 (79)	61 (53)	38 (33)	34 (69)
No pathologically confirmed tumour	31 (21)	25 (80)	23 (74)	15 (31)
Totals	146	86	61	49

Source: Jocham *et al.* (2005).

were able to demonstrate that improved detection translated into more complete patient treatment. It would be interesting to see whether this led to an improvement in overall disease-specific survival. Long-term follow-up is needed to answer this question. One worrying concern remains regarding the high number of false positives in comparison with standard white light cystoscopy. False-positive results lead to extra biopsies and an attendant increased morbidity.

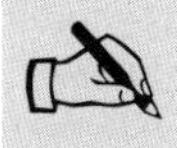

Multivariate analysis of clinical parameters of synchronous primary superficial bladder cancer and upper urinary tract tumor

Palou J, Rodriguez-Rubio F, Huguet J, *et al. J Urol* 2005; **174**: 859–61

BACKGROUND. Transitional cell carcinoma is characterized by its multifocality throughout the urinary tract simultaneously or metachronously. In cases of newly diagnosed bladder cancers, the need for systematic study of the upper urinary tract has not been fully addressed. The incidence of subsequent upper urinary tract tumour (UUTT) after a diagnosis of superficial bladder cancer has been reported to be between 1.7% and 26%. Few studies of the incidence of synchronous bladder cancer and UUTT have been reported, and most have been in relation to muscle invasive disease. In this study, the authors aimed to determine the incidence and characteristics of synchronous UUTT with primary superficial bladder cancer.

INTERPRETATION. A cohort of 1529 patients treated with TUR and random bladder biopsy for primary TCC of the bladder from November 1968 to December 1996 was reviewed. Table 9.9 lists the characteristics of the superficial tumours. Median age was 64 years. Intravenous pyelogram (IVP) was performed at the diagnosis of bladder cancer in all patients. Of the 1529 patients, 28 (1.8%) had UUTT at initial diagnosis of bladder cancer. Tumours were located more often in the lower ureter (42.9%), and 46.3% were invasive (Table 9.10). UUTT showed no preference for location, and there were multiple tumours in 17.9% of cases.

Of UUTTs, 46.3% were invasive and almost 87% were grade 2 or 3. Treatment for the 28 synchronous UUTTs was endoscopic resection in 28.6% of cases, biopsy and coagulation in 3.6%, partial ureterectomy in 10.7% and nephroureterectomy in 57.2%.

Table 9.9 Characteristics of 1529 superficial bladder tumours studied

	No. pts (%)
Sex	
Men	1357 (89)
Women	172 (11)
T stage	
Ta	547 (35.8)
T1	982 (64.2)
Associated cancer *in situ*	
Yes	284 (19)
No	1245 (81)
Grade	
1	185 (12.1)
2	942 (61.6)
3	400 (26.1)
X	2 (0.2)
Tumour size	
<1.5 cm	488 (45.1)
1.5–3 cm	360 (33.3)
>3 cm	200 (18.5)
Papillomatosis	34 (3.1)
Unknown	447 (29.2)
Bladder location	
Trigone	159 (10.7)
Posterior wall	152 (10.2)
Right wall	359 (23.5)
Left wall	369 (24.1)
Dome	16 (1.1)
Anterior wall	13 (0.9)
Bladder neck	9 (0.6)
Multiple	412 (27.7)
Unknown	40 (2.6)

Source: Palou *et al.* (2005).

Data were analysed by multivariate analysis using logistic regression. A high degree of concordance was found between bladder tumour and UUTT grades. The only variable with significance for predicting UUTT was a trigonal location of a bladder tumour (relative risk [RR] 5.8; 95% confidence interval [CI] 2.18–15.9; $P<0.0005$). Thus, the risk of synchronous UUTT was almost six times higher for a trigonal location than for other bladder tumour locations. These UUTTs represented 11 of all 159 bladder tumours (7%) at this location and corresponded to 41% of the UUTTs first diagnosed. Cox regression analysis revealed that T stage, grade, multiplicity, bladder tumour size or carcinoma *in situ* associations were not significant.

Table 9.10 Side, location, pathological stage and histological grade in 28 patients with synchronous UUTT

	No. pts (%)
Side	
Left	12 (42.8)
Right	15 (53.5)
Bilateral	1 (3.5)
Location	
Calix	2 (7.1)
Renal pelvis	8 (28.6)
Lumbar ureter	1 (3.6)
Pelvic ureter	5 (17.9)
Intramural ureter	7 (25)
Multiple	5 (17.9)
Stage	
TA	6 (21.4)
T1	5 (17.8)
T *in situ*	2 (7.1)
T2	6 (21.4)
T3A	3 (10.7)
T3B	4 (14.2)
TX	2 (7.1)
Grade	
1	1 (3.6)
2	14 (50.0)
3	10 (35.7)
Undifferentiated	2 (7.1)
GX	1 (3.6)

Source: Palou *et al.* (2005).

Comment

This important article provides an evaluation of risk factors associated with UUTT at the time of presentation of primary superficial bladder cancer. Two theories have been proposed to explain the pathophysiological mechanisms of multiplicity, namely the monoclonality hypothesis, including intraluminal seeding and intra-epithelial migration, and the field cancerization hypothesis. Most genetic studies favour a monoclonal origin of recurrent bladder tumours and primary UUTT with intraluminal seeding. The passage of tumour cells from the upper tract to the bladder, coming first into direct and closer contact with the trigone, may explain the higher incidence of tumours in that area in patients with a UUTT. The incidence of UUTT in this setting was very low (1.8%), although more than three-quarters were of a higher grade (2 or 3) and almost half were invasive. This study suggests that there is no reliable way to completely exclude patients with primary bladder tumour from an upper tract evaluation, especially those with trigonal tumours and higher grade disease.

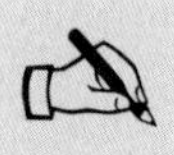

Risk factors for mucosal prostatic urethral involvement in superficial transitional cell carcinoma of the bladder

Mungan MU, Canda AE, Tuzel E, Yorukoglu K, Kirkali Z. *Eur Urol* 2005; **48**: 760–3

BACKGROUND. Multifocal development of TCC of the bladder is well known. Bladder TCC may involve the prostate, although primary prostatic TCC is rare. The exact incidence of mucosal involvement of the prostatic urethra in patients with superficial bladder TCC is not well known, and the degree of prostatic involvement has not been shown to affect the outcome. In this study, the authors evaluated the risk factors for mucosal prostatic involvement in primary superficial TCC of the bladder.

INTERPRETATION. The data from 340 consecutive male patients with the diagnosis of primary superficial TCC of the bladder treated between June 1989 and November 2004 were retrospectively reviewed. The median age was 64 years, and the median follow-up was 66 months (range 28–139 months). All patients were initially managed by TUR of the tumour. Selected site cold-cup biopsies of cystoscopically normal mucosal from lateral bladder walls, lateral to the ureteric orifices, posterior wall, dome and prostatic urethra were obtained. In case of macroscopic and/or suspected prostatic urethral involvement by TCC, TUR biopsies were obtained.

All patients underwent urine cytology and follow-up check cystoscopies every 3 months for the first year after the initial treatment, every 4 months in the second and third years, every 6 months until the fifth year and annually thereafter. Cystoscopies were performed every 3 months in the case of recurrence in the bladder. The impact of pathological stage, grade, tumour multiplicity and presence of CIS on mucosal prostatic urethral involvement was evaluated.

Of the 340 patients, 21 had mucosal involvement of the prostatic urethra at presentation. Of those, twelve (3.5%) had macroscopic involvement of the prostatic urethra, whereas nine (2.7%) had microscopic tumour on normal appearing prostatic urethra. The incidence of mucosal prostatic urethral involvement with the primary tumour characteristics was then investigated. The incidence of mucosal prostatic urethral involvement was found to be increased with stage, grade and multiplicity of the tumours of the superficial bladder cancer.

Univariate analysis showed that tumour stage, grade and multiplicity were found to be risk factors for mucosal prostatic involvement by TCC of the bladder ($P = 0.007$, $P = 0.009$ and $P = 0.001$ respectively). CIS was found to be an insignificant risk factor. On multivariate analysis, however, only tumour multiplicity was found to be an independent risk factor for mucosal prostatic urethral involvement ($P = 0.001$; risk ratio 15.832).

Comment

According to this study, the risk of mucosal urethral involvement is 16 times higher in patients with multifocal tumours of the bladder than the risk of tumour stage and grade. This result is important as it suggests the need for prostatic urethral sampling in men with multiple bladder tumours. The incidence of prostatic urethral involvement is, however, quite low, demonstrated in this study in only 6.2% of patients. TCC of the prostatic urethra is a risk factor for urethral recurrence at radical cystoprostatectomy.

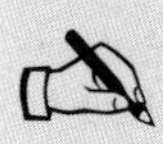

Detection of human telomerase RNA in the tumor-surrounding mucosal of bladder carcinomas as a marker for premaliganant transformation

Leuenroth S, Riethdorf S, Erbersdobler E, *et al. BJU Int* 2005; **96**: 553–7

BACKGROUND. The clinical behaviour of superficial bladder cancer is difficult to predict. The development of tumour recurrences is not completely understood; tumour recurrences may arise from tumour cells that have spread from the primary tumour or from urothelial areas outside the tumour that harbour premalignant alterations. Telomerase is a ribonucleoprotein that directs the synthesis of telomeric DNA from an RNA template. Human telomeres function to stabilize and shield the coding DNA sequences from damage (DNA degradation, chromosome loss and end-to-end-fusion), and they are important in the replication of DNA (mitotic clock). Deregulation of telomerase is pivotal for cellular immortality and oncogenesis; unlike normal somatic cells that show low or undetectable telomerase activity, germ line cells, cancer tissue and cell lines have detectable telomerase activity. Aside from germ cells in somatic tissue, telomerase activity is limited to malignant transformation and can therefore be used as a specific marker for malignant disease. The authors of this study aimed to screen non-malignant tumour surrounding bladder mucosal (NTSBM) for expression of human telomerase RNA (hTR) as a possible marker of premalignant transformation of the urothelium.

INTERPRETATION. Sixty-seven consecutive patients with primary bladder tumours underwent complete TURBT carried out using an extended resection protocol including resection of the tumour itself, the tumour ground, tumour margin and randomized biopsies of the TSBM. The mean (range) age of the patients was 66.5 (34–88) years. Mucosal tissue from 20 patients with benign urological disease served as the control. After TURB, eleven patients were diagnosed as having muscle-invasive disease or high-risk superficial TCC; seven patients were scheduled for cystectomy or cystoprostatectomy and, in four patients, this was not done due to poor performance status. Fifty-six patients were treated conservatively with curative intent and adjuvant intravesical chemotherapy (mitomycin C for 31 patients) or immunotherapy (BCG for 20 patients) in 51 patients. Five patients with small singular pTa grade I tumours were treated with TURB alone. Patients were followed for 2 years with regular cystoscopy and urine cytology assessments. A recurrent tumour was defined when cystoscopy revealed a tumour that was then confirmed on pathological evaluation.

As part of routine clinical management, biopsies were taken during TURB. At least two specimens of normal appearing (normal tissue at least >2 cm from the tumour) and two specimens of the tumour area were obtained from each patient. Sections with moderate or severe dysplasia were omitted from evaluation. Human telomerase RNA expression was detected using *in situ* hybridization with a ^{35}S-UTP-labelled riboprobe, and analysed semi-quantitatively by counting the hybridization signals.

The histopathological evaluation revealed pTa in 45 patients, pT1 in 15 patients and more than pT2 in five, with two only CIS; 10 had G1, 35 had G2 and 22 had G3 tumours. Among the 56 patients who were treated conservatively, 51 received adjuvant intravesical chemo- or immunotherapy; eight of the 56 (14.3%) had tumour recurrences.

The expression of hTR was moderate or strong in only two of 20 control tissues, but was moderate or strong in tumour tissue from 45 of 67 patients, and strong in 21 (31%). Moderate or strong hTR expression was detected in the NTSBM from 19 of 60 patients with pTa/pT1 tumours. Of the 56 patients who were treated conservatively, eight had tumour recurrence, of whom five had moderate or strong hTR expression in the TSBM, compared with only 14 of 48 patients without tumour recurrence.

Comment

The causes of tumour recurrence in patients with superficial disease are uncertain. Telomerase activity has been found in immortalized cell lines, stem cells, germ cells and in most malignant tumours, while most non-neoplastic tissues have significantly less activity. This has led to the suggestion that telomerase activation is fundamental for the development of a malignant phenotype. Recent data suggest that strong hTR expression might be an indicator of early malignant and probably also of premalignant alterations. The authors of this study found indications of an association between the strength of hTR expression in the NTSBM and tumour recurrence, but found that this association was not statistically significant, possibly because there were too few patients with tumour recurrence. Patients with tumour recurrence had moderate/strong hTR expression twice as often in the NTSBM compared with patients who did not have tumour recurrence. This finding was not a significant prognostic marker. The meticulous nature of the technique required to detect hTR expression with *in situ* hybridization makes it unlikely that it will serve as a reliable prognostic marker for each patient. However, this study supports the theory that hTR alterations might be involved in the development of tumour recurrence.

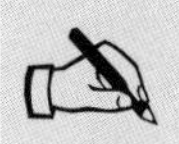

A phase-1 study of sequential mitomycin C and 5-aminolaevulinic acid-mediated photodynamic therapy in recurrent superficial bladder carcinoma

Skyrme RJ, French AJ, Datta SN, Allman R, Mason MD, Matthews PN. *BJU Int* 2005; **95**: 1206–10

BACKGROUND. Refractory superficial TCC or CIS after intravesical chemotherapy such as mitomycin C or BCG immunotherapy are common clinical dilemmas. Despite

current regimens, up to 55% of patients will develop progression to invasive disease over 5 years and require radical ablative surgery.

Photodynamic therapy (PDT) relies on the interaction between a photosensitizing agent in the target tissue and light. 5-ALA is a precursor of the photosensitizer protoporphyrin IX (PpIX). Combined therapy of mitomycin C with ALA-PDT *in vitro* gives a greater tumoricidal effect. When mitomycin C-resistant TCC cells were exposed to mitomycin C then intubated with ALA and illuminated to 635 nm, the cell kill was noted to be greater, possibly a superadditive effect. Little information is available to guide the clinical use of this therapy. The authors of this study aimed to determine the optimum dosage for sequential mitomycin with ALA-PDT, with the primary end-points being safety and patient tolerability.

Interpretation. Twenty-four patients with recurrent bladder cancer or CIS and deemed to be suitable for intravesical therapy were recruited according to the following inclusion criteria: histologically confirmed recurrent pTa, pT1 or CIS within 8 weeks of recruitment; written informed consent; performance status WHO 0–2; bladder capacity >200 ml; and normal liver function tests. Exclusion criteria included muscle invasive disease, previous pelvic radiotherapy, intravesical chemo- or immunotherapy within 12 weeks of recruitment, previous or concurrent malignancy other than non-melanoma skin cancer, a personal or family history of porphyria, or were pregnant or had a urinary tract infection (UTI). Primary end-points were safety and tolerability of combined therapy at increasing doses of ALA and light, while efficacy of the combined treatment, i.e. recurrence rates, was a secondary end-point. Frequency–volume diaries, maximum urinary free flow rates, voided volumes and post-void residual volumes were recorded, allowing the estimation of functional bladder capacity. All investigations were conducted >2 weeks before admission for PDT. The International Prostate Symptom Score (IPSS) was repeated 24 h after discharge, at 5 days and 1, 2 and 4 weeks. Patients had a follow-up cystoscopy and repeat uroflow measurements at 4 months, with subsequent follow-up being dictated both by the findings at this cystoscopy and the initial histology. Bladder capacity and post-void residuals were measured again at all visits.

Mitomycin C instillation was followed by ALA concentrations of 6%, 8% or 10%; there was no effect on toxicity. There were no episodes of skin photosensitivity or systemic toxicity. At 12–24 h, the IPSS increased in parallel with increasing total light fluence. A total fluence of 25 J/cm^2 represented the upper light dose for the tolerability of this procedure by patients. The commonest problems after PDT were urgency, frequency and suprapubic discomfort after voiding. All patients had a minimum follow-up of 2 years (range 24–33 years); there were no deaths or losses to follow-up. There were no persistently high urinary symptom scores or reduction in functional bladder capacity up to >24 months of follow-up. In this group, cumulative tumour recurrences were none at 4 months, two at 8 months, six at 12 months, nine at 18 months and 11 at 24 months after PDT. No patient had evidence of progression to muscle-invasive disease.

Comment

There is very little literature regarding the therapeutic use of ALA-PDT in bladder tumours. This study is the first to report on the use and tolerability of combined mitomycin C and ALA-PDT in bladder cancer. This study seems to suggest that mitomycin C followed by ALA-PDT is a safe and well-tolerated procedure.

Although the sample size is small and the study duration short, the recurrence rate at 2 years seems to be quite low. Further work is needed in the form of a randomized controlled trial to determine the place of this treatment in the management of bladder carcinoma.

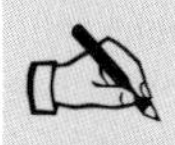

Relevance of urine telomerase in the diagnosis of bladder cancer

Sanchini MA, Gunelli R, Nanni O, *et al.* *JAMA* 2005; **294**: 2052–6

BACKGROUND. Established methods for detecting bladder cancer include urine cytology and cystoscopy, used singly or in sequence. The invasiveness of cystoscopy and the limited sensitivity of urinary cytology, especially for low-grade superficial lesions, make it of the utmost importance to develop a non-invasive, reliable and simple test to increase the rate of detection of bladder cancer. Telomerase activity in voided urine or bladder washings may be determined by the telomeric repeat amplification protocol (TRAP) assay. Using this assay, telomerase activity has been detected in almost all superficial urothelial cell carcinomas, but not in healthy urothelial. This case–control, single-blinded, prospective study was performed on urine from male individuals to validate the 50 arbitrary enzymatic units (AEUs) that had previously emerged as the best cut-off value in terms of sensitivity and specificity.

INTERPRETATION. This study was prospectively carried out in 218 men, 84 of whom were healthy and 134 of whom were patients at first diagnosis of bladder cancer, frequency matched by age (<75 years and >75 years). Median age was 62.4 years (range 22–98 years) in healthy individuals and 69.8 years (range 33–88 years) in patients. All patients underwent cystoscopy as a reference standard for bladder cancer detection, and all tumours or suspicious lesions were resected. Patients who had undergone previous treatment were excluded.

Tumour histological type and tumour cell differentiation were determined according to the World Health Organization criteria. Fifteen (11%) were well differentiated (G1), 55 (41%) were moderately differentiated (G2), and 57 (42%) were poorly differentiated. There was one carcinoma *in situ*, while no grading was available for six patients.

Urine samples were obtained from both sets of patients and processed for cytological diagnosis and TRAP assay. Forty-eight (46.6%) patients had positive cytology, 40 (38.8%) had negative cytology, eight (7.8%) patients with suspicious cytology findings had evidence of bladder cancer at histological examination, and seven (6.8%) had non-assessable cytology because of a lack of exfoliated cells (Fig. 9.3).

The population size was defined on the basis of results from a previous pilot study by the same authors, in which they obtained 93% sensitivity and 90% specificity using the 50-AEU cut-off values for the subgroup of male individuals. The threshold value for optimal sensitivity and specificity was determined using a ROC curve.

As primary end-point, the authors validated the results obtained in the pilot study using a 50-AEU cut-off value. In this series, 90% (95% CI 83–94%) sensitivity and 88% (95% CI 79–93%) specificity were observed. As secondary end-point, the diagnostic relevance of urine telomerase activity was analysed for the overall series and for the subgroups of individuals 75 years or younger and older than 75 years.

Sensitivity in the overall series ranged from 61% to 100% and specificity from 54% to 100% according to the different AEU cut-off values (Table 9.11). An increase in urine telomerase was observed from histological grades 1 to 3, but this was not statistically significant (Table 9.12). The sensitivity of urine telomerase activity in detecting bladder tumours was similar in the subgroups of patients with different tumour grades at all AEU cut-off values. In particular, at 50 AEU, the sensitivity was 93%, 87% and 89% for grades 1, 2 and 3 respectively (Table 9.13).

Table 9.11 Sensitivity and specificity of urine telomerase activity in the overall series and in individuals aged ≤75 years

				% (95% CI)
		Overall series $n = 218$		**≤75 yrs** $n = 137$
Cut-off, AEU	Sensitivity	Specificity	Sensitivity	Specificity
30	100	54 (43–64)	100	58 (45–71)
40	96 (91–98)	73 (62–81)	96 (90–99)	77 (65–87)
50	90 (83–94)	88 (79–93)	90 (82–95)	94 (85–98)
60	76 (68–83)	90 (82–95)	75 (65–83)	94 (85–98)
70	69 (61–76)	95 (88–98)	70 (60–79)	98 (90–100)
80	63 (54–70)	98 (92–99)	62 (51–72)	98 (90–100)
90	61 (53–69)	100	61 (50–70)	100

AEU, arbitrary enzymatic unit; CI, confidence interval.
Source: Sanchini *et al.* (2005).

Table 9.12 Relationship between telomerase activity and histologic grade*

	Histologic grade		
	1	**2**	**3**
Patients, no.	15	55	57
AEUs, median (range)	88 (38–382)	100 (30–265)	122 (35–344)

AEU, arbitrary enzymatic unit.
*Median test, $\chi^2 = 0.76$; $P = 0.68$.
Source: Sanchini *et al.* (2005).

Comment

Telomerase has been investigated as a potentially useful biomarker for early cancer detection and prognosis and for monitoring residual disease. The authors of this study confirmed the high sensitivity and specificity of urine telomerase levels, in particular of the 50-AEU cut-off value in detecting bladder cancer. The authors also showed that sensitivity was not age dependent, whereas specificity was higher in individuals younger than 75 years. This test represents a potential screening tool for bladder carcinoma in high-risk subgroups of patients, such as cigarette smokers.

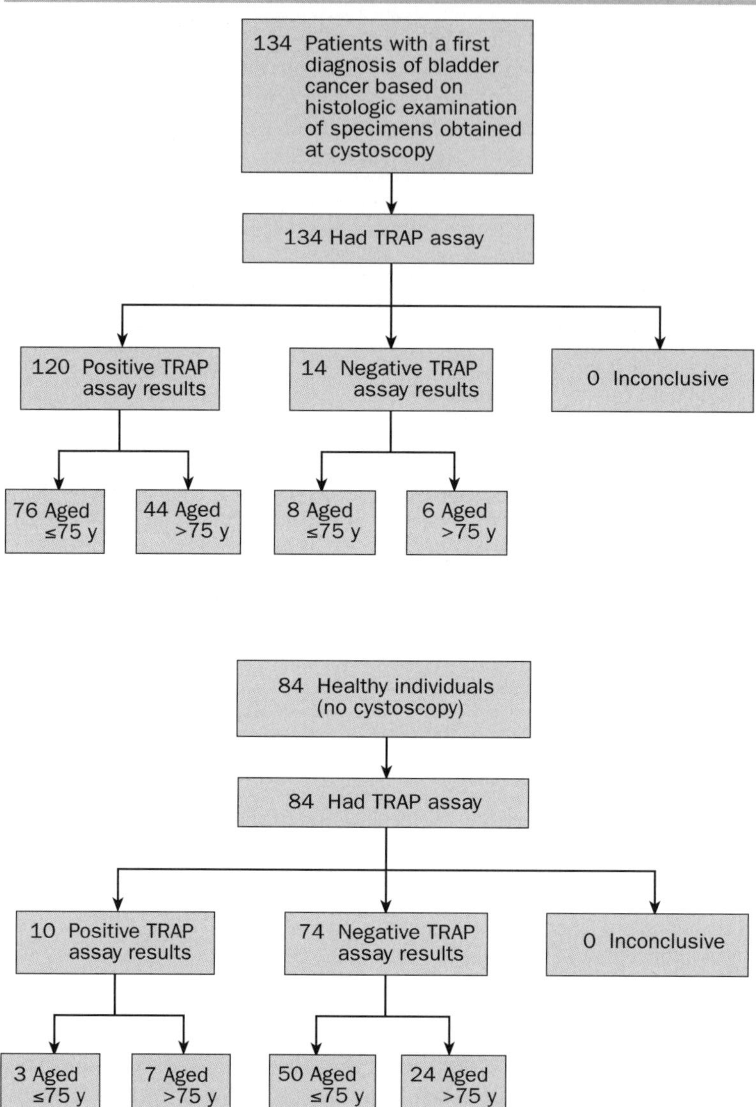

Fig. 9.3 Study flow diagram. TRAP, telomeric repeat amplification protocol. The target condition in this study was bladder cancer. Source: Sanchini *et al.* (2005).

Table 9.13 Sensitivity of urine telomerase activity in patients with different tumour grades

Cut-off, AEUs	% (95% CI)		
	Grade 1	Grade 2	Grade 3
30	100	100	100
40	93 (70–99)	96 (88–99)	95 (86–98)
50	93 (70–99)	87 (76–94)	89 (79–85)
60	73 (48–89)	71 (58–81)	79 (67–88)
70	60 (36–90)	65 (52–77)	75 (63–85)
80	53 (30–75)	60 (47–72)	68 (56–79)
90	47 (25–70)	58 (45–70)	68 (56–79)

AEU, arbitrary enzymatic unit; CI, confidence interval.
Source: Sanchini *et al.* (2005).

For this subgroup, the incidence of bladder cancer is about 10–15% and the sensitivity of urine cytology is only 30–50%. However, further prospective studies on larger patient populations are needed to assess the diagnostic role of urinary telomerase, to define the ability of this assay to detect low-grade tumours and to forecast clinical relapse.

Part III

Non-malignant conditions of the lower urinary tract

10

Urinary incontinence

HASHIM HASHIM, PAUL ABRAMS

Introduction

Urinary incontinence |**1**| has been defined by the International Continence Society as the complaint of any involuntary leakage of urine. In each specific circumstance, urinary incontinence should be further described by specifying relevant factors such as type, frequency, severity, precipitating factors, social impact, effect on hygiene and quality of life, the measures used to contain the leakage and whether or not the individual seeks or desires help because of urinary incontinence. Diagnosis and treatment of urinary incontinence (UI) should follow the International Consultation of Incontinence algorithm |**2**|.

In the diagnosis area, a few papers have been published looking at the use of frequency/volume charts, which are an indispensable part of diagnosis of lower urinary tract symptoms. The treatment area also saw many pivotal publications. In the conservative treatment arena, there were papers looking at the role of fluid manipulation and pelvic floor exercises in incontinence. In the pharmacological treatments, there were papers published looking at different antimuscarinics as well as the new selective serotonin reuptake inhibitors for stress incontinence. Finally, there were papers published in the surgical field looking at different treatment modalities for both stress and UI.

This chapter aims to summarize these interesting papers that will affect clinical practice and patient care.

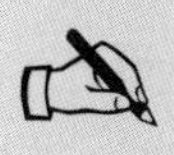

Bladder-health diaries: an assessment of 3-day versus 7-day entries

Dmochowski RR, Sanders SW, Appell RA, Nitti VW, Davila GW. *BJU Int* 2005; **96**(7): 1049–54

BACKGROUND. Bladder charts and diaries are generally the primary tool used to evaluate overactive bladder (OAB) symptoms and treatment interventions. This study assessed the reliability of symptom reports in a 3-day vs 7-day bladder diary used in two clinical drug trials, with two comparable patient groups, using transdermal oxybutynin patch. In one study, the patients filled out a 7-day diary and, in the other,

the patients filled out a 3-day diary. The internal consistency of the data from the 7-day trial was determined and then compared with the 3-day trial results. Patients in both trials were instructed on the proper methods for completing the diary, collecting and measuring urine volume and distinguishing between urgency and stress urinary incontinence episodes. The total number of UI episodes was obtained from the diaries and the number of episodes per day calculated. Also, in the 7-day trial, the change from baseline in the number of UI episodes in the 7-day diary study was re-evaluated using only the first 3 days of the diary.

INTERPRETATION. There was a statistically significant improvement in OAB symptoms in patients using the transdermal oxybutynin patch compared with placebo in both trials, as evident in the 3- and 7-day diaries. The mean change in the number of daily UI episodes in the 7-day diary was similar to that reported in the 3-day diary. Also, the results obtained using the entire 7-day diary and over the first 3 days of the same diaries were comparable. Eleven per cent of patients in the 7-day diary trial failed to document their symptoms on one or more days, compared with 0.5% in the 3-day diary trial, indicating that there is more compliance with a 3-day diary ($P < 0.001$) (Fig. 10.1).

Comment

Bladder diaries form an important first-line investigation for patients with lower urinary tract symptoms (LUTS), as they have been found to be reproducible and more accurate than patients' recall of their symptoms; however, they are under-utilized in clinical practice |3|. There have been few papers addressing the issue of

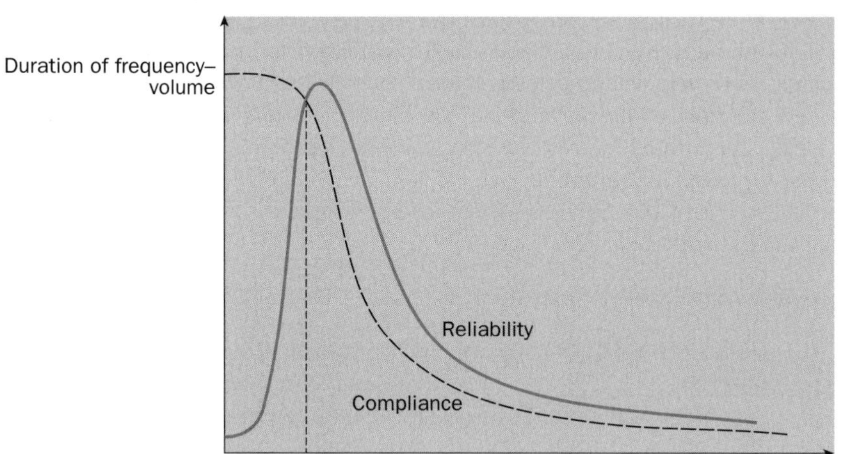

Fig. 10.1 Schematic representation of the impact of the duration of the frequency–volume chart on compliance and reliability. Theoretically, the point of intersection of the two curves projected on the abscissa will indicate the ideal compromise between the minimum number of days required while still providing acceptable reliability. Source: Dmochowski *et al.* (2005).

how many days should be recorded. Diaries can range from 1 to 14 days with 7 days being the average. The main advantage of a 7-day diary is that it would include both weekdays and weekends and thus give an overall view of patients' symptoms, as patients can change their voiding patterns between weekends and weekdays. Previous work has shown that a 4-day diary is sufficient in women **4** and a 3-day diary in men **5**. This trial did not differentiate between men and women. It can also be argued that patients in a clinical trial setting tend to comply more with protocols than those in real clinical practice, and that what is required is a trial looking at voiding diaries in patients who are attending outpatient clinics rather than those in a clinical trial setting.

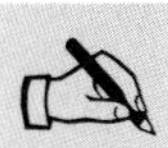

The effect of fluid intake on urinary symptoms in women

Swithinbank L, Hashim H, Abrams P. *J Urol* 2005; **174**(1): 187–9

BACKGROUND. Fluid manipulation is one of the most common methods used by women to control LUTS; however, there is little evidence in the literature to support this. This study looked at the effects of caffeine restriction and fluid manipulation on the treatment of women with urodynamic stress incontinence (USI) and idiopathic detrusor overactivity (IDO). It was a 4-week randomized, prospective, observational crossover study in 110 women with USI or IDO to determine the effect of caffeine restriction and of increasing and decreasing fluid intake on urinary symptoms. There was a baseline week (week 1), followed by 3 weeks of caffeine restriction. In the first week of caffeine restriction (week 2), women were asked to drink normally but only bland fluids. During weeks 3 and 4, women increased decaffeinated fluids to 3 l daily (week 3 or 4) or decreased decaffeinated fluids to 750 ml (five cups) daily (week 3 or 4). Women were randomized in the order in which they increased and decreased fluids.

INTERPRETATION. A total of 110 women were approached to enter the study, of whom 26 refused. There were 15 dropouts during the study, including nine women with USI and six with IDO. A total of 69 women with a mean age of 54.8 years completed the study, including 39 with USI and 30 with IDO. In the IDO group, decreasing fluid intake significantly decreased voiding frequency, urgency and wetting episodes with improved quality of life. In the USI group, there was a significant decrease in wetting episodes when fluid intake was decreased. Changing from caffeine-containing to decaffeinated drinks produced no improvement in symptoms.

Comment

Conservative measures are an integral part of the initial management of patients with incontinence. They include fluid manipulation, pelvic floor exercises and bladder training. There was little evidence in the literature on the effects of caffeine and fluid restriction on urinary incontinence. This paper provided good evidence that it is not caffeine restriction that helps control symptoms, but fluid intake as a whole. Therefore, advising patients to restrict fluid intake is a feasible measure in helping with urinary incontinence. The important thing to remember is not to restrict fluid too much, thus causing dehydration and constipation. What this paper does not address is how much should fluid restriction be and also the effects of water-containing food such as fruits and vegetables, which add on average another 500–700 ml of fluid to the diet.

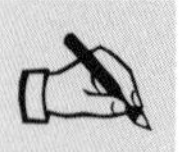

Weight loss: a novel and effective treatment for urinary incontinence

Subak LL, Whitcomb E, Shen H, Saxton J, Vittinghoff E, Brown JS. *J Urol* 2005; **174**(1): 190–5

BACKGROUND. Weight has been identified as a risk factor for UI, and evidence indicates that weight loss improves incontinence in morbidly obese women. The effect of weight loss on UI in overweight and obese women (body mass index [BMI] 25–45 kg/m^2) was evaluated in a randomized controlled trial in women aged 18 to 80 years experiencing at least four UI episodes on a 7-day frequency/volume chart. Women were randomly assigned to a 3-month low-calorie, liquid diet, weight reduction programme or a wait-list delayed intervention group. Those in the wait-list control group began the weight reduction programme in month 3 of the study. All women were followed for 6 months after completing the weight reduction programme. Quality of life was also assessed using the Incontinence Impact Questionnaire (IIQ), Urogenital Distress Inventory (UDI) and Short Form 36 (SF-36). Participants could not be blinded to their group assignment, but research investigators assessing outcomes and statistical analysts were blinded to treatment status.

INTERPRETATION. A total of 48 women were randomized and 40 were assessed 3 months after randomization. Median baseline age was 52 years, weight was 97 kg and UI episodes were 21/week. Women in the immediate intervention group had a 16-kg median weight reduction compared with 0 kg in the wait-list control group ($P<0.0001$), a 60% median reduction in weekly UI episodes (Fig. 10.2) compared with 15% in the wait-list control group ($P<0.0005$) and greater improvement in quality of life scores. Stress ($P=0.003$) and urgency ($P=0.03$) incontinent episodes decreased in the immediate intervention vs wait-list control group. Following the weight reduction programme, the wait-list control group experienced a similar median reduction in weekly UI episodes at 3, 6 and 9 months of follow-up (71%). Among all 40 women, mean weekly UI episodes decreased by 54% after weight reduction, and the improvement was maintained for 6 months. There was no change in diurnal or nocturnal micturition frequency in either group after the intervention. At 3 months, urodynamic findings were similar between the two groups, and no change was observed from baseline to 3 months in either group. However, there were significant correlations between weight change and decreased initial intravesical pressure, decreased intravesical pressure at maximum capacity and increased Valsalva leak point pressure.

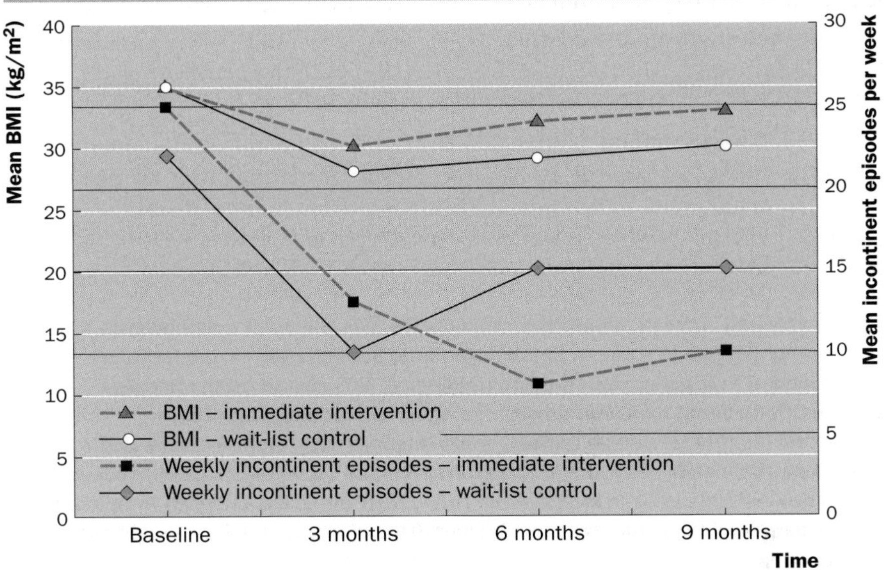

Fig. 10.2 Mean BMI and incontinence frequency by treatment group and time in cohort study. Outcomes among all participants are evaluated at 3, 6 and 9 months after initiation of weight reduction programme. Data from the end of the 3-month randomized trial were used as baseline for the wait-list control group. BMI increased during follow-up (P <0.0001 for both groups), but increases were not associated with concurrent post-intervention changes in incontinence frequency (P = 0.45). Source: Subak *et al.* (2005).

Comment

It is well known from epidemiological studies that obesity is a risk factor for stress incontinence, with some evidence that weight loss causes a reduction in stress incontinence, probably because a decrease in body weight reduces the pressure exerted on the bladder by intra-abdominal organs. Interestingly, this study also showed that weight reduction is effective in urgency incontinence, probably because an increase in intra-abdominal pressure exacerbates detrusor overactivity. During the study, it was shown that there was a decrease in intravesical pressure at follow-up with weight loss. This has support from other studies, which show that, when urodynamics is performed in the supine position, there is a lower prevalence of both detrusor overactivity and stress incontinence, indicating that, when patients are lying down, there is less provocation to the bladder |**6**|.

What this study failed to address is whether the exercise programme given to patients during the study strengthened the pelvic floor muscles causing a reduction in incontinence by a weight-independent mechanism. Nevertheless, weight reduction is a clinically feasible, safe and cheap treatment option for incontinence, with results comparable to those of other behavioural and pharmacological therapy. But, like bladder training and pelvic floor exercises, a supervised programme seems to be better than an unsupervised one.

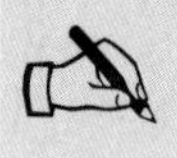

A randomized controlled trial of duloxetine alone, pelvic floor muscle training alone, combined treatment and no active treatment in women with stress urinary incontinence

Ghoniem GM, van Leeuwen JS, Elser DM, *et al.*; Duloxetine/Pelvic Floor Muscle Training Clinical Trial Group. *J Urol* 2005; **173**(5): 1647–53

BACKGROUND. Stress urinary incontinence (SUI) is the most common type of urinary incontinence in women. The International Consultation on Incontinence recommended that pelvic floor muscle training (PFMT) should be the first-line treatment for women with SUI. If that fails, then duloxetine, a serotonin norepinephrine reuptake inhibitor, can be tried before surgery. Duloxetine is believed to enhance rhabdosphincter function via the pudendal nerve, while pelvic floor muscle contraction activates the muscles of the pelvic floor but is not believed to activate the rhabdosphincter. This would imply that combination therapy would have additive effects.

A double-blind, randomized, controlled, multicentre, multinational trial was conducted in 201 women with an average of two or more incontinence episodes daily. They were randomized to one of four combinations: 40 mg of duloxetine twice-daily plus imitation PFMT (duloxetine only), duloxetine plus PFMT (combined treatment), placebo plus PFMT (PFMT only) or placebo plus imitation PFMT (no active treatment) for 12 weeks. Duloxetine and placebo were administered in double-blind fashion, but only the subject was blinded to the PFMT regimen. The variables assessed were incontinence episode frequency (IEF), the number of continence pads used and the Incontinence Quality of Life (I-QOL) questionnaire score.

INTERPRETATION. One hundred and eighty women completed post-randomization diaries and were included in the intention-to-treat IEF analysis, which included 90 women receiving placebo and 90 receiving duloxetine. Combined treatment was superior to no treatment for all outcome variables and was significantly better than PFMT alone for decrease in IEF ($P < 0.001$), but was not significantly different from duloxetine alone. Duloxetine alone had a significantly greater impact in decreasing IEF than PFMT alone, but there were no significant differences between the single treatments with respect to impact on quality of life or pad use. Duloxetine alone was significantly more effective than no treatment for the reduction in IEF ($P < 0.001$) and for the decrease in pad use ($P < 0.001$), while PFMT alone was significantly more effective than no treatment for the decrease in pad use ($P = 0.028$). There were more adverse events, especially nausea, in the two duloxetine-treated groups than in the two placebo-treated groups with greater discontinuation rates.

Comment

This is a very important trial as it shows the efficacy of combined pharmacotherapy and PFMT in the treatment of SUI. It is difficult to perform placebo PFMT, and this is probably the first trial to use 'sham' PFMT and compare it with PFMT. The authors rightly concluded from their data that the combined treatment was better than no treatment, and this was what the study was powered to show. However, they also concluded that the study provides support for the theory that combining PFMT and duloxetine may be complementary and afford greater improvement than either treatment alone, but this is not entirely correct. The combined treatment was better than PFMT alone, but it was similar to using duloxetine alone. However, as PFMT is cheap and easy to do, then there is no harm in combining it with duloxetine, especially as duloxetine has side effects that can lead to discontinuation.

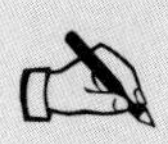

A comparison of the efficacy and tolerability of solifenacin succinate and extended release tolterodine at treating overactive bladder syndrome: results of the STAR trial

Chapple CR, Martinez-Garcia R, Selvaggi L, *et al.*; STAR Study Group. *Eur Urol* 2005; **48**(3): 464–70

BACKGROUND. The antimuscarinic class of drugs is the mainstay of oral pharmacological therapy for OAB syndrome. There is a range of antimuscarinic agents available, and this trial aimed to compare the efficacy and tolerability of two antimuscarinics in a manner that would be clinically meaningful with direct relevance to prescribers and patients. A prospective, double-blind, double-dummy, two-arm, parallel-group, 12-week study was conducted to compare the efficacy and safety of solifenacin 5 or 10 mg and tolterodine extended-release (ER) 4 mg once-daily in OAB patients. This was a multicentre, multinational trial at 117 sites in 17 European countries. After 4 weeks of treatment, patients had the option of either continuing with their original dose or requesting a dose increase based on their satisfaction with treatment efficacy and tolerability. Based on current licences, it was only possible to increase the solifenacin dose and not the tolterodine dose. Thus, for the remaining 8 weeks of the trial, the treatment regimen consisted of four arms: two groups continued with the same original dosage, one group had two 5 mg tablets of solifenacin and one group had one tolterodine tablet and one placebo.

INTERPRETATION. A total of 1355 men and women with OAB symptoms, over the age of 18 years, were screened. The safety population consisted of 1200 randomized patients (593 on solifenacin and 607 on tolterodine ER), the full analysis set consisted of 1177 patients (578 patients on solifenacin and 599 on tolterodine ER), and the per protocol set consisted of 1049 patients (525 on solifenacin and 524 on tolterodine ER). Results of the trial showed that solifenacin had superior efficacy to tolterodine ER in reducing urgency, urgency incontinence and pads used and in increasing the volume voided per void. Solifenacin was not inferior to tolterodine ER in improving nocturia or daytime frequency (Fig. 10.3). Side effects were mainly mild to moderate with higher constipation and dry mouth rates with solifenacin compared with tolterodine ER (Table 10.1). No statistical differences calculation was done in the trial on the differences in adverse events. The discontinuation rates were comparable in both drug groups.

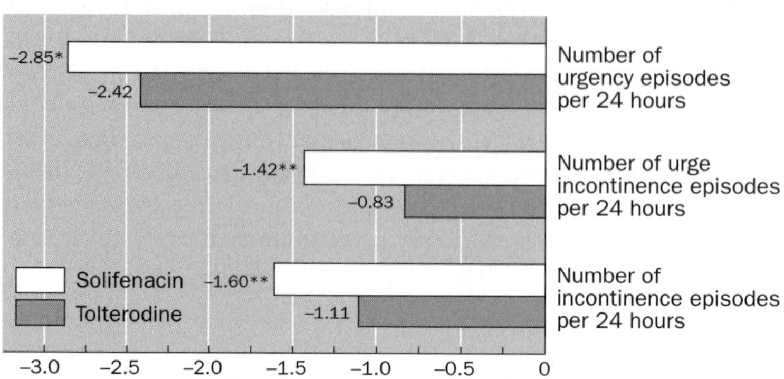

Fig. 10.3 Mean baseline to end-point change in overactive bladder symptoms. Source: Chapple *et al.* (2005).

Comment

The STAR trial mirrored clinical practice as closely as possible, as patients sometimes require a dose increase and, on the current extended release medication licences, this is not possible unless it is prescribed off licence. In the trial, the same number of tolterodine patients wanted to titrate up but could not because of licensed doses. It also provided much needed head-to-head comparative data. However, these results were the combined effects of both the 5 mg and the 10 mg doses of solifenacin and what is really needed is the comparison of each separately with respect to tolterodine ER. The trial also shows that the licensed doses are often arrived at serendipitously (almost by chance). So, the correct comparison would have been against tolterodine 6 mg or 8 mg. It should also be remembered that this was a phase IV marketing study, in which the company constructed the study to show their own drug in the best light.

The two questions that remain to be answered are: are these changes clinically relevant even though they are statistically significant and which is more important, efficacy or tolerability and side effects? Only clinical use of solifenacin will help to

Table 10.1 Total of mild, moderate and severe adverse events

Event	Adverse event (%)	
	Solifenacin	Tolterodine
Dry mouth	30	24
Constipation	6.4	2.5
Blurred vision	0.7	1.7

Source: Modified from Chapple *et al.* (2005).

answer these questions, but solifenacin will certainly increase the armamentarium of drugs available to treat OAB.

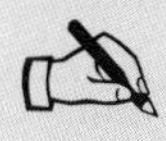

A pooled analysis of three phase III studies to investigate the efficacy, tolerability and safety of darifenacin, a muscarinic M_3 selective receptor antagonist, in the treatment of over-active bladder

Chapple C, Steers W, Norton P, *et al.* *BJU Int* 2005; **95**(7): 993–1001

BACKGROUND. Darifenacin is a new antimuscarinic that has been launched in Germany and the USA and soon around the rest of Europe to help in the treatment of OAB syndrome. It is about 60 times more selective for the M_3 receptor compared with the M_2. It has been subjected to several trials with almost identical design and enrolment of patients with OAB and, therefore, pooling these data is appropriate to look at the efficacy, tolerability and safety findings of darifenacin. The data were pooled from three phase III, multicentre, double-blind, placebo-controlled, clinical, parallel-group, fixed-dose, 12-week studies. There was a 4-week washout/run-in period, and the inclusion criteria included men and women aged ≥18 years with symptoms of OAB for ≥6 months with 5–50 episodes of incontinence per week during the run-in period and a voiding frequency ≥8 voids/24 h and urgency ≥1 episode/24 h. Electronic diaries were used throughout the studies.

INTERPRETATION. A total of 1059 patients were included in the analysis, 85% of whom were women. After 12 weeks of treatment, both doses (7.5 mg and 15 mg) of darifenacin achieved a significantly greater reduction in the median number of incontinence episodes per week, voiding frequency and number/severity of urgency episodes and increased bladder capacity compared with placebo. Consequently, there was an improvement in the proportion of patients who attained a normal voiding frequency (<8 voids/day). Some 37.1% and 52.1% of patients given darifenacin 7.5 mg or 15 mg vs 20.9% given placebo had adverse events; the most common were dry mouth and constipation. Central nervous system (CNS) side effects of dizziness and somnolence were comparable to placebo and so were the cardiovascular adverse events.

Comment

OAB negatively affects quality of life. Unfortunately, there is no 'cure' to date, and all treatments are aimed at relieving symptoms. Darifenacin seems to be an efficacious antimuscarinic in relieving OAB symptoms with minimal CNS and cardiovascular side effects. As clinical experience in using it increases, it will probably become a first-line drug in the armamentarium of antimuscarinics available. There needs to be a large head-to-head trial comparing it with oxybutynin ER or tolterodine ER.

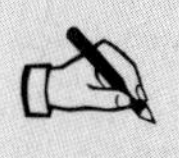

Combined use of α-adrenergic and muscarinic antagonists for the treatment of voiding dysfunction

Ruggieri MR Sr, Braverman AS, Pontari MA. *J Urol* 2005; **174**(5): 1743–8

BACKGROUND. Many patients suffer with LUTS and, therefore, a wide range and large number of patients might benefit from the combination of α-blockers and antimuscarinics. This review provides an overview of the medical literature supporting the combined use of these two drug classes for the treatment of voiding dysfunction. The Medline database (1966–2004) was searched for pertinent studies.

It was traditionally thought that α-blockers improve voiding symptoms by relaxing prostatic and urethral smooth muscle tone, which decreases outlet resistance in men with benign prostatic obstruction (BPO). However, there is increasing evidence that α-blockers also act at extraprostatic sites, such as the bladder, ganglia and spinal cord. The central facilitatory α-adrenoceptors appear to be involved in the sympathetic and somatic neural control of the lower urinary tract. The action at the CNS could increase bladder capacity and decrease the sensation to void, thereby affecting nocturia and the feeling of incomplete emptying. Also, α-adrenoceptors, which facilitate acetylcholine release, have been demonstrated at the vesical ganglia and at cholinergic nerve terminals, therefore α-blockers could decrease acetylcholine release. Other mechanisms include modulation of sensory nerves at the urothelium by evoking the release of nitric oxide, which can affect sensation and modulate sensory nerve function. Thus, α-blockers may modulate sensory responses to bladder filling. Another possible mechanism for decreasing frequency, and especially nocturia, is animal studies showing that α-antagonists decrease urine output.

As far as the antimuscarinics are concerned, the M_2 receptors contribute to about two-thirds of the muscarinic receptors in the bladder, while the M_3 receptors account for the other one-third, but it is the M_3 receptors that mediate bladder contraction, although there are several reports of M_2 contribution to bladder contraction in different pathological states. Therefore antimuscarinics can help with detrusor overactivity in patients with OAB symptoms.

INTERPRETATION. Combination therapy can be useful mainly in men with bladder outlet obstruction (BOO), as there are changes that make the α-adrenergic component of bladder function and spinal cord regulation of the bladder more important. As the changes may include upregulation of α_{1D} receptors, an α-antagonist that is effective against α_{1D} in addition to α_{1A}, which seems to be involved in BOO, would be advisable. There may be M_2-mediated contractions with BOO and, therefore, an antimuscarinic with M_2 activity as opposed to a selective M_3 antagonist may also be advisable. Combination therapy has also been used in women with LUTS, in neurogenic patients with detrusor–sphincter–dysynergia and in patients with pelvic pain syndrome including interstitial cystitis and chronic prostatitis. α-blockers can in theory cause marked hypotension, syncope, dizziness and light-headedness or vertigo, especially when the patient is standing. Antimuscarinics, on the other hand, can in theory cause hypertension but, at doses that are clinically effective for LUTS, this is rarely a reason for discontinuing the medication. Antimuscarinics are also cautioned in patients with acute angle closure glaucoma (narrow angle glaucoma) because they can cause drug-induced relaxation of the sphincter muscle and α-adrenergic-induced contraction of the dilator muscle of the pupil.

Comment

The combined use of antimuscarinics and α-blockers to treat filling and voiding symptoms, respectively, would potentially be more beneficial than either alone because they work on two different components of detrusor function. Their use may be especially effective in men with overactive bladder symptoms and bladder outlet obstruction. The main worry would be causing acute urinary retention or worsening of chronic retention, but this does not seem to be a problem from the studies already conducted. It is important that patients are aware of this potential side effect |**7**|. Although this combination has been suggested in women, using α-blockers has the theoretical risk of causing stress incontinence, and some have advised against its use in women with LUTS |**8**|.

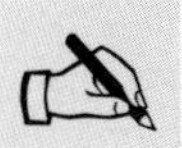

Changes in over-active bladder symptoms after discontinuation of successful 3-month treatment with an antimuscarinic agent: a prospective trial

Choo MS, Song C, Kim JH, *et al. J Urol* 2005; **174**(1): 201–4

BACKGROUND. It is not clear from the literature the point at which to discontinue antimuscarinic treatment or the time during which sustained therapeutic efficacy remains after discontinuation in patients suffering with OAB syndrome. It is up to the physician and patient to decide on a point at which to stop treatment and to see if symptoms change but, in theory, antimuscarinics should be continued for life. Women who reported improvement in OAB symptoms after 4 weeks of treatment with 20 mg of propiverine hydrochloride daily were prospectively enrolled into eight more weeks of medication and a 4-week discontinuation period. Frequency/volume charts were used to assess symptoms throughout the trial. The Indevus Urgency Severity Score was used to quantify the degree of urgency.

INTERPRETATION. Sixty-eight women were recruited. After 12 weeks of treatment, frequency, urgency and nocturia improved significantly compared with baseline. Four weeks after discontinuing treatment, all these parameters worsened significantly, but they remained improved compared with baseline. Some 35.3% of patients reported worsening of symptoms after the discontinuation of treatment and wanted further treatment. These patients were older than 55 years and had more significant urgency scores. Retreatment rates were not higher for those with detrusor overactivity (DO) on urodynamics, but those with DO did have more worsening of frequency after discontinuation. Satisfaction decreased slightly but not significantly immediately and 4 weeks after the discontinuation of treatment.

Comment

This is the first trial to look at what happens to symptoms of OAB after discontinuation of antimuscarinic therapy. The results are very interesting and clinically relevant, suggesting that patients with OAB should continue medication for longer than 3 months and that symptoms are not cured. A trial in which antimuscarinics are continued for 6 months and 12 months and longer periods needs to be conducted and medication then stopped to see what happens to symptoms. Also, this trial did not address the symptom of urgency incontinence, which would be another important factor to address. Finally, it is important to note that the Indevus Severity Score measures bladder sensation with urgency an anchor point at one end, and a scale that measures urgency is much needed to actually measure urgency in trials.

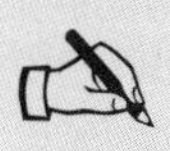

The effects of antimuscarinic treatments in over-active bladder: a systematic review and meta-analysis

Chapple C, Khullar V, Gabriel Z, Dooley JA. *Eur Urol* 2005; **48**(1): 5–26

BACKGROUND. Overactive bladder syndrome is a prevalent and debilitating condition. Treatment aims at relief of symptoms. Antimuscarinics form the cornerstone of medical treatment of patients suffering with OAB; however, they can be limited by side effects. No other drug group has shown any significant efficacy to date. This meta-analysis aimed to evaluate the tolerability, safety and efficacy of antimuscarinic drugs and to identify any differences between them. Medline, Embase, CCTR and Cinahl databases were searched for published randomized controlled trials including active and placebo-controlled trials.

INTERPRETATION. Fifty-two trials were suitable for meta-analysis. Thirty-two trials were placebo controlled and 24 trials were active controlled. All antimuscarinics were found to be efficacious in reducing urgency, frequency and urgency incontinence compared with placebo. There was also improvement in quality of life of patients receiving antimuscarinics compared with placebo. All evaluated antimuscarinic formulations (darifenacin, propiverine IR and ER, solifenacin, tolterodine IR and ER, trospium) apart from oxybutynin IR were found to be well tolerated compared with placebo. Dry mouth was the most commonly reported adverse event, and no drug was associated with an increase in any serious adverse event. This review found that antimuscarinics are safe and effective in one or more of the included outcome measures. However, there appear to be differences in the profile of the individual antimuscarinic treatments and, therefore, the choice of drug has to be tailored to the individual patient.

Comment

This is probably the most comprehensive review of antimuscarinics. It looked at different outcome measures for all the antimuscarinics individually; however, it failed to look at the decrease in nocturia as an outcome measure. Herbison *et al.* |9|

did a similar review prior to this; however, their conclusion was that the benefits of antimuscarinics are of limited clinical significance. This is refuted by this review, and the main reason for this is that the Herbison review lumped all the drugs into one while this review 'split' the drugs and analysed the data separately. One important conclusion from the meta-analysis is that there is a great need for head-to-head trials with outcomes that are meaningful to patients.

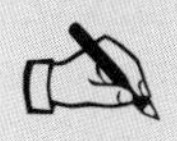

Botulinum toxin type a is a safe and effective treatment for neurogenic urinary incontinence: results of a single treatment, randomized, placebo controlled 6-month study

Schurch B, de Seze M, Denys P, *et al.*; Botox Detrusor Hyperreflexia Study Team. *J Urol* 2005; **174**(1): 196–200

BACKGROUND. Patients with neurological problems such as spinal cord injury or multiple sclerosis often suffer with urgency urinary incontinence (UUI) probably secondary to neurogenic detrusor overactivity (NDO). Botulinum toxin A (BTA) injected into the bladder via a cystoscope selectively blocks release of acetylcholine from nerve endings and had good treatment results in NDO patients, but only in non-randomized trials. This is the first double-blind, randomized, placebo-controlled, parallel-group, multicentre, multinational study performed over a 26-week period. Adult patients were included in the trial if they had UUI for at least 6 weeks caused by NDO, as demonstrated by urodynamics. They were randomized equally into a single treatment of 300 U of BTA, 200 U of BTA or placebo and followed up at weeks 2, 6, 12, 18 and 24. Under cystoscopic guidance, 30 injections of 1.0 ml each were injected intramuscularly into the detrusor, avoiding the base and trigone. The primary efficacy variable was incontinence episodes, as measured by a frequency/volume chart. Urodynamics was also performed, and the maximum cystometric capacity (MCC), reflex detrusor volume (RDV) and maximum detrusor pressure during bladder contraction (MDP) were all measured. The I-QOL questionnaire was used to assess effects on quality of life.

INTERPRETATION. A total of 59 patients (53 with spinal cord injury and 6 with multiple sclerosis) were recruited and divided equally into three treatment groups with similar demographic and baseline characteristics. In the two BTA groups, improvements were demonstrated in the daily frequency of incontinence episodes and urodynamic parameters. Improvements occurred from 2 weeks post treatment and were generally maintained for the 24-week duration of the study. The decrease in incontinence episodes was better for the 300-U group at 2 weeks ($P < 0.015$) and for the 200-U group at week 24 ($P < 0.019$). Urodynamically, there were significant increases from baseline in mean MCC and RDV and significant decrease in MDP in both BTA groups at all post-treatment time-points ($P < 0.020$), compared with the placebo group. There were significant improvements in quality of life in the active treatment groups compared with the placebo group. Urinary tract infections and injection site pain were the main adverse events.

Comment

Both UUI and NDO can have a significant impact on the quality of life of patients with neurological problems. The main treatments include antimuscarinics and intermittent self-catheterization. BTA has been used to treat strabismus and spasmodic torticollis for many years. It has been used recently as second-line treatment by some urologists to treat NDO. In non-randomized trials, botulinum toxin has shown subjective and objective significant improvements for at least 6 months and up to 14 months.

The main problem with botulinum toxin is that it is not known how much and what dose to inject, where in the bladder to inject, how often to inject and what type of botulinum toxin to inject (A or B). Long-term effects on the bladder are also not known.

This is the first study to look at the effects of BTA compared with placebo, but what is required is longer term studies with larger patient numbers to address the uncertainties. Also, to date, there are no randomized, double-blind, placebo-controlled trials to look at the effects of BTA in idiopathic detrusor overactivity. Preliminary reports suggest that it may useful in IDO, but no trials have been conducted comparing it with placebo in such patients.

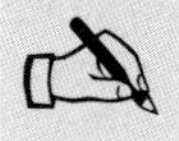

An open, multicentre study of NASHA/Dx Gel (Zuidex™) for the treatment of stress urinary incontinence

Chapple CR, Haab F, Cervigni M, Dannecker C, Fianu-Jonasson A, Sultan AH.
Eur Urol 2005; **48**(3): 488–94

BACKGROUND. There is a great need for an office procedure to bridge the gap between conservative treatment for SUI and surgery. Urethral injection of a non-animal stabilized hyaluronic acid/dextranomer (NASHA/Dx) gel via the Implacer™ device into the mid-urethral submucosa is a minimally invasive therapy that can potentially obviate the need for surgery. It is presumed to work by increasing outlet resistance and therefore theoretically reducing SUI. Women aged ≥18 years with a history of SUI for ≥12 months were recruited into this open, non-comparative, multicentre study.

INTERPRETATION. One hundred and forty-two women were recruited into the study, and 34 patients (24%) withdrew prematurely due to lack of efficacy. At month 12, 77% of patients demonstrated ≥50% decrease in provocation test leakage. At 8 weeks, before retreatment, the corresponding proportion was 68%. Sixty-two per cent of patients were essentially dry at 12 months. There was minimal decrease in the response rate between week 12 and month 12. There was also subjective improvement in 8/9 domains on the King's Health Questionnaire at month 6 and 6/9 domains at month 12. Adverse events were mainly mild or moderate and were of a nature expected with injection therapy including urinary retention, injection site pseudocyst and urinary tract infections.

Comment

Until recently, surgery, in the form of urethral bulking agents, low-tension slings or colposuspension, was the main treatment offered for women with SUI. Surgery is invasive and may require general, regional or local anaesthesia. Duloxetine, a selective serotonin reuptake inhibitor, in the form of oral tablets has been launched recently to help bridge the gap between pelvic floor exercise treatment and surgery. However, some patients cannot tolerate the tablets because of nausea, and it is only indicated in moderate to severe incontinence. The option of having an office-based procedure that can offer relatively good efficacy results of about 60% dry rates at 12 months, which are comparable to those of other periurethral and transurethral bulking agents |**10,11**|, such as silicon particles, carbon particles and collagen, with little distress to patients, is a feasible option. Injection therapy may be considered as a first-line treatment option for patients who have failed conservative therapy such as pelvic floor exercises and who decline surgery, or decline or have a contra-indication for pharmacological treatment. The safety and durability of these agents will need to be looked at long term.

The main problem with this trial is that it is an open-label trial with no blinding. What is required is a double-blind, multicentre trial against placebo, or perhaps against a minimally invasive operation such as tension-free vaginal tape (TVT).

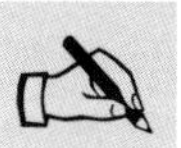

Detrusor overactivity and urge urinary incontinence following midurethral versus bladder sling procedures

Botros SM, Abramov Y, Goldberg RP, *et al. Am J Obstet Gynecol* 2005; **193**(6): 2144–8

BACKGROUND. Retropubic urethropexies and bladder neck slings were the standard method of treatment of SUI until a few years ago when midurethral tension-low slings were introduced and are rapidly becoming the standard treatment for SUI. One of the problems with SUI surgery is the development of *de novo* DO and UUI following SUI surgery or worsening of these symptoms in patients with mixed urinary incontinence (MUI). This retrospective study of patients selected with SUI or MUI, confirmed by urodynamics, was looking at the rates of resolution and of new-onset UUI and DO following either transvaginal midurethral slings (TVT or SPARC) vs transvaginal bladder neck slings made of allograft material anchored to Cooper's ligament.

INTERPRETATION. Three hundred and forty women were identified. In those who had DO preoperatively, more had resolution of DO and UUI at 3 months in the midurethral sling group compared with the bladder neck sling group (Table 10.2). Bladder neck slings also significantly increased the risk of persistent DO and post-void residue over midurethral slings. There was no difference in the development of *de novo* subjective UUI between both procedures, in those patients who did not report UUI pre-operatively. Pre-operative DO and having a bladder neck sling procedure were the only independent predictors of post-operative DO.

Table 10.2 Rates of pre-operative and post-operative DO and UUI

	Pre-operative		3 months post-operative				1 year post-operative
	DO	**UUI**	**Resolution of DO**	**Resolution of UUI**	***De novo* UUI**	***De novo* UUI**	***De novo* UUI**
Bladder neck slings ($n = 195$)	143/188 (76%)	166/195 (85%)	18/123 (15%)	45/139 (32%)	26/42 (62%)	8/28 (29%)	7/25 (28%)
Midurethral slings ($n = 145$)	84/138 (61%)	96/141 (68%)	23/61 (38%)	36/75 (48%)	13/45 (29%)	9/43 (21%)	10/38 (26%)
P-value	0.005	<0.001	0.025	0.03	0.002	0.461	0.883

Source: Botros *et al.* (2005).

Comment

This is one of very few studies that looked at DO and UUI following SUI surgery. Operating on patients with SUI and MUI poses a dilemma for the operating surgeon, as there is a risk of developing DO and UUI which affects quality of life drastically. In this study, midurethral tension-free slings seem to be better at decreasing the rates of developing *de novo* DO and better for the resolution of UUI when compared with bladder neck slings, but were not different for the onset of *de novo* UUI symptoms.

The patients in this study had higher rates of pre-operative DO than reported in the literature, and this may be due to the fact that filling of these patients was continued beyond the maximum cystometric capacity as defined by the International Continence Society (volume at which the patient feels she can no longer delay micturition), thus demonstrating DO more frequently. The authors also suggest that the high rate of *de novo* DO post-operatively in the bladder neck slings group may be due to an increase in the urethral closure pressure and intrinsic urethral resistance following the procedure, thus allowing the detection of low-pressure DO that was not detectable before the procedure.

The most important factor is to counsel patients adequately regarding post-operative complications. What is needed is a prospective, large, randomized, double-blind, multicentre trial looking at this issue. It is, however, important to remember that, in patients with MUI, treatment should be aimed at the most bothersome symptom.

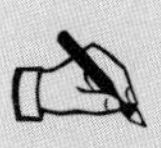

Detrusor myectomy: long-term results with a minimum follow-up of 2 years

Kumar SPV, Abrams PH. *BJU Int* 2005; **96**(3): 341–4

BACKGROUND. Detrusor myectomy (DM) is a surgical technique that attempts to bridge the gap between the medical and the surgical treatment alternatives for refractory DO. An extraperitoneal approach is used via a Pfannenstiel incision. The bladder is distended with 250 ml of saline mixed with methylene blue, and the peritoneum is dissected off the dome and the superoposterior aspect of the bladder and a disc of detrusor muscle of 8–12 cm is excised. The mucosa is left intact to develop into a broad-based superiorly situated diverticulum. After excising the detrusor muscle, the peritoneum is opened and the omentum brought down and sutured anteriorly and laterally to the detrusor edge. Short-term results for DM have been encouraging, but very few studies have published long-term results.

INTERPRETATION. Thirty consecutive patients (median age 33 years) had DM over a 10-year period. Twenty-four patients (80%) had idiopathic DO (six males and 18 females) and six (20%) had neurogenic DO (four males and two females). All these patients had failed on antimuscarinic treatment and were confirmed to have DO on urodynamics before surgery, and 26 (87%) had urodynamics afterwards. All patients were taught clean intermittent self-catheterization before surgery just in case they needed it afterwards. The median (range) follow-up was 79 (28–142) months. Nineteen (79%) of those with idiopathic DO and two with NDO showed a continued overall improvement. Of those who showed improvement, 14 (67%) had no evidence of DO on cystometry after DM. The cystometric capacity improved in 80% of patients after surgery by a mean of 165 ml ($P<0.001$), while the detrusor pressure at maximum flow and the bladder contractility index decreased in 60% ($P<0.25$) and 78% ($P<0.06$) of the patients respectively. Ten patients (45%) had to start clean intermittent self-catheterization after surgery mainly due to recurrent urinary tract infections. Eight patients (27%) required secondary procedures, five of whom had NDO.

Comment

At the moment, conservative measures including antimuscarinics form the basis of treatment of patients with overactive bladder symptoms. If this fails, then urodynamics is performed to look for detrusor overactivity. If this is confirmed, then the treatment options include botulinum toxin injections into the bladder detrusor or resiniferatoxin instillation, if available, into the bladder. If these fail, then neuromodulation is the next step, although this remains a very expensive procedure. If that fails, then surgery is the last option which, until 1989, was mainly in the form of urinary diversion or enterocystoplasty. Detrusor myectomy, as shown in this study, is a simple but tedious operation to perform, especially if perforations occur. It seems to give satisfactory results with minimal complications in patients with IDO. It is also less morbid than enterocystoplasty and certainly does not preclude subsequent surgery if required. Although it is less expensive than neuromodulation, it causes more complications, but will probably help to bridge the gap between neuromodulation and enterocystoplasty. Careful patient selection and further evaluation of this technique is required in patients with NDO.

Conclusion

When reading this chapter, it is intended that the reader gets a flavour of the exciting developments in the field of urinary incontinence and the potential for future research and development. Every part of the management algorithm has new things being researched, and it could hopefully stimulate the reader to participate and collaborate in future projects. It was also aimed to be evidence based and thus can help with clinical practice dilemmas.

References

1. Abrams P, Cardozo L, Fall M, Griffiths D, Rosier P, Ulmsten U, van Kerrebroeck P, Victor A, Wein A; Standardisation Sub-committee of the International Continence Society. The standardisation of terminology of lower urinary tract function: report from the Standardisation Sub-committee of the International Continence Society. *Neurourol Urodyn* 2002; **21**(2): 167–78.
2. Abrams P, Andersson KE, Brubaker L, Abrams P, Andersson KE, Brubaker L, Cardozo L, Cottenden A, Denis L, Donovan J, Fonda D, Fry C, Griffiths D, Hanno P, Herschorn S, Homma Y, Hu T, Hunskaar S, van Kerrebroeck P, Khoury S, Madoff R, Morrison J, Mostwin J, Newman D, Nijman R, Norton C, Payne C, Richard F, Smith A, Staskin D, Thuroff J, Tubaro A, Vodusek DB, Wall L, Wein A, Wilson D, Wyndaele JJ; Members of the Committtees. Recommendations of the International Scientific Committee: Evaluation and treatment of urinary incontinence, pelvic organ prolapse and faecal incontinence. In: Abrams P, Cardozo L, Khoury S, and Wein A (eds). *Incontinence.* Paris: Health Publication Ltd, 2005; 1589–630.
3. Abrams P, Klevmark B. Frequency volume charts: an indispensable part of lower urinary tract assessment. *Scand J Urol Nephrol Suppl* 1996; **179**: 47–53.
4. Schick E, Jolivet-Tremblay M, Dupont C, Bertrand PE, Tessier J. Frequency–volume chart: the minimum number of days required to obtain reliable results. *Neurourol Urodyn* 2003; **22**(2): 92–6.
5. Belal M, Al-Hayek S, Harris S, Dark E, Swithinbank L, Abrams P. Shortest number of days required to obtain reliable results from frequency–volume charts in men. *Prog Urol* 2006; **14**(Suppl 3): 17.

6. Shukla A, Johnson D, Bibby J. Impact of patient position on filling phase of urodynamics in women. *Int Urogynecol J Pelvic Floor Dysfunct* 2005 Jul 7; [Epub ahead of print].
7. Reynard JM. Does anticholinergic medication have a role for men with lower urinary tract symptoms/benign prostatic hyperplasia either alone or in combination with other agents? *Curr Opin Urol* 2004; **14**(1): 13–16.
8. Menefee SA, Chesson R, Wall LL. Stress urinary incontinence due to prescription medications: alpha-blockers and angiotensin converting enzyme inhibitors. *Obstet Gynecol* 1998; **91**(5 Pt 2): 853–4.
9. Herbison P, Hay-Smith J, Ellis G, Moore K. Effectiveness of anticholinergic drugs compared with placebo in the treatment of over-active bladder: systematic review. *BMJ* 2003; **326**(7394): 841–4.
10. Pickard R, Reaper J, Wyness L, Cody DJ, McClinton S, N'Dow J. Periurethral injection therapy for urinary incontinence in women. *Cochrane Database Syst Rev* 2003; (**2**): CD003881.
11. Meulen H, van Kerrebroeck E. Injection therapy for stress urinary incontinence in adult women. *Expert Rev Med Devices* 2004; **1**(2): 205–13.

11

Lower urinary tract symptoms and suspected benign prostatic obstruction in the ageing man

ALUN THOMAS, MAHMOOD SHAFEI

Introduction

Lower urinary tract dysfunction (LUTD) produces a huge burden on sufferers in particular and on society in general, with lower urinary tract symptoms (LUTS) having a high prevalence within the community. It has been clearly shown that the incidence of LUTS increases with age. It has been reported that more than 50% of men aged 65 years and over have LUTS [1]. As the population ages, especially with the ever increasing life expectancy, it is clear that the number of patients with LUTS seen by general practitioners, urologists, continence advisers and other healthcare professionals is likely to increase. In conjunction with this, the number of patients seeking advice will increase with greater patient awareness and expectation, partly due to widespread media coverage and publicity events. The increase in the number of consultant urologists in the UK reflects the escalating demand for appropriate patient management. As a consequence, the demand for treatment will increase.

The mechanisms by which benign prostatic hyperplasia (BPH), a histological process, causes LUTS are not fully understood. BPH gives rise to benign prostatic enlargement (BPE) with the possible subsequent complication of benign prostatic obstruction (BPO). However, there are poor correlations between the presence and severity of LUTS and the anatomical and urodynamic measures of the severity of BPE and BPO, which suggests a more complex process. Even so, symptoms are what bring the patient to the clinician, and reliable methods of measuring LUTS are important in the process of understanding the impact of symptoms in men with BPO, and in evaluating the efficacy of treatments for these symptoms.

The interpretation of a patient's symptoms is modified by many factors. The limits of normality are not adequately defined and, for an individual case, it may be what the patient, rather than the doctor, considers as being normal. The adequacy of communication is important, as are many preconceived ideas of the medical staff. With regard to more complex symptom assessment, symptom indices have been used extensively in clinical urology. Symptom indices are scientifically validated instruments that allow reproducible objective evaluation of the patient's symptoms. The aim has been two-fold. First, to predict prognosis by measurement of symptom severity and, secondly, to evaluate changes over a period of time, with or without treatment intervention. Symptom indices within urology have been developed mainly for use in patients with LUTS suggestive of BPO, although more recently there have been developments in the assessment of women with urinary incontinence. The presence and degree of symptoms constitute only one component when evaluating the impact of LUTS on men's lives. Patients respond differently to similar symptom levels. Hence, evaluation of how bothered men are by their symptoms is an important part of the assessment. To complicate matters further, LUTS and its treatments can affect other domains of the patients' lives. Principal examples are continence and sexual function, and the impacts of these domains on a patient's life require careful evaluation.

Treatment decisions depend on knowledge of the natural history of LUTD. There has been a widely held view that patients inevitably deteriorate relatively quickly, thereby justifying early treatment. There are few data on the natural history of LUTD on which healthcare professionals can make decisions that ultimately affect the patients' health and quality of life. This lack of information may be the cause of the wide disparity in prostatectomy rates in England: district rates varying from 2.8 to 29.2 per 10 000 population. The most recent data indicate that the rates of prostatectomy have climbed, from 25 000 in 1975 to 42 000 in 1990, with a slight drop more recently (40 000 in 1999) |**2**|. Prostatectomy is clearly indicated in acute urinary retention (AUR) or urinary tract damage due to chronic retention: however, these indications constitute only a small proportion of prostatectomies, approximately 10–15% for acute retention plus a significantly smaller percentage for obstructive nephropathy. The majority of operations are performed electively to relieve urinary symptoms, assumed to be caused by bladder outlet obstruction (BOO) related to the presence of BPH. In the UK, of these men with uncomplicated symptoms, 38% are treated surgically, 33% with drugs and 29% conservatively |**2**|.

Within the last 10–20 years, there has been a revolution in the treatment options for BPO. Studies examining the natural history of the disorder suggest that symptoms do not necessarily deteriorate with time to a level at which intervention is mandatory. This allows a 'watchful waiting' policy for those who are minimally symptomatic or unbothered by their symptoms. Pharmacological therapies now offer an alternative to surgery for some men, with numerous randomized controlled trials (RCT) demonstrating reduction in symptoms and improvements in flow. However, not all men are suitable for medical therapy. First, significant proportions do not respond to such treatment. Secondly, such tablets have side effects that some men find intolerable and, finally, complications of BPO such as urinary retention are an indication for surgical intervention from the outset.

Until recently, invasive treatment has principally comprised transurethral resection of the prostate (TURP). This operation has been performed for many years and is one of the most common procedures performed in the NHS today. It is considered the 'gold standard' treatment against which all other therapies are compared, preferably in a RCT. However, there has been a relatively recent explosion in 'minimally invasive' therapies, driven by the medical equipment companies' desire to produce an alternative to TURP. The term 'minimally invasive' is an expression that has flourished without a consensus as to what it actually means. The principle of treatment is the same as for TURP, that is to remove excess prostatic tissue to relieve the obstruction, but in a way that limits or removes the need for hospital stay and reduces the peri- and post-operative complications associated with TURP.

The armamentarium of minimally invasive treatment modalities has increased constantly over the last decade. The energy sources used range from micro-/radiofrequency waves to high-intensity focused ultrasound, laser vaporization/coagulation/resection and electrosurgical techniques. Each of these devices has its own particular advantages and disadvantages. A convenient way of classifying these therapies is according to the therapeutic temperature that they generate. Transurethral microwave therapy (TUMT) can be used in both low-energy (45–60°C) and high-energy (60–80°C) forms. Transurethral needle ablation (TUNA) causes prostate ablation by delivering low-level radiofrequency energy (80–200°C) to the prostate via needles inserted transurethrally. Transrectal high-intensity focused ultrasound (HIFU; 100°C) causes thermocoagulation by generation of high temperatures within the beam focus. Transurethral electro-vaporization (TUVP; 200–400°C) is a technique that has gained increasing popularity in recent years and works by combining two electrosurgical effects (tissue vaporization and desiccation), allowing prostate tissue removal with minimal bleeding at the same time. Finally, several laser devices are being used with promising results, including interstitial laser coagulation (ILC), visual laser ablation (VLAP) and holmium–laser resection. These are different devices that use different laser energies.

The following recently published papers highlight the contemporary issues related to the evaluation and treatment of BPH and LUTS.

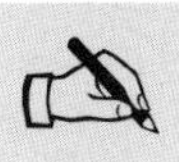

EAU 2004 guidelines on assessment, therapy and follow-up of men with lower urinary tract symptoms suggestive of benign prostatic obstruction (BPH guidelines)

Madersbacher S, Alivizatos G, Nordling J, Sanz CR, Emberton M, de la Rosette JJ. *Eur Urol* 2004; **46**: 547–54

BACKGROUND. BPH and BPE are two of the most common problems affecting the ageing male population, which can lead to LUTS. The relationship between BPH/BPE and LUTS is complex, as not all patients with prostatic enlargement go on to develop symptoms. As we improve our understanding of the disease process and its natural history, new treatment modalities and techniques are going to be pioneered. With ever expanding technology and urologists' ambitions to open new frontiers, guidelines

are put in place to guide us in choosing the best evidence-based practice for our patients.

Interpretation. Recent findings on the natural history of the disease, its progressive nature and new treatment modalities have prompted the European Association of Urology (EAU) to publish this update, especially in view of the development of 5-alpha reductase type 1 and 2 inhibitors and data from the Medical Therapy of Prostatic Symptoms (MTOPS) trial. Systematic literature review using Medline from 1999 to 2003 was conducted. This, in combination with expert opinions, led to recommendations on the usefulness of diagnostic tests, therapeutic options and patient follow-up (Tables 11.1 and 11.2). Compared with the 2001 guidelines, only a few modifications were made.

Comment

The current guidelines are the first update of the 2001 version. The EAU recommends regular updates of such guidelines every 2–4 years, so that the latest evidence-based information can be taken into account. With the exception of the recommendation for serum creatinine measurement, it correlates closely with the 2003 American Urological Association (AUA) update guidelines, which included a variety of meta-analytic techniques and peer reviewing by 58 experts.

Table 11.1 EAU 2004 recommendations regarding initial assessment for elderly men with LUTS suggestive of BPO

Assessment	EAU 2004 recommendations
Medical history	Recommended
Symptom score	Recommended
Physical examination including DRE	Recommended
Prostate-specific antigen	Recommended
Creatinine measurement	Recommended
Urinalysis	Recommended
Flow rate	Recommended
Post-void residual volume	Recommended
Pressure flow studies	Optional
Endoscopy	Optional
Imaging of the upper urinary tract	Optional
Imaging of the prostate	Optional
Voiding charts (diaries)	Optional
Excretory urography	Not recommended
Filling cystometry	Not recommended
Retrograde urethrogram	Not recommended
Computed tomography	Not recommended
Transrectal magnetic resonance imaging	Not recommended

Source: Madersbacher *et al.* (2004).

Table 11.2 EAU 2004 recommendations regarding treatment for elderly men with LUTS suggestive of BPO

Treatment	EAU 2004 recommendations
Watchful waiting	Recommended
Medical therapy	
α1-blocker	
Alfuzosin	Recommended
Doxazosin	Recommended
Tamsulosin	Recommended
Terazosin	Recommended
5ARI	
Dutasteride	Recommended
Finasteride	Recommended
Combination therapy	
α1-blocker plus 5ARI	Recommended
Plant extracts	Not recommended
Minimally invasive therapies	
High-energy TUMT	Recommended
TUNA*	Recommended
Prostatic stents†	Recommended
Surgical therapies	
TUIP	Recommended
TURP	Recommended
Open prostatectomy	Recommended
Transurethral holmium laser enucleation	Recommended
Transurethral laser vaporization*	Recommended
Interstitial laser coagulation*	Recommended
Transurethral laser coagulation*	Recommended
Emerging therapies	
Ethanol injection	
High-intensity focused ultrasound	
Water-induced thermotherapy	
PlasmaKinetic™ tissue management	

*Not as a first-line treatment.
†Only for high-risk patients as an alternative for permanent catheterization.
Source: Madersbacher *et al.* (2004).

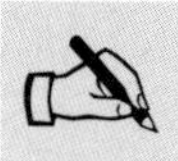

The natural history of lower urinary tract dysfunction in men: minimum 10-year urodynamic follow-up of untreated detrusor underactivity

Thomas AW, Cannon A, Bartlett E, Ellis-Jones J, Abrams P. *BJU Int* 2005; **96**(9): 1295–300

BACKGROUND. Detrusor underactivity (DUA) in men is responsible for LUTS in a significant minority of patients, its symptomatology being indistinguishable from that seen in BOO. There have been few long-term follow-up data on men with DUA. This study aimed to assess the long-term symptomatic and urodynamic outcomes of men with untreated DUA.

INTERPRETATION. From a historical cohort of 224 neurologically normal men with LUTS, over 18 years of age at presentation between 1972 and 1986, with a diagnosis of DUA, 137 (61.2%) were still alive at the time of this follow-up study, a mean of 13.6 years later. Of those still alive, 84 (61.3%) were reassessed; 64 (76.2%) with full re-evaluation, six (7.1%) with uroflowmetry and for symptoms, and 14 (16.7%) with symptomatic appraisal only. Of the 69 men who initially opted for a conservative (non-surgical) approach and attended for repeat assessment, 58 (84%) remained untreated. No significant changes in symptoms were noticed over the follow-up period. The only significant urodynamic finding was an increased proportion of patients exhibiting detrusor overactivity, with worsening chronic retention not seen.

Comment

Detrusor underactivity has been shown to occur in men of all ages. Despite this, there have been few long-term follow-up data on this condition. Short-term studies suggest that neither LUTS nor DUA inevitably progresses to the stage at which intervention is required. Nevertheless, in the long term, if DUA were to be progressive, it may be accompanied by several serious long-term complications, including urinary tract infections, chronic urinary retention and, possibly, renal failure. This study has followed patients with DUA for a minimum of 10 years. It did not demonstrate any significant change in voiding as judged by uroflowmetry. This was corroborated by the pressure flow data, with no significant changes in voiding efficiency, despite an increase in prostate size. A significant increase in the proportion of patients exhibiting detrusor overactivity was seen on follow-up, but there was no deterioration in storage symptoms. Neither objective changes in daytime and night-time voiding nor increase in subjective reporting of urgency/urge incontinence was observed. Overall, for those with untreated DUA, there was no significant urodynamic or symptomatic deterioration with time. These results provide insights into the changes in both the severity of LUTS and urodynamic parameters in men with DUA. It provides valuable information on how to advise patients about treatment. In men with DUA presenting with LUTS, it presents evidence of minimal urodynamic change and no symptomatic deterioration with time. Previous hypotheses regarding worsening chronic retention with time do not hold true.

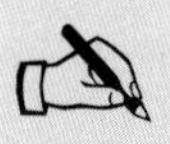

The natural history of lower urinary tract dysfunction in men: minimum 10-year urodynamic follow-up of untreated bladder outlet obstruction

Thomas AW, Cannon A, Bartlett E, Ellis-Jones J, Abrams P. *BJU Int* 2005; **96**(9): 1301–6

BACKGROUND. There is little information regarding the natural history of untreated BOO and LUTS in men. Studies to date clearly suggest that neither BOO nor LUTS inevitably progresses to a stage at which prostatectomy is required. This study aimed to assess the long-term outcomes of untreated BOO, on the assumption that, if little or no deterioration was seen, then a conservative approach to management would be justified.

INTERPRETATION. Men over 45 years old presenting with LUTS, investigated initially between 1972 and 1986, diagnosed with BOO, who opted initially for no specific treatment were invited for repeat symptomatic and urodynamic evaluation. Identical methods of assessment were used, so allowing direct comparison of results. Of the 170 men who initially opted for a conservative approach and attended for repeat assessment, 141 (83%) remained untreated, with a mean follow-up time of 13.9 years. The only significant urodynamic changes seen were a reduction in detrusor contractility and an increased prevalence of detrusor overactivity. The majority of patients reported no change in their symptoms, but a significant minority experienced a gradual deterioration. Of those who failed the conservative approach ($n = 29$), 22 proceeded to surgery for LUTS, and seven for urinary retention.

Comment

Long-term outcome data, especially from pressure flow studies, regarding the natural history of LUTS and BOO have been lacking. These results provide insights into the changes in the severity of LUTS and urodynamic parameters in men with BOO, and provide valuable information as to how to advise patients on treatment and its timing. In men with outlet obstruction presenting with LUTS, this study presents evidence of minimal urodynamic and symptomatic deterioration with time. The small urodynamic deterioration that occurs is related to deterioration in detrusor function and not an increase in obstruction. Therefore, one can reassure those men who do not wish to be treated surgically that they are unlikely to deteriorate either quickly or significantly even over a long period. These findings justify a conservative approach to men with LUTS associated with BOO.

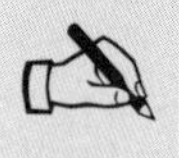

Efficacy and safety of two doses (10 and 15 mg) of alfuzosin or tamsulosin (0.4 mg) once daily for treating symptomatic benign prostatic hyperplasia

Nordling J. *BJU Int* 2005; **95:** 1006–12

BACKGROUND. Alpha-blockers are considered the first-line treatment for managing LUTS associated with BPH and suggestive of BOO. Alfuzosin 2.5 mg tds and the 5 mg bd dosages have been available in most countries since 1988. Once daily, extended release alfuzosin has a better pharmacokinetic profile and better patient compliance, and was developed and launched in Europe in 2000 and the USA in 2003.

INTERPRETATION. This study was an 18-month randomized, double-blind, placebo-controlled, multicentre trial involving 625 patients. The objective of this study was to evaluate the benefit-to-risk profile of alfuzosin 10 and 15 mg daily compared with placebo for treating LUTS. A tamsulosin arm at 0.4 mg dose was included as an active reference group. This study was one of three pivotal studies considered by the Food and Drug Administration (FDA) in the USA before granting approval for alfuzosin 10 mg extended release. Both alfuzosin at 10 mg dose and tamsulosin at 0.4 mg dose significantly improved urinary symptoms and maximum flow (Qmax) compared with placebo and were well tolerated. The incidence of sexual function adverse events seemed to be higher with tamsulosin than with alfuzosin, compared with placebo. The benefit-to-risk ratio of alfuzosin 10 mg appeared to be reduced at the 15 mg dose.

Comment

This paper compared two of the most commonly used alpha-1 adrenoceptor blockers worldwide. The results of this study show that the extended release alfuzosin at 10 mg and tamsulosin at 0.4 mg are equally effective in alleviating urinary symptoms and bring about improvement in Qmax. They were also seen to be well tolerated. It is also interesting to see that tamsulosin has higher sexual function adverse events compared with alfuzosin 10 mg extended release.

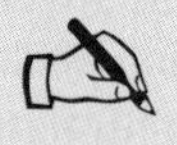

The natural history of lower urinary tract dysfunction in men: minimum 10-year urodynamic follow-up of transurethral resection of prostate for bladder outlet obstruction

Thomas AW, Cannon A, Bartlett E, Ellis-Jones J, Abrams P. *J Urol* 2005; **174**(5); 1887–91

BACKGROUND. Despite long-term symptomatic and uroflowmetry studies following TURP, there are few pressure flow (PFS) data. Consequently, there is minimal information to account for the long-term symptomatic failure and flow rate reduction seen with time following the early improvements after surgery.

INTERPRETATION. Men over 45 years old investigated at the Bristol Urological Institute between 1972 and 1986, diagnosed with bladder outlet obstruction, who opted for surgical intervention were invited for repeat symptomatic and urodynamic assessment. Identical methods were used, so allowing direct comparison of results.

A total of 217 of the men followed up underwent TURP, with a mean follow-up time since surgery of 13.0 years. A significant sustained reduction in the majority of symptoms and improvements in urodynamic parameters were seen. Long-term symptomatic failure and flow rate reduction were principally associated with the development of DUA rather than obstruction. Presentation predictive factors for the future development of DUA included reduced detrusor contractility and a lesser degree of obstruction.

Comment

The selection biases associated with retrospective studies notwithstanding, the results of this study have provided valuable long-term information about surgically treated BOO. This study demonstrates a long-term sustained improvement in almost all urodynamic and symptomatic parameters following surgery. Uroflow and pressure flow data show significant improvement in most urodynamic parameters. Interestingly, despite reports of resolution of detrusor overactivity (DO) in the short term following TURP, this study demonstrates that it recurs on long-term follow-up. Symptomatically, the results show significant sustained objective and subjective improvements in the long term. The results highlight that LUTD and LUTS following TURP are principally detrusor in origin, and not related to re-obstruction, with a BOO rate of only 17.5% found in those re-presenting with problems. This demonstrates that those who remain symptomatic after operation are not commonly obstructed and should be urodynamically investigated to determine the aetiology of their voiding dysfunction before repeating surgery. However, our faith in the long-term efficacy of TURP is justified.

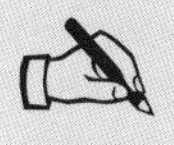

The natural history of lower urinary tract dysfunction in men: the influence of detrusor underactivity on the outcome from TURP with a minimum 10-year urodynamic follow-up

Thomas AW, Cannon A, Bartlett E, Ellis-Jones J, Abrams P. *BJU Int* 2004; **93**(6): 745–50

BACKGROUND. There exist virtually no data evaluating the efficacy of TURP in men with DUA, a cause of LUTS in a significant minority of men. This study aimed to assess the long-term outcomes of this approach.

INTERPRETATION. Neurologically intact men with LUTS, urodynamically investigated between 1972 and 1986, diagnosed with DUA, who underwent surgical intervention were invited for repeat symptomatic and urodynamic assessment. Identical methods were used, so allowing direct comparison of results. A total of 224 men were initially diagnosed with DUA. Eighty-seven (39%) of these died in the interim. Twenty-two of the men followed up underwent TURP, with a mean follow-up time since surgery of 11.3 years. No significant sustained reduction in any symptoms was seen. A small but significant reduction of questionable clinical significance in the BOO index was noted, but this was not translated into an improvement in flow rate. Comparison with 58 age-matched DUA patients who remained untreated revealed no significant advantage, in the long term, of surgical intervention; on the contrary, a greater degree of chronic retention was seen in those who had been operated on.

Comment

There are few data evaluating the efficacy of TURP in those with DUA, although men with lower voiding pressures have been shown to have a less favourable symptomatic outcome following elective TURP. This is a very important consideration as the majority of men in the UK undergo a TURP for LUTS on the basis of symptoms and uroflowmetry only, and it is well recognized that DUA and BOO are indistinguishable on the basis of these two parameters. An operation designed to relieve outlet obstruction, where detrusor failure is the underlying pathology, would seem unlikely to produce any changes in voiding efficiency, although it has been suggested that a reduction in outlet resistance may produce more efficient emptying by straining.

The data from this study demonstrate that, following TURP for DUA, despite a clinically non-relevant reduction in outlet obstruction, there are no long-term urodynamic or symptomatic gains to be made, compared with the improvements seen in those with BOO. Intermittent self-catheterization (ISC) for chronic retention secondary to detrusor failure, despite minimizing the attendant complications of this disorder, produces no long-term change in voiding function. These results suggest that DUA is a contraindication for TURP, and that DUA should be distinguished from BOO pre-operatively: this necessitates pressure flow studies.

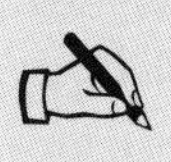

Evaluation of male sexual function in patients with lower urinary tract symptoms (LUTS) associated with benign prostatic hyperplasia treated with phytotherapeutic agent (permixon), tamsulosin or finasteride

Zlotta AR, Teillac P, Raynaud JP, Schulman CC. *Eur Urol* 2005; **48**: 269–76

BACKGROUND. With increasing use of medical therapy for treatment of BPH and associated LUTS, the sexual function aspect of these medications had often been ignored until recently. This has now increasingly gained attention. Both tamsulosin and finasteride are known to affect sexual function adversely. Tamsulosin causes retrograde ejaculation and erectile dysfunction, and low-volume ejaculates have been associated with the use of finasteride. An extract of *Serenoa repens* (permixon) has been studied extensively and approved for treatment of LUTS. Permixon has been shown to be as effective in both reducing LUTS and improving flow rates when

compared with tamsulosin. Similarly, permixon has also been shown to be as effective in reducing symptom scores and improving peak flows when compared with finasteride, although placebo arm comparators have been lacking. The aspect of sexual function after permixon use compared with finasteride or tamsulosin has not been studied before.

Interpretation. A total of 2511 patients from three double-blinded, randomized, controlled studies were included in this database: permixon vs finasteride, permixon vs tamsulosin and permixon 160 mg vs 320 mg. The International Prostate Symptom Score (IPSS) was measured. The male sexual function questionnaire (MSF-4) was also used, exploring four domains: patients' interest in sex, the quality of erection, achievement of orgasm and ejaculation. Peak urinary flow and prostate volume were also measured. Data from the two permixon dosages were later combined, as no difference was seen in terms of outcome between these groups.

These results showed that there was no statistically significant difference between all treatment options in terms of IPSS score and maximum flow at 3 months (Table 11.3). permixon had no effect on any of the MSF-4 domains. However, a very modest decrease in global sexual function was seen with finasteride and tamsulosin after 6 months (Table 11.4).

Table 11.3 Evolution in IPSS, *Q*max and prostate volume in patients receiving permixon, finasteride or tamsulosin

	Permixon 160 mg	**Permixon 320 mg**	**Finasteride**	**Tamsulosin**	***P*-value**
	(*n* = 914)	**(*n* = 698)**	**(*n* = 545)**	**(*n* = 354)**	
IPSS change at 3 months mean (SD)	–4.4 (4.5)	–4.0 (4.4)	–5.4 (4.9)	–4.1 (4.6)	>0.05
*Q*max evolution from baseline at 3 months mean ml/sec (SD)	+2.67 (5.48)	+2.34 (5.09)	+2.62 (6.22)	+1.73 (5.07)	>0.05
Prostate volume decrease from baseline at 3 months mean cm^3 (SD)	–2.58 (12.65)	–3.59 (10.28)	–6.73 (11.10)	Non-available	0.001*

*Comparing permixon vs finasteride and tamsulosin for IPSS and *Z*max, permixon vs finasteride for prostate volume.
Source: Zlotta *et al.* (2005).

Table 11.4 Changes in MSF-4 global score at 3 and 6 months of therapy compared with baseline values

	Permixon (*n* = 1609)	**Finasteride** (*n* = 545)	**Tamsulosin** (*n* = 354)
MSF-4 total score at baseline mean (SD)	8.2 (5.1)	8.5 (5.5)	7.9 (5.1)
Change in MSF-4 total score at 3 months mean (SD)	0.0 (2.8)	+0.5 (3.5)	+0.3 (2.9)
Change in MSF-4 total score at 6 months mean (SD)	–0.2 (3.1)*	+0.8 (3.8)	+0.3 (3.4)
% of patients improved at 3 months	30.2%	28.2%	31.0%
% of patients aggravated at 3 months	27.1%	32.0%	39.9%
% of patients stable at 3 months	42.7%	39.8%	29.1%
% of patients improved at 6 months	31.8%*	27.5%	34.4%
% of patients aggravated at 6 months	29.5%*	38.6%	40.7%
% of patients stable at 6 months	38.7%*	33.9%	24.9%

*Analysis performed on 902 patients treated with permixon.
Source: Zlotta *et al.* (2005).

Comment

There are some limitations to this study. Longer follow-up is desirable to assess the effect of finasteride on LUTS associated with BPH. Furthermore, there was no placebo or watchful waiting arm to this study. However, this paper shows permixon to be as effective as both finasteride and tamsulosin, but with no adverse effect on sexual function. The reported sexual adverse effects of finasteride and tamsulosin are rare and in line with previous studies.

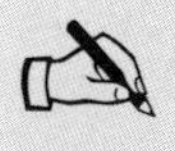

Tamsulosin in the management of patients in acute urinary retention from benign prostatic hyperplasia

Lucas MG, Stephenson TP, Nargund V. *BJU Int* 2005; **95**(3): 354–7

Background. Acute urinary retention is one of the more serious complications of benign prostatic hyperplasia. AUR is relatively common and is both distressing and painful for the patient. Patients are managed in the acute phase with catheterization. Management following this is a matter of great debate. Depending on the clinical scenario, options include trying trials without catheter (TWOCs) or surgery to the prostate. LUTS in men can be alleviated by alpha-blockers, presumably by reducing outlet resistance by relaxation of muscle fibres in the bladder neck and prostatic stroma. By the same token, the same medication may also improve TWOC rates. This study aimed to assess the efficacy of modified-release tamsulosin hydrochloride (0.4 mg daily) vs placebo in the management of patients with AUR who were suitable for a TWOC.

INTERPRETATION. One hundred and forty-nine men presenting with AUR were included in this double-blinded, randomized, controlled trial to either tamsulosin or placebo. TWOC was undertaken between 3 and 8 days after commencement of medication. A successful void was deemed as a post-void residual of less than 200 ml.

Forty-eight per cent (34/71) of the tamsulosin group and 26% (18/70) of the placebo group did not require recatheterization ($P = 0.011$) (Fig. 11.1). Overall, the incidence of adverse events was similar in the two groups.

Comment

This elegant study looks at a common urological condition faced by most urologists in their day-to-day practice. It demonstrates the efficacy of this alpha-blocker in the management of AUR. There are, however, still unanswered questions from this study, which do need further evaluation to clarify an optimum strategy for this group of patients. What is the optimum timing to undertake a trial without catheter, and how many doses of alpha-blocker are required for maximum effect? Which groups of patients are most likely to benefit from tamsulosin therapy, and what is the long-term outcome for the patients managed in this fashion? Even though this is a good study, it is not designed or powered enough to answer these important questions.

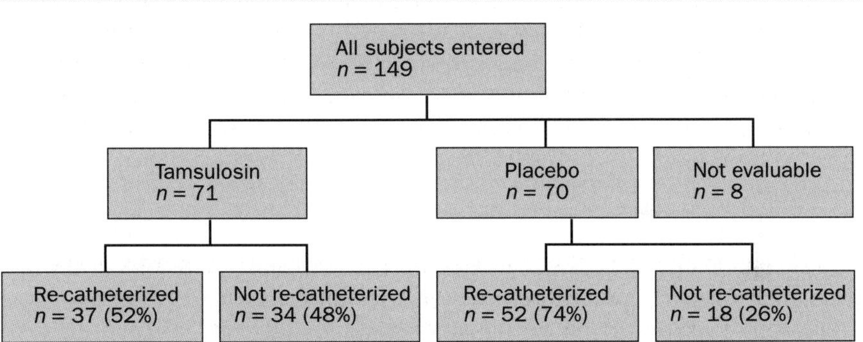

Fig. 11.1 Patient outcomes for catheterization at visit 2 for the intent-to-treat population. Source: Lucas *et al.* (2005).

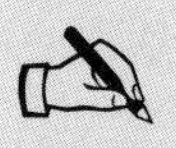

Transurethral microwave thermotherapy versus transurethral resection for treating benign prostatic hyperplasia: a systematic review

Hoffman RM, MacDonald R, Monga M, Wilt TJ. *BJU Int* 2004; **94**: 1031–6

BACKGROUND. Several minimally invasive surgical techniques have been developed in recent years for treating BPH in order to try and reduce the morbidity associated with TURP. TURP remains the gold standard however. Direct comparative studies between TURP and other minimally invasive techniques are limited. TUMT has gained popularity as a treatment and can be delivered in a single session on an outpatient basis. It delivers high microwave energy heating the prostate to produce coagulation necrosis. It has fewer complications compared with TURP and reduces hospital stay. The AUA (2003) guidelines on managing BPH concluded that TUMT is effective in partially relieving symptoms, and the EAU (2004) recommends that it should be reserved for those who prefer to avoid surgery or who are not fit for anaesthesia.

INTERPRETATION. This is a systematic review of six RCTs involving 540 patients, evaluating the efficacy and safety of TUMT compared with TURP. Medline, Cochrane Library and other reference lists of retrieved studies were used to identify RCTs of >6 months' duration with >10 patients in each treatment arm. The mean difference for the symptom score at follow-up was –1.83 favouring TURP. The pooled mean peak urinary flow (PUF) increased by 70% with TUMT and 119% for TURP. Retrograde ejaculation, transfusion and retreatment for stricture were significantly lower for TUMT. However, incidence of retreatment for BOO, the occurrence of urinary retention and the symptom of dysuria were significantly less following TURP.

Comment

This study clearly demonstrates the superiority of TURP over TUMT with regard to improvement in PUF and IPSS in the long term. However, TUMT carries less adverse events, and the procedure can be delivered on an outpatient basis. There are, however, a few criticisms of the RCTs used for this review. First, none of the trials clearly had adequate concealment of randomization. The follow-up of some of the trials was short (6 months only). Furthermore, one important complication, thermal injury, was not consistently reported. The American FDA has published a public health notification because they have received 16 reports of severe thermal injuries associated with the use of TUMT (ten fistulas and six reports of tissue damage to the urethra and penis). This study can be a useful tool in guiding patients and physicians in weighing the short-term relative risks and benefits of TUMT and TURP. Further research and longer follow-up of TUMT trials are desirable to assess the safety and also to determine the best energy settings for TUMT.

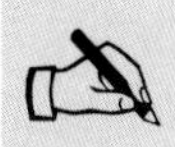

Acute urinary retention: what is the impact on patients' quality of life?

Thomas K, Oades G, Taylor-Hay C, Kirby RS. *BJU Int* 2005; **95**: 72–6

BACKGROUND. Acute urinary retention is a urological emergency characterized by sudden inability to pass urine and lower abdominal pain. Studies such as The Olmsted County cohort have examined the natural history of men with LUTS, and have identified increased age as a risk factor for developing acute retention. This implies that the prevalence of AUR is likely to increase in an ageing population. Although our understanding of the natural history and incidence of AUR has increased, very little has been done to study the impact on patients' quality of life.

INTERPRETATION. This study was designed to evaluate the impact of admission for AUR on patients' health-related quality of life (HRQoL), compared with the impact of elective BPH-related surgery, and also renal colic. Self-completed HRQoL questionnaires were administered at 72 hours after admission and then at 1, 2, 3 and 6 months follow-up. The authors have shown that the AUR group had a mean pain score on admission of 7.7 compared with 5.6 for elective patients and 8.3 for renal colic patients. AUR patients had most investigations and recurrent attendances at a casualty department, and their mean hospital stay was longer. Furthermore, 15% had extra help at home at a mean cost of £430 for 6 months. As for emotions, overall mental state and the general health domains, there were no differences between AUR and elective patients.

Comment

Far more studies have evaluated the QOL issues in an oncological setting compared with benign conditions. This study shows what impact a single episode of AUR has on the quality of life of patients. What is alarming is what goes on beyond the initial presentation at hospital, which is not appreciated by the urologist. The economic burden to the healthcare system and patients alike is potentially huge. This study provides a rationale for preventative measures in at-risk patients using pharmacotherapy. Clearly, more work is needed to evaluate other strategies that could improve a patient's journey when affected by AUR.

Conclusion

These reviews highlight the ongoing controversies and research surrounding the treatment of older men with lower urinary tract symptoms suggestive of benign prostatic obstruction. With time, our understanding of the disease processes are improving, and therefore treatment options are increasing. With the guidelines that are now available, we can offer better advice to the patient so that he is able to make a more informed decision between the therapeutic choices available.

References

1. Lytton B, Emery JM, Harvard BM. The incidence of benign prostatic obstruction. *J Urol* 1968; **99**: 639–45.
2. Yang Q, Abrams P, Donovan J, Mulligan S, Williams G. Transurethral resection or incision of the prostate and other therapies: a survey of treatments for benign prostatic obstruction in the UK. *BJU Int* 1999; **84**(6): 640–5.

12

Andrology and erectile dysfunction

CHI-YING LI, DAVID RALPH

Introduction

In the field of andrology, there have been many recent advances.

Dapoxetine, the first medication (currently under development) for the treatment of premature ejaculation (PE) [1], has stolen the limelight long dominated by research into erectile dysfunction (ED) since the licensing of sildenafil. Results from the phase III clinical trials of dapoxetine demonstrated that on-demand dapoxetine is more effective than placebo in increasing the intravaginal ejaculatory latency time (IELT) [1]. However, the latest press release from ALZA corporation [2] states that the new drug application for dapoxetine to the US Food and Drug Administration (FDA) was not approved. Nevertheless, the company plans to address issues raised by the FDA and continues to invest in the global development programme.

In the research arena of ED, there are continued challenges to the boundaries of 'gold standard' therapy, with the increased flexibility and superiority of daily dosing regimes for phosphodiesterase (PDE) 5 inhibitors and the potential benefits in endothelial dysfunction [3].

The management of Peyronie's disease, specifically extracorporeal shock wave therapy (ESWL), has been under scrutiny at the National Institute of Clinical Excellence (NICE). The publication of interventional guidance on ESWL therapy for Peyronie's disease [4] states that the specialist advisers found difficulty in evaluating efficacy for ESWL from comparative studies, because of lack of control data and agreement regarding end-points. They also noted placebo responses and that the current evidence does not support the use of this procedure. Future non-surgical treatment options for Peyronie's disease will have to demonstrate safety and efficacy through prospective, placebo-controlled, multi-institutional clinical trials.

Androgen deficiency in the ageing male has dominated debate between andrologists and endocrinologists for quite a while; what is new is the suggestion that hypogonadism may be an additional component of metabolic syndrome [5], a diagnosis in itself even more vigorously debated among our expert medical colleagues.

Although the diagnostic criteria for metabolic syndrome and thus the validity of the diagnosis itself is contentious, what is certain is that the most up-to-date accepted diagnostic criteria |6| share similar risk factors to ED and that the goal of validating the diagnosis of metabolic syndrome and diagnosing ED is to predict and prevent cardiovascular disease. We shall no doubt be hearing more of this diagnosis.

Within andrological surgery, organ-preserving surgery in the treatment of penile cancer has continued to gain confidence and support among surgeons, with the emergence of long-term oncological control data (Minhas *et al.* 2005 reviewed below).

Basic science research on corporal smooth muscle physiology and thus the pathophysiological process underlying priapism (Muneer *et al.* 2005 reviewed below) has been translated into clinical practice, whereby patients with acute priapism showing signs of irreversible corporal smooth muscle damage should be offered the insertion of penile implants |7|.

The aim of this chapter is to provide an overview of some of the 'hot topics' discussed, agreed or debated in the field of andrology through ten selected original research/review articles.

Peyronie's disease

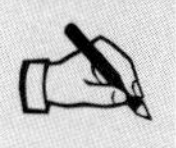

The relationship between the type of penile abnormality and penile vascular status in patients with Peyronie's disease

Kendirci M, Nowfar S, Gur S, Jabren GW, Sikka SC, Hellstrom WJ. *J Urol* 2005; **174**(2): 632–5

BACKGROUND. The aim of this paper was to assess penile vascular status, using penile duplex Doppler ultrasound (PDDU), and its correlation with penile abnormality/curvature in men with Peyronie's disease (PD). A total of 523 patients with PD were included in this study. PDDU was carried out following injections of 10–15 μg of prostaglandin E1 intracavernosally to evaluate penile blood flow. The definition values used for different arterial status are shown in Table 12.1. Objective evaluation of penile curvature was made using a protractor during maximum erection. Penile curvatures were divided into seven groups based on the characteristics of the abnormalities. The correlation between PDDU findings was compared statistically among the seven groups.

INTERPRETATION. Mean peak systolic velocity (PSV) in the ventrolateral group was the highest ($P<0.05$), while the lowest PSV was noted in the hourglass abnormality group ($P<0.05$). The rate of arterial status and its correlation with the curvature types are shown in Table 12.2. The hourglass group had the highest rate of pure arterial insufficiency, while veno-occlusive dysfunction was seen most commonly in the ventral

Table 12.1 The definition values used for different arterial status

Pure arterial insufficiency	PSV <25 cm/s
Borderline arterial insufficiency	PSV 25–30 cm/s
Pure veno-occlusive dysfunction	PSV >30 cm/s, EDV >5 cm/s and RI <0.8
Mixed vascular disorder	PSV <25 cm/s and EDV >5 cm/s
Non-vascular aetiology	PSV >30 cm/s, EDV <5 cm/s and RI >0.8

PSV, peak systolic velocity.
EDV, end diastolic velocity.
RI, calculated resistive index.
Source: Kendirci *et al.* (2005).

Table 12.2 The rate of arterial insufficiency (AI), borderline AI, veno-occlusive disease (VOD), mixed vascular disease and non-vascular status according to curvature type

Direction	**% vascular abnormalities**				
	AI	**Borderline AI**	**VOD**	**Mixed vascular disease**	**Non-vascular status**
Dorsal	24.56	7.02	23.24	4.82	40.35
Lateral	26.15	12.30	16.54	6.53	38.46
Ventral	20.69	3.45	30.17	8.62	37.07
Dorsolateral	12.07	12.06	22.41	3.45	50.00
Ventrolateral	3.12	6.25	12.50	3.12	75.00
Indentation	20.59	5.88	17.65	7.35	48.53
Hourglass	35.71	3.57	10.71	8.92	41.07

Source: Kendirci *et al.* (2005).

curvature group. The ventrolateral group showed the most normal vascular status parameters. This study demonstrates that there is a correlation between the type of penile curvature and penile vascular status in patients with PD; although patients in the hourglass abnormality group were the youngest, it was associated with the poorest penile vascular status, whereas patients with ventrolateral curvature had the best penile haemodynamics.

Comment

PD is a condition that may adversely affect male sexual function; it has no known cause.

Previous studies have demonstrated that a stable deformity is best corrected, with the least post-operative ED, by a Nesbit procedure and that plaque incision and grafting should be reserved for men with good erectile function and those concerned with penile shortening as there is a slightly higher incidence of post-operative ED. Implantation of a penile prosthesis is an excellent option for men with concomitant ED **|8|**.

Based on these recommendations, the state of the penile vasculature plays a significant role in decision making for the type of surgery that patients should receive.

This paper very nicely demonstrated a significant correlation between cavernosal PSV and the type of penile curvature present: that hourglass deformities are associated with the lowest PSV and thus the highest rate of arterial insufficiency, and that this group of patients would benefit most from a penile implant insertion from the outset.

Another interesting finding in this paper is that the hourglass group with the lowest PSV did not correlate with the highest percentage of clinical ED (61%) [assessed using the International Index of Erectile Function (IIEF) after 1997 and a sexual function questionnaire before], but the group with the highest PSV, namely the ventrolateral group, had the second highest percentage of ED (75%). This group of patients were also older than the others; however, they had significantly fewer comorbidities ($P<0.05$), i.e. diabetes, hypertension, smoking, hyperlipidaemia and coronary artery disease – all risk factors for ED. Furthermore, the mean angle of penile curvature in this group was not significantly different from the others.

The observed vascular abnormalities in PD may have resulted from the PD itself, as suggested by the authors; however, it may also be true that patients with vascular insufficiency are predisposed to penile trauma as a consequence of inadequate rigidity on erection.

The pathophysiological process underlying PD is complex, and the cause–effect relationship needs to be clarified with further scientific research.

Penile prosthesis

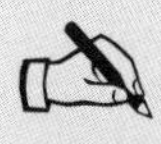

Antibiotic coating reduces penile prosthesis infection

Droggin D, Shabsigh R, Anastasiadis AG. *J Sex Med* 2005; **2**(4): 565–8

BACKGROUND. The aim of this study was to evaluate the efficacy of a new antibiotic-coated (rifampicin + monocycline) penile prosthesis in preventing penile prosthesis infection. A retrospective comparison was made of patients who had penile implantation of non-antibiotic-coated inflatable penile prostheses (between July 1990 and June 2001) with those receiving antibiotic-coated penile implants (between July 2001 and November 2003). All implants were American Medical Systems (AMS) inflatable penile prostheses. A total of 152 men aged 27–79 years with erectile dysfunction were included in the study; 58 patients received the antibiotic-coated prosthesis, and 94 patients received the non-antibiotic-coated prosthesis.

INTERPRETATION. In the non-antibiotic-coated prosthesis group, three developed implant infection requiring reoperation, translating to an implant infection rate of 3.2%. The antibiotic-coated prosthesis group had no infection of the penile prosthesis (infection rate 0%), although the follow-up period is not comparable to the non-antibiotic-coated group. The authors conclude that antibiotic locally delivered from the prosthesis coating may be effective in preventing prosthesis-related infection.

Comment

Over the years, penile implantation has remained the gold standard treatment for erectile dysfunction in those who have failed conservative treatments.

The overall satisfaction rate ranges between 69% and 92% |**9,10**|, and the most devastating complication is implant infection as prosthesis infection invariably results in removal despite aggressive antibiotic therapy. Reimplantation risks further episodes of infection if carried out early and penile fibrosis and shortening if left for too long. The only way to minimize this potentially disastrous complication is to prevent infection occurring in the first place.

There are two main penile implant manufactures, namely Mentor Corp and AMS. Each of these manufacturers has developed implants with hydrophilic/ antibiotic coating, respectively, in an attempt to minimize the risk of penile implant infections.

Mentor Corp currently markets an inflatable penile prostheses called Titan™, with a hydrophilic coating. This hydrophilic coating reduces the chance of bacterial attachment to the implant and, furthermore, if pre-soaked in an antibiotic solution, it absorbs the antibiotic on to its surface. Studies have demonstrated that the hydrophilic coating in 2357 Titan™ compared with 482 Alpha-1 (Mentor non-hydrophilic-coated) implants has an infection rate of 1.06% as opposed to 2.07% without the hydrophilic coating |**11**|.

AMS currently markets penile prostheses with an optional external coating of Inhibizon™, which is an antibiotic treatment containing rifampicin and minocycline.

This paper demonstrated that the antibiotic-coated penile implants resulted in a lower rate of implant infection. However, in the group without the antibiotic coating, there was also a higher rate of reimplant for reasons other than infection, and this category of patients is also prone to increased risks of infection as previous studies have demonstrated that clinically uninfected implants have become colonized with organisms |**12**|.

Further long-term, and preferably prospective, trials should be carried out.

Erectile dysfunction

An evaluation of an alternative dosing regimen with tadalafil, 3 times/week, for men with erectile dysfunction: SURE study in 14 European countries

Mirone V, Costa P, Damber JE, *et al. Eur Urol* 2005; **47**(6): 846–54

BACKGROUND. This aim of this study was to assess patient preference between two dosing regimes, namely on-demand versus three times weekly, for tadalafil, which

has a duration of action of up to 36 h in men with ED. This is a multicentre, crossover, open-label study, involving men with ED (*n* = 4262) from 14 European countries. They were randomized to tadalafil 20 mg on demand (before sexual activity) or three times per week for 5–6 weeks. At the end of this, a 1-week washout period takes place, followed by the alternative regimen for 5–6 weeks. Patient preference was assessed using a treatment preference question (TPQ).

INTERPRETATION. At the end of the study, 3861 men completed the TPQ, which showed that 57.8% preferred the on-demand regimen and 42.2% preferred the three times a week regime. Both were efficacious in treating ED and well tolerated. The authors conclude that, although the majority prefer the on-demand regime, a large proportion prefer the three times per week regime; in other words, there is no significant difference in preference between these two regimes. The study demonstrates that the three times per week regime is efficacious in treating ED, allowing the option of dosing flexibility with tadalafil.

Comment

This study has demonstrated that the long half-life of tadalafil has given patients with ED the flexibility of a regular, three times per week regime, with the same level of efficacy. Although there are no significant differences in preference between the on-demand group and the regular dosing, what is more important is that the safety and tolerability of the regular regime are comparable with that of the on-demand regime, leaving the choice to patient preference.

What is not reported in this paper, but was later published from this study, is the pattern of sexual behaviour |**13**|. Some 47% of the sexual attempts in the on-demand regimen and 71% in the three times per week regime took place more than 4 h after dosing. The efficacy of tadalafil was 70% mean-per-patient success regardless of the time interval after dosing. Studies have demonstrated daily tadalafil to be superior to on-demand tadalafil |**14**|; furthermore, patients previously unresponsive to on-demand tadalafil may respond to daily tadalafil |**15**|. The potential benefit of improving endothelial function |**3**| will ensure that daily dosing will have a role in future ED management.

One must also bear in mind the potential cost implication to both patients and our healthcare system |**16**|.

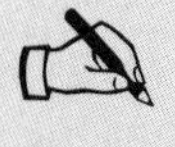

Development and evaluation of a prostate sexual rehabilitation clinic: a pilot project

Davison BJ, Elliott S, Ekland M, Griffin S, Wiens K. *BJU Int* 2005; **96**(9): 1360–4

BACKGROUND. The aim of this paper is to evaluate a sexual health service for men with prostate cancer and to development a framework for future care. One hundred and fifty-five men with prostate cancer were recruited for this study; 78.1% were treated with radical prostatectomy. Of the 155 men who were recruited, 90 completed

the 4-month evaluation. Among the attendees, the partners of 58 were present and 35 completed the evaluation. Questionnaires to assess sexual function and feelings towards the partner were completed before and at 4 months after the clinic visit and, at the later stage, satisfaction with treatments was also assessed.

Interpretation. The main concerns of patients were the changes that may occur to their sexual function as a result of the prostate cancer treatment, therapeutic options for erection enhancement and issues regarding their relationships. Patients were significantly more positive towards their partners and more satisfied with their treatment than their partners. The ED treatments employed with these patients were PDE5 inhibitors and intracavernosal injections. The total scores on sexual function were higher at 4 months; however, this was not clinically significant as the overall score remains poor. This paper concludes with the proposal that partners should be included routinely as part of men's sexual rehabilitation and a structured follow-up programme is needed to monitor the success of treatment.

Comment

This paper raises a very important issue in the management of ED in patients with prostate cancer, in that there is scope for improvement in practice and the multi-disciplinary team involving the partner approach to 'prostate sexual rehabilitation'.

The message from this paper is generally echoed in other studies [**17–19**]. The Prostate Cancer Outcome Study carried out by the National Cancer Institute in the US involving 1977 and 1282 patients with clinically localized prostate cancer treated with radical prostatectomy/radiotherapy, at 60 months follow-up, found that only a small proportion of these men were treated for ED, despite high proportions suffering from ED. It also found that the treatment of ED in prostate cancer, post-radical prostatectomy/radiotherapy, is generally poor in both the numbers treated and the effectiveness of the treatments available.

Regarding the effectiveness of treatments available, other studies have shown that both newer on-demand PDE5 inhibitors, tadalafil and vardenafil, demonstrated promising success [**20–22**]. Furthermore, there is evidence to support ED 'prophylaxis' in patients undergoing radical prostatectomy, using intracavernosal alprostadil injections or daily PDE5 inhibitors, started early in the post-operative period [**23**].

The important take-home message from this study and others is a more planned and structured approach to the management of this group of patients, who have a high risk of developing ED.

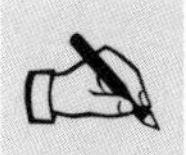

Subclinical coronary artery atherosclerosis in patients with erectile dysfunction

Chiurlia E, D'Amico R, Ratti C, Granata AR, Romagnoli R, Modena MG. *J Am Coll Cardiol* 2005; **46**(8): 1503–6

Background. ED has been associated with ischaemic heart disease; however, it is unknown whether it represents a marker of subclinical coronary atherosclerosis. The

aim of this study was to assess the prevalence and extent of coronary artery atherosclerosis in asymptomatic patients with vascular ED. A total of 70 consecutive patients with vascular ED were included in this study. All were evaluated by penile Doppler. An age-, race- and coronary risk score-matched control group of 73 subjects was also evaluated. Coronary risk factors, circulating levels of C-reactive protein (CRP), endothelial function by ultrasound of brachial artery and coronary artery calcification by multislice computerized tomography were measured.

INTERPRETATION. Patients with ED had significantly higher high-sensitivity CRP levels ($P < 0.001$), more impaired flow-mediated dilation of the brachial artery ($P < 0.001$) and more frequent coronary artery calcification ($P = 0.01$) compared with the control subjects. Multiple logistic regression analysis showed that patients with ED had an overall odds ratio of 3.68 for having calcium score above the 75th percentile, compared with the control subjects. The authors conclude that coronary atherosclerosis is more severe in patients with vascular ED, who are clinically asymptomatic for coronary artery disease (CAD), and ED predicts the presence and extent of subclinical atherosclerosis independently of traditional risk factors for cardiovascular disease. Thus, ED may be considered an early warning sign of coronary atherosclerosis.

Comment

It has been demonstrated in many previous studies that ED no doubt shares many similar risk factors to CAD **|24,25|**, namely diabetes, hypertension, hyperlipidaemia and smoking, with a proposed common underlying pathophysiological pathway of endothelial dysfunction; however, the exact relationship between these two disease entities is not clear.

This study has demonstrated that the prevalence of atherosclerosis is significantly higher in patients with ED compared with control subjects.

This is an excellent study; with the concurrent evaluation of matched control subjects, it gives a stronger claim that ED is not only a vascular disorder, but its presentation precedes that of CAD.

These findings are supported by another study **|26|** which, by assessing brachial artery flow-mediated vasodilatation, demonstrated that patients with ED but no clinical cardiovascular disease have an impaired endothelium vasodilatation compared with normal matched subjects.

It has been proposed that ED is a manifestation of a generalized vascular disorder affecting the penile arteries. As the penile arteries are of smaller diameter compared with that of the coronary arteries, the clinical symptoms of ED present a golden opportunity for a 'diagnostic lead time' for the more sinister CAD, which leads to the current recommendation that all patients with ED should be screened for cardiovascular diseases **|27|**.

Premature ejaculation

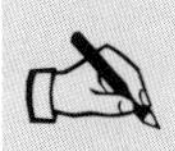

On-demand SSRI treatment of premature ejaculation—pharmacodynamic limitations for relevant ejaculation delay and consequent solutions

Waldinger MD, Schweitzer DH, Olivier B. *J Sex Med* 2005; **2**: 121–31

BACKGROUND. On-demand serotonin reuptake inhibitors (SSRI) have been proposed to be effective in the treatment of premature ejaculation in delaying ejaculation, compared with daily use, without the adverse effects of chronic drug administration. The aim of the authors was to provide evidence that SSRI-induced ejaculation delay is mainly dependent on the pharmacodynamic rather than the pharmacokinetic properties. Based on this hypothesis, combining an SSRI with a specific 5-hydroxytryptamine (5-HT) receptor antagonist would lead to further ejaculation delay compared with on-demand SSRI administration alone. The authors conducted a detailed analysis of serotonin neurotransmission and a detailed literature review of current publications on clinical studies of on-demand SSRI, including current debates on the definition of PE, as well as animal research on the concomitant use of SSRI and 5-HT receptor antagonists.

INTERPRETATION. The clinical effects of on-demand SSRI cannot be explained by current knowledge of neuropharmacological mechanisms because, based on the current understanding, acute SSRI administration leads to only a mild increase in 5-HT neurotransmission and, thus, stimulation of post-synaptic 5-HT receptors. Prolonged daily treatment demonstrates better prolonged ejaculatory delay. If on-demand SSRI were to be effective, concomitant administration of a 5-HT_{1A} receptor antagonist is required, based on *in vitro* animal studies. The authors conclude that on-demand SSRI treatment gives less ejaculation delay than chronic SSRI treatment. The development of SSRIs with a shorter half-life is unlikely to be more effective. Based on animal research, the combined use of a 5-HT_{1A} receptor antagonist with on-demand SSRI is likely to increase ejaculation delay. The authors acknowledge the current lack of consensus in the diagnostic criteria for PE and propose that the definition of PE should be based on large-scale stopwatch-assessed epidemiological study on IELT.

Comment

On-demand SSRI has been a topic of great interest. This review paper summarized the current literature surrounding on-demand SSRI for the treatment of PE. The author argues against the use of on-demand SSRI, based on the current insight into the negative feedback mechanisms of serotonin neurotransmission and, on this principle and animal research, proposes the concomitant use of on-demand SSRI with a 5-HT receptor antagonist.

The authors' proposition is excellent using scientific principles and our current understanding of the mechanisms underlying the process of ejaculation. On-demand SSRI has been proposed clinically to be superior to a daily regime because of the adverse effects associated with chronic administration. Dapoxetine, the new SSRI developed specifically for the treatment of PE, has demonstrated increase in IELT and, more importantly, patient satisfaction |**1**|.

What is generally agreed is that the issue of diagnostic criteria for PE is a source of contentious debate at all times. The lack of disease definition and measurable parameters make the design and methodology between clinical studies inconsistent and, consequently, interpretation and comparison between clinical trials is impossible.

The current consensus from an international consultation with over 200 multidisciplinary experts from 60 countries issued a report in 2004 |**28**|, which proposed a multivariant definition of PE as 'persistent or recurrent ejaculation with minimal stimulation before, on, or shortly after penetration and before the person wishes it, over which the person has no voluntary control, which causes the person and/or his partner bother or distress'. It is debated that this definition has no objective measurable criteria, such as the IELT, and therefore lacks standardization. Despite the current lack of consistency and objective measurable parameters, one must bear in mind that the target outcome is patient and partner satisfaction |**29**|, which cannot ultimately be quantified using IELT.

Penile cancer

What surgical resection margins are required to achieve oncological control in men with primary penile cancer?

Minhas S, Kayes O, Hegarty P, Kumar P, Freeman A, Ralph D. *BJU Int* 2005; **96**(7): 1040–3

BACKGROUND. Organ-sparing surgery in penile cancers has dramatically improved the quality of life for men with penile cancer, who would previously have had to undergo radical penile amputation. The aim of this study was to evaluate the surgical excision margin required for local control in penile cancers as the optimum surgical excision margin to achieve oncological control is currently unknown. Fifty-one patients (mean age 61 years) with squamous cell carcinoma of the penis were included in the study in which histopathological features of the tumours, including type, grade, stage and distance from the surgical excision margin, were evaluated. All patients were staged before surgery using magnetic resonance imaging (MRI).

INTERPRETATION. The histopathological review analysed 102 surgical margins with 48% within 10 mm of the tumour edge and 90% within a <20-mm resection margin. Six per cent had tumour involvement at the surgical margin and had further surgery, whereas 4% developed local tumour recurrence and were treated successfully with partial penectomy. The authors conclude that a traditional 2-cm excision margin for penile cancer is unnecessary, and that conservative techniques, involving excision margins of only a few millimetres, appear to offer excellent oncological control.

Comment

The ultimate goal of penile surgery treatment is to achieve oncological control/cure with maximum organ preservation.

Previous radical surgical (subtotal or total penile amputation) advising a >2-cm macroscopic excision tumour margin has no doubt achieved >90% oncological control; it has, however, also been associated with significant psychological and functional impairment.

Various organ-preserving techniques have been proposed, including laser photocoagulation, intratumoral chemotherapy, radiotherapy and Moh's micrographic surgery. These are unfortunately associated with high recurrence rates.

Previous studies |**30**| have demonstrated that most patients with penile carcinoma can be offered organ-preserving surgery; this is further confirmed by the promising result of this paper that large resection is not required in achieving cure in penile cancer. In addition, a few selected cases have been successfully treated with wide local excision and skin grafting, resulting in excellent cosmetic outcomes |**31**|.

This paper has demonstrated a low 4% recurrence rate with conservative surgical techniques.

This has a significant implication for the management of penile cancer, as radical surgery has a significant psychological impact for patients suffering from penile cancer, and the future of penile cancer management will be dominated by organ- and sexual function-preserving surgery.

Priapism

Investigation of cavernosal smooth muscle dysfunction in low flow priapism using an *in vitro* model

Muneer A, Cellek S, Dogan A, Kell PD, Ralph DJ, Minhas S. *Int J Impot Res* 2005; **17**(1): 10–18

Background. Low-flow priapism is characterized by a prolonged period of ischaemia in the corporal smooth muscle environment. Corporal aspirates obtained from patients with low-flow priapism demonstrate hypoxia and acidosis. Rapid treatment leading to detumescence reverses this insult, but untreated, prolonged priapism ultimately results in irreversible erectile dysfunction. The degree of insult required to initiate irreversible tissue damage is not known. By using *in vitro* rabbit penis, the effects of hypoxia (po_2: 50 mmHg), acidosis (pH 6.9) or glucopenia

(absence of glucose) on the tone of corpus cavernosum were investigated. The recovery of smooth muscle contractility following exposure to these conditions was also assessed.

Interpretation. This study demonstrated that hypoxia, acidosis or glucopenia alone or in combination induced a reduction in the corporal smooth muscle tone, which produced complete reversible recovery upon reperfusion of the tissue. However, if hypoxia and glucopenia were combined or when hypoxia, glucopenia and acidosis were used in combination, this reduction in smooth muscle tone became irreversible. The implication is that, following an episode of hypoxia and acidosis in priapism, removal of the blood by aspiration followed by reperfusion of normoxic blood is likely to resume smooth muscle function, and administration of an intracavernosal alpha-agonist at this stage is likely to cause tumescence. However, if glucopenia was allowed to develop, together with hypoxia and acidosis, cell death is likely to be initiated. In the clinical setting, if after aspiration and reperfusion, an alpha-agonist fails to induce detumescence, it is likely to represent the presence of irreversible smooth muscle damage.

Comment

Low-flow priapism is considered to be a state of acute ischaemia with rapidly progressive hypoxia and acidosis. If persistent, this leads to smooth muscle fibrosis and, finally, penile failure with loss of function. This occurs in approximately 57% of patients |**32**|, who may subsequently require penile implant.

The last international consultation published guidance on the management of ischaemic priapism |**33**|, including urgent intracavernosal aspiration followed by alpha-agonist. If all these conservative measures fail, surgery should be considered. Traditionally, shunt surgery was the initial management choice; however, disappointing outcomes have been reported in which approximately 50% required repeated procedures to achieve detumescence |**34**|.

This led to the notion of placing a penile prosthesis in patients with prolonged ischaemic priapism |**35**|. A small series of eight patients with mean duration of prolonged priapism of 91 h (range 33–192 h) were studied prospectively, all of whom have had failed conservative treatment and some failed shunt surgery. All these patients were satisfied with the outcome of surgery, with return to normal sexual function and preservation of penile length.

This paper has demonstrated that neither acidosis nor hypoxia alone ultimately lead to irreversible tissue damage. However, in combination with the resultant development of glucopenia, this leads to cell death and irreversible smooth muscle damage. Once the ischaemic blood has been aspirated and the corporal cavernosum reperfused, failure to respond to alpha-agonist therapy is a reliable indicator that irreversible damage has taken place. This provides a useful clinical indication for the insertion of a penile prosthesis. Another advantage of placing an implant early is that the surgery is relatively easier before penile fibrosis and shortening has developed.

This research has influenced our current practice, whereby all patients with failed conservative management of ischaemic priapism would be offered the option of immediate penile prosthesis insertion |**7**|.

Androgen deficiency/hypogonadism

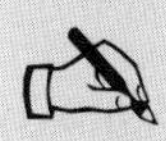

Does sildenafil combined with testosterone gel improve erectile dysfunction in hypogonadal men in whom testosterone supplement therapy alone failed?

Greenstein A, Mabjeesh NJ, Sofer M, Kaver I, Matzkin H, Chen J. *J Urol* 2005; **173**(2): 530–2

BACKGROUND. The aim of this study was to evaluate the efficacy of testosterone gel, alone and in combination with sildenafil, in patients with ED and hypogonadism for 20.2 months. A total of 49 men with ED and hypogonadism (total testosterone <400 ng/dl) were included. Sexual function was assessed using the IIEF questionnaire and a global assessment question (GAQ). Lower urinary tract symptoms (LUTS) were assessed using the International Prostate Symptom Score (IPSS). Serum investigations included total, bioavailable testosterone and prostate-specific antigen (PSA). After treatment with testosterone gel for 3 months, men who were not satisfied with their erectile function had sildenafil added to their regime for a further 3 months.

INTERPRETATION. At 3 months, all the patients achieved normal total testosterone and free testosterone levels, and all experienced improvement in their sexual desire score ($P<0.001$); only 31 reported significant improvement in the erectile function (EF) ($P<0.001$) domain following treatment with testosterone supplement alone. The remaining 17 patients proceeded to have combined testosterone supplement and sildenafil. After 3 months, all had significant improvement in their EF ($P<0.001$). One patient was excluded from the study after developing urinary retention. The authors concluded that testosterone supplement normalized serum testosterone levels in hypogonadal men and demonstrated a beneficial effect on ED in these patients. In those in whom treatment with testosterone supplement alone failed, combined therapy with sildenafil improved EF significantly.

Comment

Androgen deficiency/hypogonadism in ageing men has recently been a topic of great debate among both andrologists and endocrinologists, especially after the recent suggestion of its potential links with metabolic syndrome |**5**|.

This paper has clearly demonstrated testosterone supplements to be beneficial in improving sexual desire in men and improving erectile function in some (63.2% in this series). It is worth noting that the group who were dissatisfied with their sexual function using testosterone alone had a lower EF score at the beginning of the study

(13 vs 15 in the satisfied group). What is encouraging was that there was no change in serum PSA and, clinically, IPSS, although one patient had worsened LUTS and another developed urinary retention.

Hypogonadism or, more specifically, late-onset hypogonadism (LOH) is defined as a clinical and biochemical syndrome characterized by typical symptoms, including depressed mood, irritability, decreased cognitive function, sleep disturbances, loss of lean body mass, decreased body hair, bone mineral density, resulting in osteoporosis and fractures, as well as loss of libido and erectile dysfunction.

Biochemically, there is a general agreement between early morning (7am–11am) total testosterone <8 nmol/l (<231 ng/dl) and free testosterone <180 pmol/l (<5.2 ng/dl).

An international panel of experts in the study of ageing males and andrologists met in 2004 and made a list of recommendations on the investigations, treatment and monitoring of LOH |**36**|, which some may find useful.

Infertility

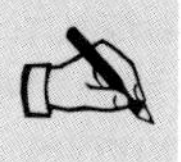

Outcome and late failures compared in 4 techniques of microsurgical vasoepididymostomy in 153 consecutive men

Schiff J, Chan P, Li PS, Finkleberg S, Goldstein M. *J Urol* 2005; **174**(2): 651–5

BACKGROUND. The aim of this study was to assess the outcome of four different surgical techniques employed to perform vasoepididymostomies (VE), namely end-to-end (EE), end-to-side (ES) and intussusception end-to-side, three-suture triangulation intussusception (TIVE) and two-suture longitudinal intussusception (LIVE). A total of 153 consecutive VEs done by one surgeon (MG) were included in this study. The parameters evaluated were patency, pregnancy, late failures (defined as disappearance of sperm after initial return of sperm to the ejaculate), sperm density, motility and morphology (World Health Organization [WHO] 1992 criteria).

INTERPRETATION. TIVE and LIVE display a comparable patency rate, a slightly improved pregnancy rate and a significantly lower late failure rate. The results are summarized in Table 12.3. The authors conclude that, although a technically demanding microsurgical procedure, recent technical innovations in TIVE and LIVE offer better or comparable outcomes compared with EE and ES procedures. Furthermore, the late failure rate is lower with the use of the intussusception techniques (LIVE and TIVE) with only one late failure in 22 men compared with 11 out of 30 in the non-intussusception groups ($P = 0.006$).

Table 12.3 Results of vasoepipidymostomy outcome

Groups	No. of men	Post-operative follow-up period in months	Return of intact sperm	Motile sperm in men with sperm analysis data (%)	Mean months of return of sperm to ejaculate (range)	Pregnancies in men with return of sperm to ejaculate (%)	Disappearance of sperm after initial patency (%)
LIVE	17	17.2	12/15 (80)	10/15 (67)	2.9 (1–6)	4/9 (44)	0/9 (0)
TIVE	38	70.8	16/19 (84)	13/19 (68)	2.8 (1–11)	6/13 (46)	1/13 (7.6)
ES	32	116.7	20/27 (72)	10/27 (37)	2.8 (1–13)	4/10 (40)	5/10 (50)
EE	66	140.2	30/41 (73)	20/41 (49)	3.5 (1–17)	4/20 (20)	6/20 (30)
Chi-squared *P*-value			0.95	0.2	0.94	0.07	0.04

Source: Schiff *et al.* (2005).

Comment

A vasectomy is commonly performed surgery. Although patients are counselled to regard this as an irreversible procedure, vasovasostomy (VV) is a procedure that has earned a reputation for being highly successful with patency rates ranging between 90% and 99%.

However, it is often not possible to regain vasal patency with vasovasostomy if an epididymal obstruction is present; a VE will then be required.

It may be possible to predict pre-operatively, with the age of the patient and the interval between vasectomy and its reversal, but more often the decision to proceed to VE is made intra-operatively. If VE will be required, the general consensus is that surgeons who carry out vasectomy reversal/vasovasostomy should be able to perform VE, as a large proportion of men in VV failure have epididymal obstruction.

When carrying out microsurgical VE, various techniques have been described.

This paper examined four techniques employed in carrying out VE, EE, ES, TIVE and LIVE, and demonstrated that the newer TIVE and LIVE techniques simplify the anastomotic process with fewer sutures, yet still display a comparable patency rate, a slightly improved pregnancy rate and a significantly lower late failure rate.

The main weakness of this study, especially when referring to late failure rates, is that the follow-up period in these four techniques were not similar, with the LIVE group having the shortest post-operative follow-up period of 17 months compared with the EE group of 140 months. More important than the technique is probably the surgical expertise with the use of microsurgery.

Conclusion

Recent developments are encouraging, with the publication of excellent practice-changing research, some of which has already been mentioned in this chapter.

The importance of sexual health, previously centred on male but, more recently, female sexual health, is becoming more widely recognized by the medical community and healthcare-delivering bodies.

In the future, andrology will continue to be a dynamic and rapidly evolving speciality; some basic science research on the pathophysiology of PE is keenly anticipated. Dapoxetine looks set to be of particular importance in the near future.

Previous research has demonstrated the safety, tolerability and efficacy of chronic/daily PDE5 inhibitor; there is a risk of unnecessary overprescription, and one must bear in mind the financial constraints imposed on both the patient and the NHS.

Studies thus far have demonstrated that the link between ED and cardiovascular diseases is overwhelming; future research will not only concentrate on treatment but also on prevention of ED. Thus, cardiovascular disease and gene therapy will have a significant role in the future, not only in ED but across urological subspecialities.

In the past, urologists/andrologists have become disinterested in the management of infertility. They are encouraged to take an active role in the field of infertility especially in cases of obstructive azoospermia, in which technically challenging microsurgical skill is required.

Since the establishment of NICE, there have been multiple urological guidelines, appraisals and extensive guidance on urological interventions published and more are under development. Our clinical practice, clinical audits and research have never been more closely linked with NICE guidance and recommendations.

Limitations of space necessitate choosing ten articles from the plethora of literature published, which is a hard task in view of the large amount of excellent research/reviews published. We would like to take this opportunity to congratulate all those who have undoubtedly produced a high standard of work and apologize if we have not included your articles on account of the limited space available.

References

1. Pryor JL, Althof SE, Steidle C, Miloslavsky M, Kell S. Efficacy and tolerability of Dapoxetine in the treatment of premature ejaculation. *J Urol* 2005; **173**(4 Suppl): 201.
2. Dapoxetine news release. http://www.jnj.com/news/jnj_news/20051026_164127.htm, 2006.
3. Rosano GM, Aversa A, Vitale C, Fabbri A, Fini M, Spera G. Chronic treatment with tadalafil improves endothelial function in men with increased cardiovascular risk. *Eur Urol* 2005; **47**(2): 214–20.
4. ESWL for Peyronie's disease – NICE guideline. http://www.nice.org.uk/distributionlist, 2006.
5. Makhsida N, Shah J, Yan G, Fisch H, Shabsigh R. Hypogonadism and metabolic syndrome: implications for testosterone therapy. *J Urol* 2005; **174**(3): 827–34.
6. Alberti KG, Zimmet P, Shaw J. The metabolic syndrome: a new worldwide definition. *Lancet* 2005; **366**(9491): 1059–62.
7. Kumar P, Agrawal V, Kayes O, Christopher N, Ralph D, Minhas S. Ischaemic priapism: acute versus delayed penile implant insertion results in fewer complications. *J Sex Med* 2006; **3**(s3): 188.
8. Ralph DJ, Minhas S. The management of Peyronie's disease. *BJU Int* 2004; **93**(2): 208–15.
9. Brinkman MJ, Henry GD, Wilson SK, Delk JR 2nd, Denny GA, Young M, Cleves MA. A survey of patients with inflatable penile prostheses for satisfaction. *J Urol* 2005; **174**(1): 253–7.

10. Montorsi F, Rigatti P, Carmignani G, Corbu C, Campo B, Ordesi G, Breda G, Silvestre P, Giammusso B, Morgia G, Graziottin A. AMS three-piece inflatable implants for erectile dysfunction: a long-term multi-institutional study in 200 consecutive patients. *Eur Urol* 2000; **37**(1): 50–5.

11. Wolter CE, Hellstrom WJ. The hydrophilic-coated inflatable penile prosthesis: 1-year experience. *J Sex Med* 2004; **1**(2): 221–4.

12. Henry GD, Wilson SK, Delk JR 2nd, Carson CC, Silverstein A, Cleves MA, Donatucci CF. Penile prosthesis cultures during revision surgery: a multicenter study. *J Urol* 2004; **172**(1): 153–6.

13. Moncada I, Damber JE, Mirone V, Wespes E, Casariego J, Chan M, Varanese L. Sexual intercourse attempt patterns with two dosing regimens of tadalafil in men with erectile dysfunction: results from the SURE study in 14 European countries. *J Sex Med* 2005; **2**(5): 668–74.

14. McMahon C. Comparison of efficacy, safety, and tolerability of on-demand tadalafil and daily dosed tadalafil for the treatment of erectile dysfunction. *J Sex Med* 2005; **2**(3): 415–25.

15. McMahon C. Efficacy and safety of daily tadalafil in men with erectile dysfunction previously unresponsive to on-demand tadalafil. *J Sex Med* 2004; **1**(3): 292–300.

16. Sun P, Seftel A, Swindle R, Ye W, Pohl G. The costs of caring for erectile dysfunction in a managed care setting: evidence from a large national claims database. *J Urol* 2005; **174**(5): 1948–52.

17. Matthew AG, Goldman A, Trachtenberg J, Robinson J, Horsburgh S, Currie K, Ritvo P. Sexual dysfunction after radical prostatectomy: prevalence, treatments, restricted use of treatments and distress. *J Urol* 2005; **174**(6): 2105–10.

18. Penson DF, McLerran D, Feng Z, Li L, Albertsen PC, Gilliland FD, Hamilton A, Hoffman RM, Stephenson RA, Potosky AL, Stanford JL. Five-year urinary and sexual outcomes after radical prostatectomy: results from the prostate cancer outcomes study. *J Urol* 2005; **173**(5): 1701–5.

19. Stephenson RA, Mori M, Hsieh YC, Beer TM, Stanford JL, Gilliland FD, Hoffman RM, Potosky AL. Treatment of erectile dysfunction following therapy for clinically localized prostate cancer: patient reported use and outcomes from the Surveillance, Epidemiology, and End Results Prostate Cancer Outcomes Study. *J Urol* 2005; **174**(2): 646–50.

20. Brock G, Nehra A, Lipshultz LI, Karlin GS, Gleave M, Seger M, Padma-Nathan H. Safety and efficacy of vardenafil for the treatment of men with erectile dysfunction after radical retropubic prostatectomy. *J Urol* 2003; **170**(4 Pt 1): 1278–83.

21. Nehra A, Grantmyre J, Nadel A, Thibonnier M, Brock G. Vardenafil improved patient satisfaction with erectile hardness, orgasmic function and sexual experience in men with erectile dysfunction following nerve sparing radical prostatectomy. *J Urol* 2005; **173**(6): 2067–71.

22. Montorsi F, Nathan HP, McCullough A, Brock GB, Broderick G, Ahuja S, Whitaker S, Hoover A, Novack D, Murphy A, Varanese L. Tadalafil in the treatment of erectile dysfunction following bilateral nerve sparing radical retropubic prostatectomy: a randomized, double-blind, placebo-controlled trial. *J Urol* 2004; **172**(3): 1036–41.

23. Montorsi F, Briganti A, Salonia A, Rigatti P, Burnett AL. Current and future strategies for preventing and managing erectile dysfunction following radical prostatectomy. *Eur Urol* 2004; **45**(2): 123–33.

24. Seftel AD, Sun P, Swindle R. The prevalence of hypertension, hyperlipidemia, diabetes mellitus and depression in men with erectile dysfunction. *J Urol* 2004; **171**(6 Pt 1): 2341–5.

25. Sun P, Swindle R. Are men with erectile dysfunction more likely to have hypertension than men without erectile dysfunction? A naturalistic national cohort study. *J Urol* 2005; **174**(1): 244–8.

26. Kaiser DR, Billups K, Mason C, Wetterling R, Lundberg JL, Bank AJ. Impaired brachial artery endothelium-dependent and -independent vasodilation in men with erectile dysfunction and no other clinical cardiovascular disease. *J Am Coll Cardiol* 2004; **43**(2): 179–84.

27. Montague DK, Jarow JP, Broderick GA, Dmochowski RR, Heaton JP, Lue TF, Milbank AJ, Nehra A, Sharlip ID; Erectile Dysfunction Guideline Update Panel. Chapter 1: The management of erectile dysfunction: an AUA update. *J Urol* 2005; **174**(1): 230–9.

28. McMahon CG, Abdo C, Incrocci L, Perelman M, Rowland D, Waldinger M, Xin ZC. Disorders of orgasm and ejaculation in men. *J Sex Med* 2004; **1**(1): 58–65.

29. Montague DK, Jarow J, Broderick GA, Dmochowski RR, Heaton JP, Lue TF, Nehra A, Sharlip ID; AUA Erectile Dysfunction Guideline Update Panel. AUA guideline on the pharmacologic management of premature ejaculation. *J Urol* 2004; **172**(1): 290–4.

30. Pietrzak P, Corbishley C, Watkin N. Organ-sparing surgery for invasive penile cancer: early follow-up data. *BJU Int* 2004; **94**(9): 1253–7.

31. McDougal WS. Phallic preserving surgery in patients with invasive squamous cell carcinoma of the penis. *J Urol* 2005; **174**(6): 2218–20, discussion.

32. El-Bahnasawy MS, Dawood A, Farouk A. Low-flow priapism: risk factors for erectile dysfunction. *BJU Int* 2002; **89**(3): 285–90.

33. Pryor J, Akkus E, Alter G, Jordan G, Lebret T, Levine L, Mulhall J, Perovic S, Ralph D, Stackl W. Priapism. *J Sex Med* 2004; **1**(1): 116–20.

34. Nixon RG, O'Connor JL, Milam DF. Efficacy of shunt surgery for refractory low flow priapism: a report on the incidence of failed detumescence and erectile dysfunction. *J Urol* 2003; **170**(3): 883–6.

35. Rees RW, Kalsi J, Minhas S, Peters J, Kell P, Ralph DJ. The management of low-flow priapism with the immediate insertion of a penile prosthesis. *BJU Int* 2002; **90**(9): 893–7.

36. Nieschlag E, Swerdloff R, Behre HM, Gooren LJ, Kaufman JM, Legros JJ, Lunenfeld B, Morley JE, Schulman C, Wang C, Weidner W, Wu FC; International Society of Andrology (ISA); International Society for the Study of the Aging Male (ISSAM); European Association of Urology (EAU). Investigation, treatment and monitoring of late-onset hypogonadism in males. ISA, ISSAM, and EAU recommendations. *Eur Urol* 2005; **48**(1): 1–4.

Part IV

New techniques and experimental developments

13

Trends in investigative urology

JOHN PROBERT

Introduction

Once again, this is deliberately the most disparate of chapters in this volume, attempting to provide a sample of the vast amount of work that has been performed in the field of investigative urology over the past year. Again, several hundred papers have been reviewed, and the aim has been to provide the interested clinician with a taster of some of the different fields of research currently in vogue. Genetic polymorphisms in prostate cancer, functional bladder studies, testicular torsion, surgery for stress incontinence, drug treatment of erectile dysfunction, catheter blockage, stone formation, chemotherapy for bladder cancer, laparoscopic partial nephrectomy and urethral reconstruction are just some of the subjects touched on in the following pages. As with the previous two volumes, the subject matter of some of the papers reviewed may soon have clinical relevance. Others have been chosen because their subject matter will hopefully be of interest to those not familiar with some of the current techniques and findings in this field.

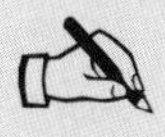

Genetic polymorphism of glutathione *S*-transferase genes (GSTM1, GSTT1 and GSTP1) and susceptibility to prostate cancer in Northern India

Srivastava DS, Mandhani A, Mittal B, Mittal RD. *BJU Int* 2005; **95**: 170–3

BACKGROUND. Phase II metabolizing enzymes are involved in the detoxification of chemical carcinogens. One subgroup of these enzymes is the glutathione *S*-transferase (GST) family, which is involved in detoxification and also in the activation and deactivation of carcinogenic compounds implicated in prostate carcinogenesis. Members of this family of enzymes that have been most extensively studied include the GSTM1 null, the GSTP1-313A/G substitution and the GSTT1 null polymorphism. This study aims to determine the genotypic frequency of these polymorphisms in a population in Northern India and to look at possible associations with sporadic prostate cancer.

INTERPRETATION. One hundred and twenty-seven patients with prostate cancer and 144 age-matched control subjects were assessed. GST polymorphisms were determined

Table 13.1 The distribution, as *n* (%), of GST genotypes in the patients with prostate cancer and control subjects

Genotype	Controls	Patients	*P*	OR (95% CI)
n patients	144	127		
GSTM1	93 (64.6)	57 (44.9)	1.0	
Null	51 (35.4)	70 (55.1)	0.001	2.24 (1.37–3.65)
GSTT1	115 (79.9)	86 (67.7)	1.0	
Null	29 (20.1)	41 (32.3)	0.026	1.89 (1.09–3.28)
GSTP1				
I/I	83 (57.6)	46 (36.2)	1.0	
I/V	56 (38.9)	77 (60.6)	<0.001	2.48 (1.51–4.08)
V/V	5 (3.5)	4 (3.2)	0.598	1.44 (0.37–5.64)
Double				
GSTM1 and GSTT1				
Both	76 (52.8)	39 (30.7)	1.0	
Either null	56 (38.9)	65 (51.2)	0.002	2.26 (1.34–3.83)
Both null	12 (8.3)	23 (18.1)	0.001	3.73 (1.68–8.29)
GSTM1 and GSTP1				
M1 (+/+) and P1 (I/I)	57 (39.6)	19 (15.0)	1.0	
M1 (+/+) and P1 (I/V or V/V)	36 (25.0)	38 (29.9)	0.001	3.17 (1.59–6.32)
M1 (–/–) and P1 (I/I)	26 (18.1)	29 (22.8)	0.001	3.35 (1.59–7.02)
M1 (–/–) and P1 (I/V or V/V)	25 (17.4)	41 (32.3)	<0.001	4.92 (2.40–10.10)
GSTT1 and GSTP1				
T1 (+/+) and P1 (I/I)	70 (48.6)	31 (24.4)	1.0	
T1 (+/+) and P1 (I/V or V/V)	46 (32.0)	55 (43.3)	0.001	2.70 (1.52–4.80)
T1 (–/–) and P1 (I/I)	14 (9.7)	16 (12.6)	0.026	2.58 (1.22–5.93)
T1 (–/–) and P1 (I/V or V/V)	14 (9.7)	25 (19.7)	<0.001	4.03 (1.85–8.79)
Triple				
M1 and T1 (+/+) and P1 (I/I)	47 (32.6)	13 (10.2)	1.0	
M1 and T1 (+/+) and P1 (I/V or V/V)	29 (20.1)	26 (20.5)	0.004	3.24 (1.44–7.29)
M1 (–/–), T1 (+/+) and P1 (I/I)	21 (14.6)	18 (14.2)	0.012	3.10 (1.29–7.47)
M1 (–/–), T1 (+/+) and P1 (I/V or V/V)	18 (12.5)	29 (22.8)	<0.001	5.83 (2.49–13.63)
M1 (+/+), T1 (–/–) and P1 (I/I)	10 (7.0)	6 (4.7)	0.200	2.17 (0.66–7.09)
M1 (+/+), T1 (–/–) and P1 (I/V or V/V)	7 (4.9)	12 (9.5)	0.001	6.20 (2.03–18.93)
M1 (–/–), T1 (–/–) and P1 (I/I)	5 (3.5)	9 (7.1)	0.003	6.51 (1.86–22.80)
M1 (–/–), T1 (–/–) and P1 (I/V or V/V)	7 (4.9)	14 (11.0)	<0.001	7.23 (2.42–22.63)

Source: Srivastava *et al.* (2005).

by polymerase chain reaction (PCR) or PCR/RFLP (restriction fragment length polymorphism). There was a significant association in null alleles of GSTM1 and GSTT1 with prostate cancer risk, and also in the GSTP1-313 G polymorphism. The distribution of GST genotypes in the patients with prostate cancer and control subjects is shown in Table 13.1. Table 13.2 summarizes the association of genetic polymorphisms of GST subtypes and the risk of prostate cancer according to nationality.

Comment

These observations concur with data obtained from a Japanese population, whereas in Austrian, German and American studies, no relationship with the GSTM1 genotype could be shown. This study showed a greater risk of developing prostate cancer in individuals who possessed several risk alleles: combining the three risk genotypes increased the risk to seven times. GST enzymes detoxify a large number of potentially carcinogenic compounds, and it is interesting to note that it is the inactive forms of these enzymes that confer the higher risk. GSTs are also important for the control of the synthesis of proteins that modulate DMA repair and, therefore, it may be for multiple reasons that the inactive form of these enzymes results in increased cancer risk.

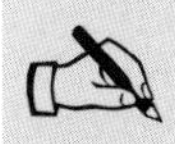

Volume-induced effects on the isolated bladder: a possible local reflex

Lagou M, Drake MJ, Gillespie JI. *BJU Int* 2004; **94**: 1356–65

BACKGROUND. In the bladder of the guinea pig, autonomous activity (transient rises in intravesical pressure propagating contraction waves) is augmented by muscarinic and nicotinic agonists to produce larger rises in intravesical pressure and more dynamic waves and local stretches. This activity is also seen in the filling phase of the human bladder. It is therefore suggested that the mechanisms generating phasic activity in the bladder receive excitatory and inhibitory impulses. The aim of this study was to determine the effects of changing the intravesical volume on autonomous activity in the guinea pig bladder, to indemnify the mechanisms that might contribute to the induced changes and to explore the concept that changes in bladder volume affecting phasic activity may be part of a local bladder wall reflex arc.

INTERPRETATION. Female guinea pig bladders were isolated, cannulated via the urethra, maintained *in vitro* in Tyrode's solution and exposed to drugs while the intravesical pressure was monitored. The isolated unstimulated bladder generated small rises in pressure. Increases in volume increased autonomous activity. Muscarinic agonists augmented autonomous activity. Reduced bladder volume inhibited phasic activity. Tetrodotoxin had no effect on volume-induced changes. Capsaicin, which stimulates and eliminates sensory fibres, produced a complex change in phasic activity. Oxadiazolo-[4,3-a]quinoxalin-1-one (ODQ), an inhibitor of guanyl cyclase in the interstitial cells of the bladder, did not affect the volume-induced rise in frequency but did produce a reduced inhibition on volume reduction.

Table 13.2 The association of genetic polymorphisms of GSTM1, GSTT1 and GSTP1 and prostate cancer risk according to nationality

Gene/population	Cases	Controls	Comparison	OR (95% CI)
GSTM1				
North Indian	127	144	Null vs non-null	2.2 (1.37–3.65)
American	276	499	Null vs non-null	1.0 (0.73–1.36)
Japanese	115	204	Null vs non-null	1.6 (0.84–2.99)
Danish	153	288	Null vs non-null	1.3 (0.9–1.9)
German	91	127	Null vs non-null	1.2 (0.71–2.05)
Austrian	166	166	Non-null vs null	0.86 (0.55–1.36)
GSTT1				
North Indian	127	144	Null vs non-null	1.89 (1.08–3.28)
American	276	499	Non-null vs null	1.61 (1.14–2.28)
Danish	153	288	Null vs non-null	1.3 (0.8–2.2)
German	91	127	Null vs non-null	2.31 (1.17–4.59)
Japanese	115	204	Null vs non-null	1.6 (0.84–2.99)
Austrian	166	166	Non-null vs null	0.78 (0.43–1.42)
GSTP1				
North Indian	127	144	A/A vs A/G	2.48 (1.51–4.08)
Austrian	166	166	A/A vs A/G	0.65 (0.38–1.09)
Danish	153	288	A/G plus G/G vs A/A	0.8 (0.54–1.19)
German	91	127	A/G plus G/G vs A/A	1.08 (0.66–1.77)
Swedish	171	148	A/A vs A/G plus G/G	0.85 (0.54–1.32)
Scottish	36	155	A/A vs A/G plus G/G	0.4 (0.02–3.3)
Japanese	81	105	A/A vs A/G plus G/G	9.31 (0.47–18.4)

Source: Srivastava *et al.* (2005).

Comment

This study demonstrates that distension stimulates components of the bladder wall to affect phasic activity. Motor or sensory nerves are not directly involved in the local reflex, although sensory nerves can affect phasic activity. The diagrams illustrate the effects of the various substances tested on the guinea pig bladders. Figure 13.1 proposes a way in which the central nervous system (CNS) may interact with the urothelium via the network of sensory afferents, stretch receptors and interstitial cells that may be found within the bladder wall. The work presented here also suggests that bladder sensations may be modulated in the periphery, contrary to the widely accepted concept that this kind of information is processed at the spinal and supraspinal levels.

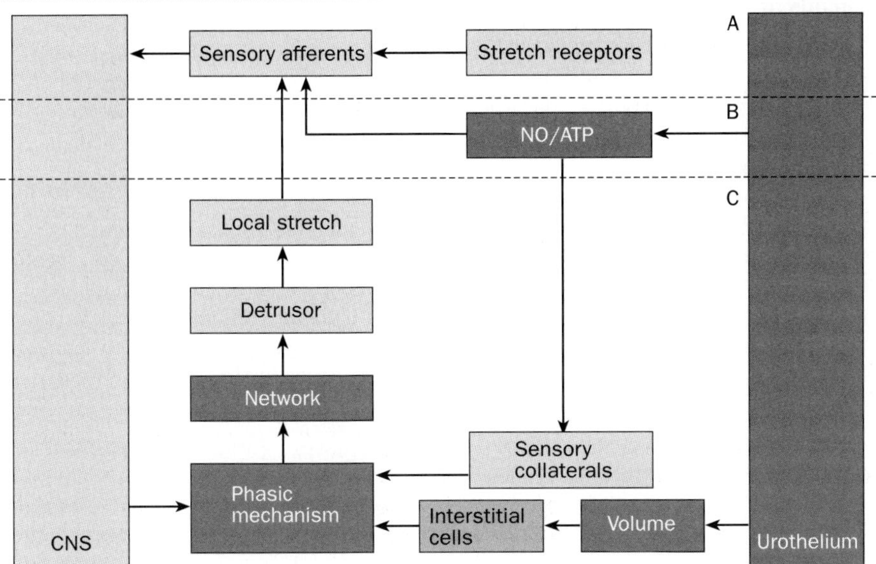

Fig. 13.1 A schematic diagram of the mechanisms that might contribute to the generation of sensation in the bladder. A. Represents the 'classical' view of a sensory nerve ending, deformed by stretch in the bladder wall, sending signals to the central nervous system (CNS). B. Represents an extension to this concept, whereby substances released by the urothelium (nitric oxide, adenosine triphosphate *inter alia*) act directly on the afferent nerve ending to modulate discharge. C. Represents the system outlined in the present report, proposing the existence of specific mechanisms within the bladder wall capable of generating phasic activity. This phasic activity or pacemaker controls a network of cells resulting in detrusor activation, which comprises contraction waves and local stretches. These stretches may activate afferent discharge |**1**|. The amplitude and frequency of the phasic activity can be influenced by different mechanisms, including the intravesical volume (IVV), possibly via local reflexes, collaterals of sensory fibres and by excitatory and inhibitory inputs from the CNS. In this way, such a complex mechanism could function as a modulated motor/sensory system. Source: Lagou *et al.* (2004).

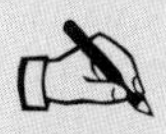

Allopurinol provides long-term protection for experimentally induced testicular torsion in a rabbit model

Kehinde EO, Anim JT, Mojiminiyi OA, *et al.* *BJU Int* 2005; **96**: 175–80

Background. The sequelae of testicular torsion may currently be explained as a consequence of ischaemia/reperfusion (I/R) injury. Previous studies have reported, in animal models, the efficacy of antioxidants in reducing the short-term damage incurred by testicular torsion. However, these studies have only looked at the short-term follow-up of the effects of drugs such as superoxide dismutase (SOD), catalase, allopurinol and aspirin. The aim of this study was to examine the effects of five different antioxidants, namely acetyl salicylic acid, ascorbic acid, allopurinol,

quercetin and SOD, on the exocrine function of rabbit testes twenty-four hours and three months after experimental torsion.

Interpretation. The left testes of pre-pubertal rabbits were clamped for 60 minutes to simulate torsion, after which the clamps were removed to allow reperfusion. In each rabbit, the right testis served as an internal control. The groups studied are summarized in Tables 13.3 and 13.4. In each group, the testes of four rabbits were harvested at either 24 hours of reperfusion or three months. Each harvested testis underwent histological examination and was assessed for levels of testicular malondialdehyde (MDA), which acts a measure of free radical damage. Twisted viable testes had higher levels of MDA than controls, and the torted testes of rabbits given allopurinol had lower MDA levels than those of untreated rabbits and rabbits given other antioxidants. The other drug groups had lower MDA levels than untreated rabbits, except for the acetyl salicylic acid-administered group, which had even higher levels.

Table 13.3 Experimental rabbit groups

Group	Procedure
A	Sham-operated
B	60-minute ischaemia followed by reperfusion
C	60-minute ischaemia followed by left orchidectomy
D	60-minute ischaemia plus reperfusion plus drugs as shown in Table 16.4

Source: Kehinde *et al.* (2005).

Table 13.4 Experimental rabbit groups subgroup 'D' drug groups

Group	Drug administered
D1	Acetyl salicylic acid
D2	Ascorbic acid
D3	Allopurinol
D4	Quercetin
D5	Superoxide dismutase (SOD)

Source: Kehinde *et al.* (2005).

Comment

In this study, the reasoning behind harvesting the rabbit testes at three months is that three months corresponds to 6–8 years in human terms, which is apparently the approximate time at which humans marry after torsion of the testis and attempt to have a family. The only drug shown to confer an improvement in testicular viability was allopurinol, but the doses used in this study (200 mg/kg) were high. The paper suggests that giving humans doses of allopurinol of up to 300 mg should produce serum levels that produce an antioxidant effect without causing toxicity.

On the basis of the results shown, the proposal of this study that the outcome of testicular torsion could be improved by the use of effective antioxidants such as allopurinol seems a valid one.

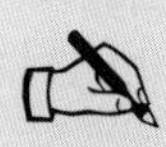

A tissue-engineered suburethral sling in an animal model of stress urinary incontinence

Cannon TW, Sweeney DD, Conway DA, *et al.* *BJU Int* 2005; **96**: 664–9

BACKGROUND. A suburethral sling is one of the surgical methods of treatment of stress urinary incontinence (SUI). Current options for the type of material from which the sling can be made include: autograft tissue, such as rectus fascia and tensor fascia lata; allograft tissue, such as dura mater; xenografts; and artificial materials such as polytetrafluoroethylene (PTFE), polypropylene and polyester. None of these is ideal, each having their own advantages and disadvantages. An autograft has the inherent advantage of minimizing the risk of adverse tissue reaction but requires harvesting from another site and is therefore at risk of infection. Synthetic materials are stronger, last longer and avoid the need for harvesting. Therefore, the ideal sling would be a combination of the two. This study looks at the functional effects of a tissue-engineered sling in a rat model of SUI.

INTERPRETATION. Sprague–Dawley rats were divided into the following groups: the tissue-engineered sling was created using cells obtained from the gastrocnemius muscle, minced and then seeded for two weeks on a small intestine submucosal (SIS) scaffold (see Fig. 13.2). The leak point pressures (LPPs) in each group were measured as shown in the figure. Figures 13.2 and 13.3 show the experimental set-up. LPPs from both sling groups were not significantly different from untreated controls.

Table 13.5 Study groups

Group	Procedure
C (control)	No intervention
D (denervated)	Bilateral proximal sciatic nerve transaction (PSNT)
S (sling)	Bilateral PSNT and suburethral sling of small intestinal submucosa
M	Bilateral PSNT and tissue-engineered sling

Source: Cannon *et al.* (2005).

Comment

As mentioned above, the concept of autograft tissue-engineered sling with the tensile properties of one of the synthetic implants commonly used is an attractive one. The tissue-engineered slings in this study produced results similar to the untreated or SIS groups. Therefore, incorporating muscle cells into SIS slings does not appear to alter the sling's mechanical properties, although obviously, if it were

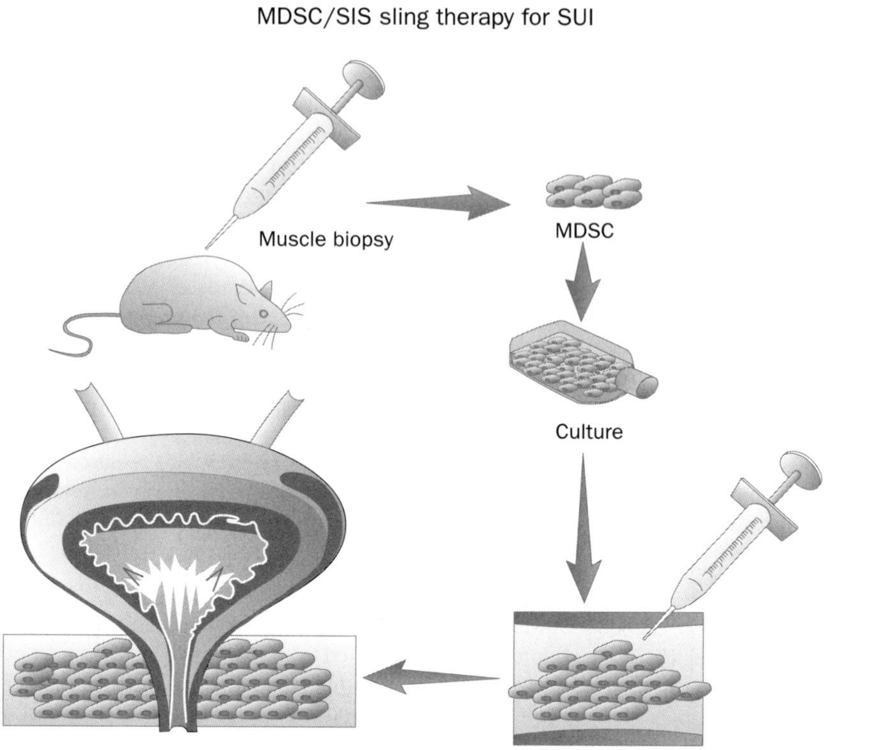

Fig. 13.2 A model of the life cycle of a tissue-engineered sling. Source: Cannon *et al.* (2005).

to make no difference at all long term, then the use of such a technique is questionable. As the paper concludes, further functional studies of such tissue-engineered sling materials need to be performed.

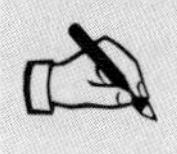

Sildenafil inhibits the formation of superoxide and the expression of gp47 NAD[P]H oxidase induced by the thromboxane A2 mimetic, U46619, in corpus cavernosal smooth muscle cells

Koupparis AJ, Jeremy JY, Muzaffar S, Persad R, Shukla N. *BJU Int* 2005; **96**: 423–7

Background. Relaxation of the corpus cavernosum leads to penile erection and is mediated by an increase in nitric oxide (NO) formation. The superoxide ion reacts with NO to form peroxynitrite among others, decreasing NO's bioavailability and affecting

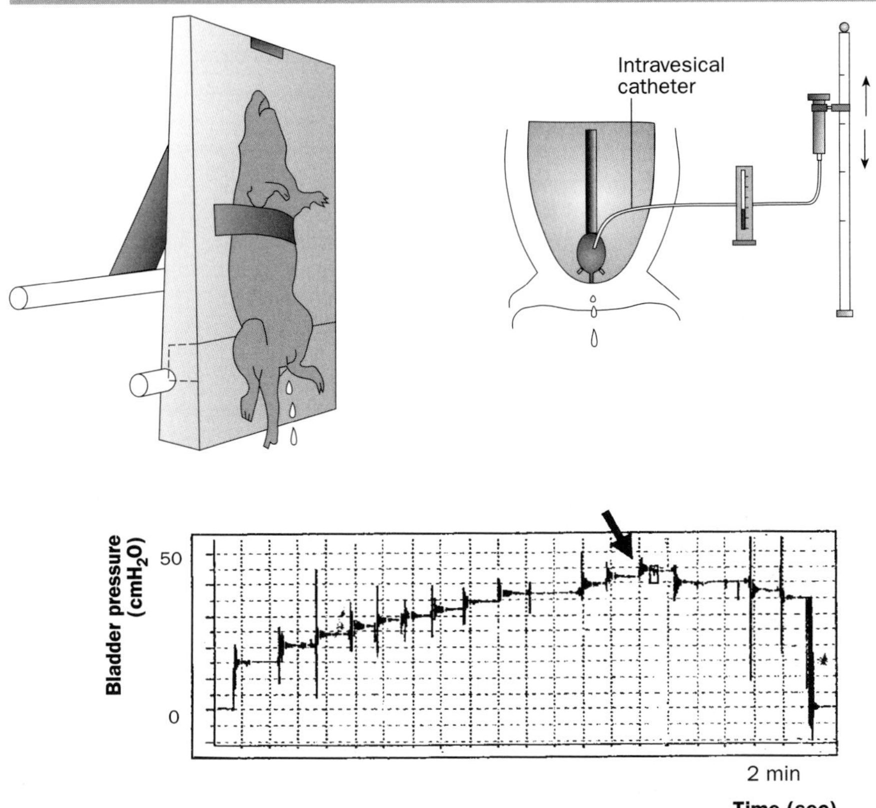

Fig. 13.3 The LPP was measured with the rat vertical, using a cystostomy catheter. The lower tracing illustrates a typical study, with the *arrow* denoting the LPP. Source: Cannon *et al.* (2005).

the normal erectile response. It has been suggested that excess production of the superoxide ion is caused by the overexpression of endogenous vascular nicotinamide adenosine dinucleotide phosphate (reduced form) (NAD[P]H) oxidase, whose upregulation may contribute to erectile dysfunction (ED). Thromboxane A2 constricts the cavernosal vessels and also contributes to ED, and its pathogenic effect may be due to upregulation of NAD[P]H oxidase expression. gp47^{phox} is an active component of NAD[P]H oxidase. The aim of this study was to examine the effect of sildenafil, a type 5 phosphodiesterase inhibitor, on superoxide formation and gp47^{phox} expression in cultured corpus cavernosal smooth muscle cells (CVSMCs) using U46619, which is a thromboxane A2 analogue.

INTERPRETATION. Rabbit penile CVSMCs were incubated with U46619 with or without sildenafil, and superoxide formation was assessed using spectrophotometric reduction of ferricytochrome *c* and Western blot analysis of gp47^{phox}. Superoxide

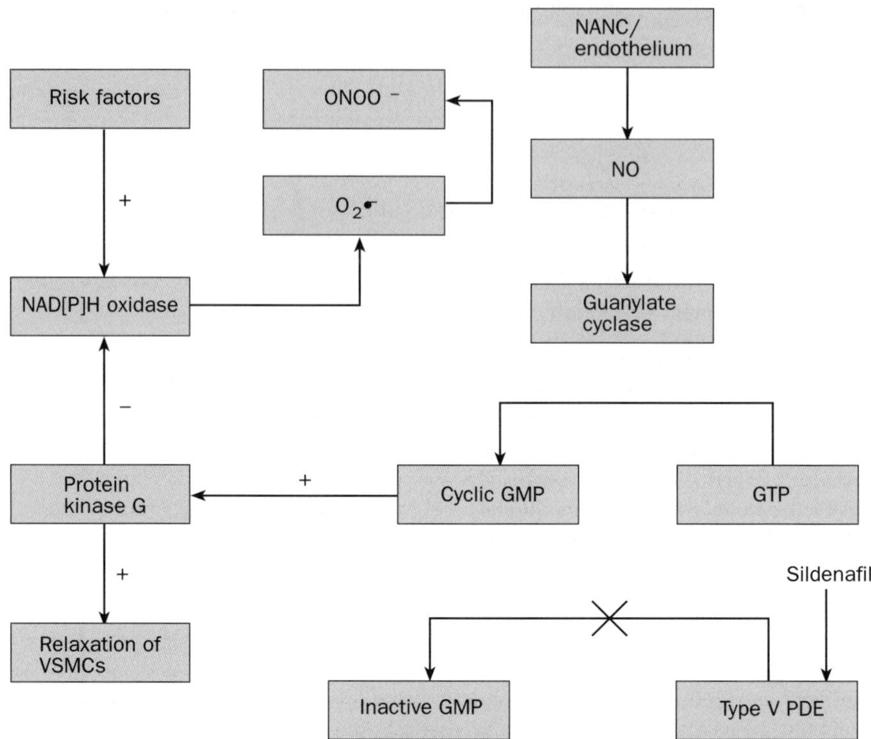

Fig. 13.4 The proposed mechanism underlying the antioxidant effect of sildenafil and its effect on erectile function. Risk factors for ED promote the endogenous expression of NAD[P]H oxidase, which generates O_2•− in penile tissue, the increased formation of which negates the pro-erectile activity of NO through direct chemical reactions to form pro-inflammatory species such as peroxynitrite (ONOO−). As sildenafil inhibits PDE-5, the hydrolysis of cyclic guanosine monophosphate (cGMP) is blocked. Increased cGMP promotes erection by augmenting smooth muscle cell relaxation, despite reduced NO formation. However, as the NO–cGMP axis also inhibits NAD[P]H oxidase expression/activity, it follows that augmentation of cGMP levels would also promote the inhibition of this enzyme. Reduced O_2•− would further augment NO bioavailability, which would feed back into the loop to enhance the inhibition of NAD[P]H oxidase expression and activity. Source: Koupparis *et al.* (2005).

formation was found to be greater in cells incubated with U46619 than in controls. This effect was blocked by NAD[P]H oxidase inhibitors. The effects of U46619 were inhibited by sildenafil.

Comment

Since its release onto the international market, oral sildenafil has rapidly become a popular and acceptable method of treating erectile dysfunction. This study serves to show that, as well as a phosphodiesterase inhibitor, it is also a potent inhibitor of superoxide formation, which is a new, previously unreported pharmacological action of this drug.

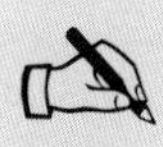

Does the valve-regulated release of urine from the bladder decrease encrustation and blockage of indwelling catheters by crystalline *Proteus mirabilis* biofilms?

Sabbuba NA, Stickler DJ, Long MJ, Dong Z, Short TD, Feneley RJC. *J Urol* 2005; **173**: 262–6

BACKGROUND. Long-term indwelling catheterization of the bladder remains a major cause of morbidity in patients requiring bladder drainage. The bacteriuria such patients inevitably acquire is often asymptomatic, but can lead to pyelonephritis, renal and bladder calculi and life-threatening sepsis. Many such episodes are triggered by catheter encrustation and blockage. The aim of this study was to examine whether valve-controlled intermittent release of urine reduces the rate of catheter blockage and encrustation by crystalline bacterial biofilms.

INTERPRETATION. A laboratory model of the bladder was utilized (see Fig. 13.5), with artificial urine, which was infected with *Proteus mirabilis*. Urine was allowed to either drain continuously through the catheters or drain intermittently at regular intervals through the use of valves. The time taken for the catheters to block was recorded, and they were subsequently examined using the electron microscope for encrustation. It was found that catheters on free drainage became blocked significantly more quickly than catheters drained at two-hourly or four-hourly intervals. Electron microscopic examination confirmed that the quantity of crystalline biofilm present was substantially less on the valve-regulated catheters.

Comment

This study suggests that the use of a valve to regulate urine drainage from the bladder reduces the rate at which encrustation occurs, thus increasing the length of time that the catheter can remain *in situ* and reducing the frequency of catheter changes, which are potential sepsis-inducing events in themselves. The use of a valve may of course not be possible for patients with poor eye–hand coordination. The urine used was artificial, and it would be interesting to see the results of a repeat study using genuine infected urine. The concept of bacterial interference would also be an interesting model to investigate in this setting to determine whether or not regular drainage combined with a suitable 'inhibiting' organism might help to reduce encrustation rates still further.

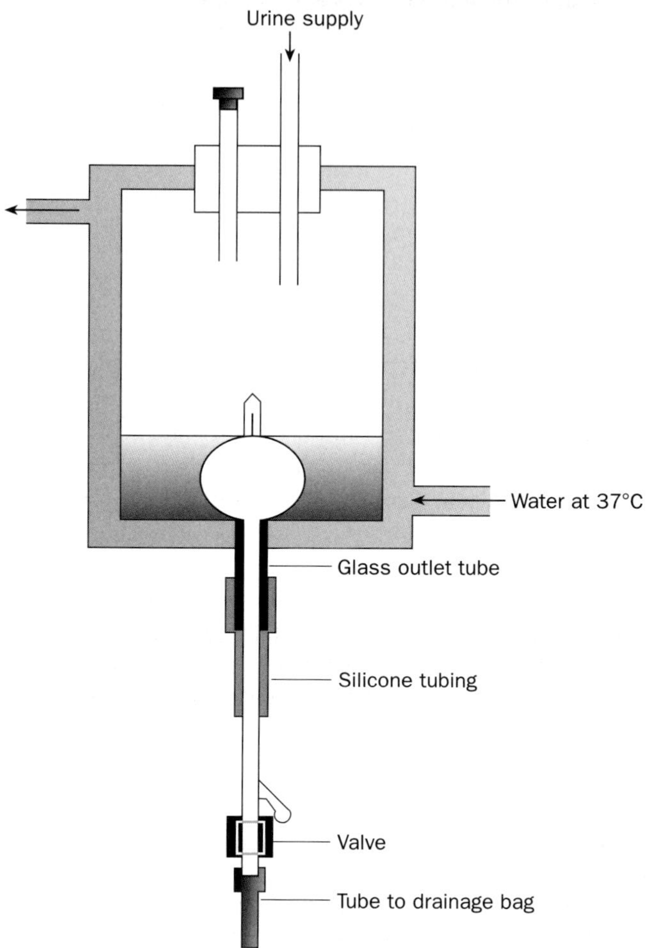

Fig. 13.5 *In vitro* laboratory bladder model. Source: Sabbuba *et al.* (2005).

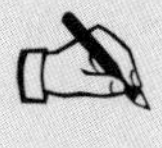

Citrate provides protection against oxalate and calcium oxalate crystal-induced oxidative damage to renal epithelium

Byer K, Khan SR. *J Urol* 2005; **173**: 640–6

Background. Oxalate and calcium oxalate crystals injure renal epithelial cells by the production of reactive oxygen species (ROS). Citrate is a calcium chelator, alkalinizes urine and decreases urinary supersaturation for calcium oxalate. It also increases reduced nicotinamide adenine dinucleotide phosphate formation, thus

helping to maintain cellular antioxidant defences. This study hypothesizes that exogenously administered citrate should act as an antioxidant and protect cells from oxalate-induced injury

Interpretation. LLC-PK1 and MDCK cells were exposed to either oxalate or calcium oxalate for 30, 60 and 180 minutes with or without 3 mg/ml citrate. Cell viability was determined by the release of lactate dehydrogenase (LDH), involvement of ROS by measuring hydrogen peroxide levels and peroxidation of lipid by measuring levels of 8-isoprostane. Cells incubated with citrate were found to have a significant decrease in LDH release, hydrogen peroxide production and 8-isoprostane secretion.

Comment

This study concludes that citrate protects cells from the damaging effects of oxalate and calcium oxalate crystals by decreasing ROS production, thus preventing the peroxidation of lipids. Citrate is already a commonly prescribed treatment in the management of calcium oxalate stone disease for the reason mentioned above. The results of this study provide another reason for its administration in stone formers.

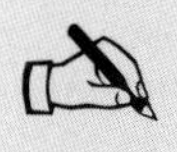

Effect of hyperthermia on the cytotoxicity of four chemotherapeutic agents currently used for the treatment of transitional cell carcinoma of the bladder: an *in vitro* study

van der Heijden AG, Verhaegh G, Jansen CF, Schalken JA, Witjes JA. *J Urol* 2005; **173**: 1375–80

Background. Thermo-chemotherapy of the bladder has been studied for nearly forty years. The mechanism of its action is not understood, but previous results have suggested that this therapeutic option is worthy of further study. The aim of this paper was to investigate the cytotoxicity of the chemotherapeutic agents mitomycin-C, epirubicin, gemcitabine and EO9 at temperatures of 37°C and 43°C.

Interpretation. RT4, RT112, 253J and T24 human transitional cell carcinoma (TCC) cell lines were treated with increasing concentrations of mitomycin-C, epirubicin, gemcitabine and EO9 at temperatures of 37°C and 43°C. The effect of these factors on cell survival was determined by MTT (3-(4,5-dimethylthiazol-2-yl)-2, 5-diphenyltetrazoliumbromide) assay. As the concentration of the drugs was increased, decreased cell proliferation was observed. Hyperthermia alone had no effect. EO9 was the most potent agent at both temperatures. There was some evidence of synergism between temperature and concentration with each of the agents used, with what appeared to be an optimum concentration for some of the agents to work synergistically with the raised temperature.

Comment

Raising the temperature of the tumour cells alone did not result in a reduction in their proliferation. It is possible that the drugs concerned work better at higher temperatures, either because they react with the cells more quickly or because the cells themselves become somehow more receptive to the drugs. A raised temperature might also promote apoptosis once the cell has been damaged by drug action. Ideally, such a study should incorporate normal bladder urothelial cells as well to determine whether or not thermo-chemotherapy has increased adverse effects on normal tissue. Obviously, further work on this technique needs to be performed before such issues as how the drug could be kept at the required temperature in the bladder can be addressed.

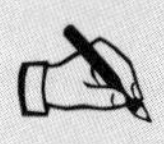

Water jet-assisted laparoscopic partial nephrectomy without hilar clamping in the calf model

Moinzadeh A, Hasan W, Spaliviero M, *et al. J Urol* 2005; **174**: 317–21

BACKGROUND. Haemostasis can represent a considerable challenge during laparoscopic partial nephrectomy (LPN), often requiring hilar vessel clamping to minimize bleeding. This means that surgery then has to be performed under warm ischaemia. The Hydro-Jet device (Fig. 13.6) is a device with adjustable pressure setting capable of delivering a jet of normal saline that can dissect renal parenchyma without causing damage to associated structures such as blood vessels and the pelvicaliceal system. The aim of this study was to evaluate the use of this device in LPN in the calf model.

INTERPRETATION. It was intended that ten male calves undergo bilateral Hydro-jet-assisted LPN of the lower/mid pole of the kidney without control of the hilar vessels. The Hydro-jet device is illustrated in Fig. 13.6. Resection of approximately 20% of each of the twenty kidneys was attempted using a high-velocity, ultracoherent saline stream at 450 psi. Table 13.6 illustrates the effects of different pressure settings on renal tissue. Bipolar diathermy was used on exposed intrarenal blood vessels before transaction was attempted. No cases required open conversion. Eighteen out of the twenty cases were eventually performed without hilar clamping. Mean nephrectomy time ranged from 13 to

Table 13.6 Hydro-Jet pressure setting with resultant effect on renal tissue

Hydro-Jet pressure setting (psi)	Result
<400	Non-reliable parenchymal cutting with waterlogging
400–600	Precise parenchymal incision with preservation of intrarenal vessels and caliceal system
600–850	Cutting of small blood vessels
>850	Cutting of large blood vessels + collecting system

Source: Moinzadeh *et al.* (2005).

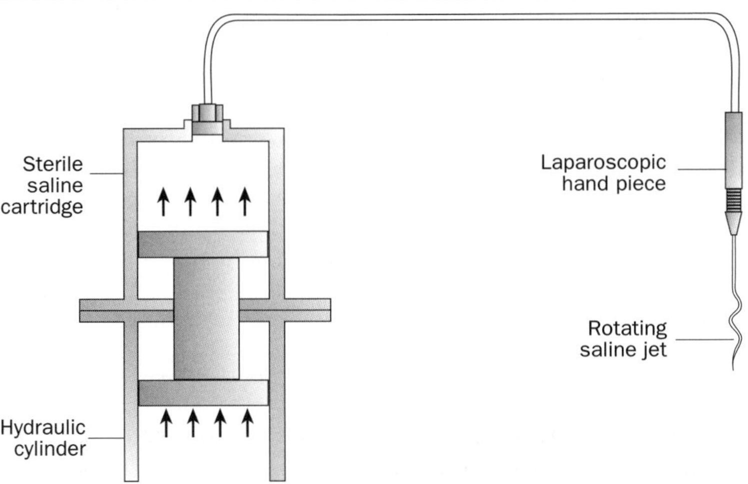

Fig. 13.6 Helix Hydro-Jet® device components. Source: Moinzadeh *et al.* (2005).

150 minutes. Mean blood loss ranged from 20 to 750 ml. No cases suffered post-operative urinary leak.

Comment

Hydro-Jet technology has been used previously for cutting, among other things, ceramic, glass, metal and dog liver. This study suggests that the use of this device for LPN is feasible. Technical concerns included backsplatter on the laparoscope lens, but this could be kept to a minimum as long as the saline jet did not strike a metallic object. Puddle formation and frothing was avoided by keeping the instrument tip close to the working area to allow the integrated suction device to prevent these. The avoidance of vessel clamping is an obvious advantage of this technique, which requires further evaluation regarding its use as a technique in the treatment of solid renal parenchymal tumours.

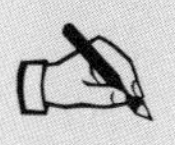

The tunica vaginalis dorsal graft urethroplasty: experimental study in rabbits

Calado AA, Macedo A Jr, Delcelo R, de Figueiredo LF, Ortiz V, Srougi M. *J Urol* 2005; **174**: 765–70

Background. Urethroplasty in which a straightforward anastomosis is not possible requires tissue interposition. Typical areas for harvest of such tissue include buccal or vesical mucosa, vascularized skin flaps or full thickness skin grafts. In some cases, such tissue may not be available. The aim of this study was to study the

histological and radiological characteristics of free graft dorsal-only urethroplasty using the tunica vaginalis as graft tissue in a rabbit model.

Interpretation. In twenty New Zealand rabbits, part of the dorsal surface of the urethra was excised to create a defect. The tunica vaginalis of the left testis was freed from its attachments and sutured in place using 6/0 polydioxanone sutures (Fig. 13.7). Animals were sacrificed at 2, 4, 8 and 12 weeks post surgery, with retrograde urethrography being performed at autopsy and the penis being sent for histological examination. Urethrograms showed no evidence of fistula or stricture formation. As time went on post surgery, it was noted that the mesothelial lining of the tunica vaginalis became replaced by an epithelial lining similar to the normal urethral urothelium.

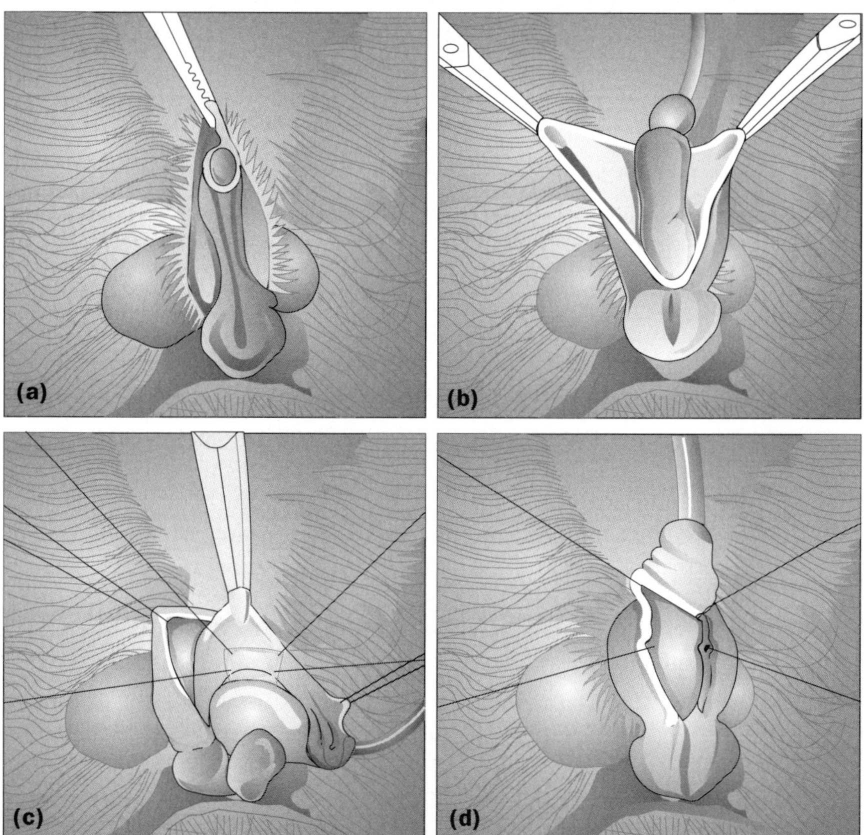

Fig. 13.7 Surgical technique. (a) Normal penile anatomy; (b) midline skin incision exposed urethra; (c) tunica vaginalis graft was placed dorsally over corpora cavernosa and tied with four interrupted sutures; (d) mucosal margin of urethral defect was sutured to graft edges. Source: Calado *et al.* (2005).

Comment

One of the main advantages of a tunica vaginalis graft is that, compared with tissue obtained from the mouth, bladder or elsewhere, it is relatively easy to harvest, causing few complications to the donor site. Also important is that, once placed in the urinary tract, it undergoes metaplasia to normal urothelium. This study suggests that tunica vaginalis can act as a successful urethral substitute in the animal model. The paper points out that there was no control group, but that the workers intend to remedy this situation.

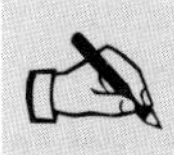

Effects of pneumoperitoneal gases and pressures on transitional cell carcinoma adhesion, growth, apoptosis and necrosis: an *in vitro* study

Tan BJ, Dy JS, Chiu PY, *et al. J Urol* 2005; **174**: 1463–7

BACKGROUND. Tract recurrence and port site metastasis following laparoscopic nephroureterectomy and cystectomy for TCC can be as high as 4.0%. Carbon dioxide (CO_2) is the gas most commonly used for insufflation of the peritoneum, and the question has been raised as to whether or not this gas may in fact increase the incidence of port site metastases. The aim of this study was to study the effects of CO_2, nitrogen (N_2) and helium (He) in terms of both type of gas used and the pressure exerted on the adhesion, growth, apoptosis and necrosis of TCC in an *in vitro* model.

INTERPRETATION. AY-27 rat TCC cells were incubated with CO_2, N_2 and He for 3 hours at pressures of 0, 10 and 15 mmHg *in vitro*. After this, the effects of these exposures on tumour cell adhesion, growth, apoptosis and necrosis were compared. It was found that the tumour adhesion rate was lowest in the cells exposed to CO_2, and highest in the N_2-exposed group. If the gas pressure was increased, the adhesion rates decreased in the CO_2- and He-exposed groups, but increased in the N_2 group. He and CO_2 caused an increase in cellular proliferation to begin with but, by 24 hours, tumour growth had decreased. Rates of apoptosis and necrosis were highest for He compared with the other gases.

Comment

This study shows that the type of gas and degree of pressure of insufflation affect tumour growth and cell adhesion. CO_2 tends to be the insufflation gas of choice for laparoscopy, despite such reported adverse reactions as hypercarbia, acidosis and gut ischaemia. An inert gas such as helium might be less likely to cause these complications, while at the same time promoting tumour apoptosis and necrosis, and thus reducing the risk of tumour spread. As this paper quite rightly points out in its conclusion, *in vivo* studies are needed to help in the understanding of the complex inter-relationships between insufflation gas, tumour cell growth and survival, and the effect of these on the host and the local environment.

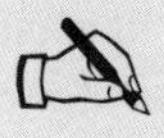

Intraoperative recordings of electroneurographic signals from cuff electrodes on extradural sacral roots in spinal cord-injured patients

Kurstjens GA, Borau A, Rodriguez A, Rijkhoff NJ, Sinkjaer T. *J Urol* 2005; **174**: 1482–7

BACKGROUND. Inhibition of the micturition reflex can be achieved by stimulating the pudendal afferents, thus inhibiting unwanted contractions of the detrusor muscle. Conditional stimulation, i.e. stimulation only when a detrusor contraction occurs, can be as effective as continuous stimulation. For this to work, the intravesical pressure needs to be monitored. Whole nerve electroneurographic (ENG) signals recorded from cuffs placed in the pelvic nerves of animals such as cats and pigs have been shown to reflect changes in bladder pressure. The aim of this study was to determine the feasibility of recording afferent nerve activity related to mechanical activity of the detrusor muscle from the extradural sacral nerve root in humans.

INTERPRETATION. Six spinal cord-injured patients underwent implantation of the extradural Fine-Tech-Brindley bladder system (Fig. 13.8). Nerve cuff electrodes were placed on the extradural root of S3 in each patient, and the dorsal penile or clitoral nerve was stimulated. ENG signals were recorded during mechanical stimulation of the dermatome, rapid bladder filling and rectal distension, and also during bladder contraction. It was found that ENG responses during stimulation of the dermatome and rectum were produced in all six patients. Five patients had recordable responses during bladder filling. The responses recorded from the bladder and rectum were small. Four patients out of five who were stimulated had nerve responses following bladder contractions.

Comment

This small study suggests that it may be possible to detect afferent nerve activity from the dermatome, bladder and rectum using the cuff electrodes used, but further work needs to be done on improving the quality of the recordings and also on methods of processing the signals obtained.

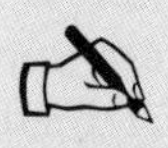

Effects of the selective acetylcholinesterase inhibitor TAK-802 on the voiding behaviour and bladder mass increase in rats with partial bladder outlet obstruction

Hashimoto T, Nagabukuro H, Doi T. *J Urol* 2005; **174**: 1137–41

BACKGROUND. Impaired bladder emptying is a common urological problem with a number of causes, including bladder outlet obstruction (BOO) and impaired detrusor contraction. Intermittent self-catheterization (ISC) is advocated for cases in which detrusor contraction is impaired, but this can lead to urinary tract infection (UTI) and

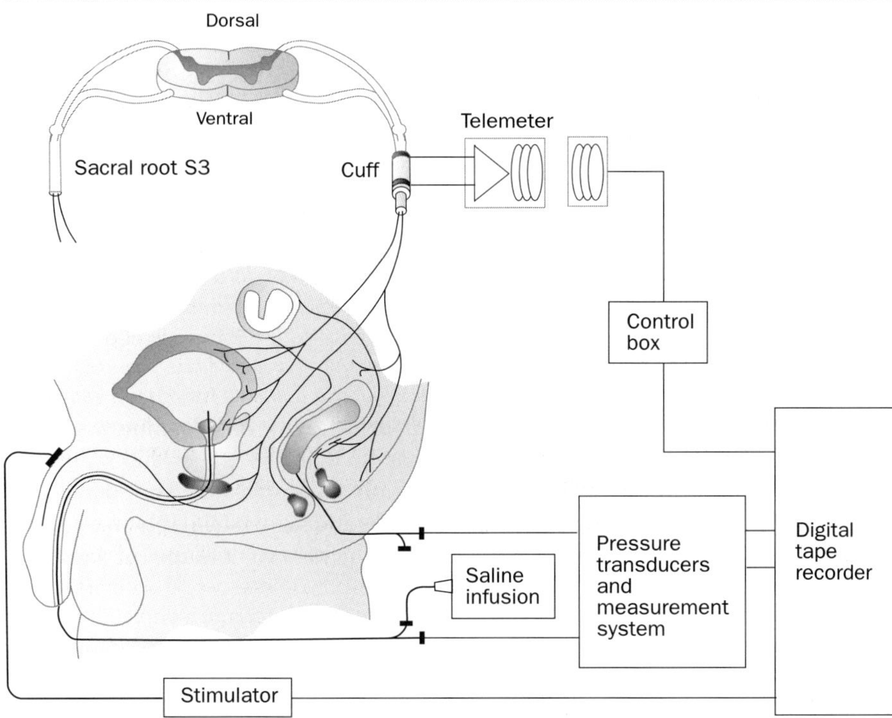

Fig. 13.8 Experimental set-up. Source: Kurstjens *et al.* (2005).

bladder injury. Cholinomimetic drugs such as muscarinic agonists and acetylcholinesterase (AChE) inhibitors may improve bladder contractions via the parasympathetic nervous system. Such drugs are not commonly used for the condition of impaired detrusor contractility. The aim of this study was to look at the effect of a selective AChE inhibitor TAK-802 on voiding behaviour and residual urine volumes in rats with partial BOO compared with rats that had been administered the non-selective AChE inhibitor distigmine and bethanechol, a muscarinic agonist.

Interpretation. Male Wistar rats underwent a procedure to produce partial BOO. Six to eight days after this, voiding behaviour was observed. The rats were then administered one of the above drugs orally, and voiding frequency and volume voided were measured for three hours. It was found that TAK-802 and distigmine increased the average voided volume without causing a change in frequency. Bethanechol increased voiding frequency without affecting voided volume. All three drugs reduced the residual urine volume, with TAK-802 yielding the best results. In a separate experiment, bladder weight was assessed in rats with BOO after doses of TAK-802, which was found to prevent the increase in bladder mass seen in the control group.

Comment

Drugs such as distigmine bromide used to be more widely used but have fallen out of favour. This study shows that AChE inhibition can decrease residual urine volumes in rats with BOO by restoring voiding function. Bethanechol also decreased residual urine volumes, but the voiding frequency in this group was increased. Further clinical studies of these drugs would be worthwhile, particularly if they would be of benefit to certain patients who are either unable physically to perform ISC, or in whom it is difficult or contraindicated because of, for example, recurrent false passage and stricture formation.

Conclusion

As mentioned in the introduction, there is deliberately little common ground between the papers discussed here, save that they all fall under the banner of 'investigative urology', and it is hoped that the often complicated work detailed in these papers has been summarized in a readable and understandable manner for the clinician with little time to plough through the vast amount of literature produced every year in this field.

Reference

1. Gillespie JI. The autonomous bladder: a view of the origin of bladder overactivity and sensory urge. *BJU Int* 2004; **93**: 478–83.

14

New developments in cancer biology

MARTO SUGIONO, TOBY PAGE, MALCOLM CRUNDWELL

Introduction

The human genome project was completed more than 2 years ago and heralded exciting possibilities in the diagnosis and treatment of many diseases including cancer. However, it was apparent from the start that mapping the genome was only the first step in a long journey in understanding complex disease mechanisms. The field of proteomics and epigenetics has expanded more recently in an effort to understand these molecular pathways. This has led to the discovery of novel therapeutic targets in cancer, which has resulted in several molecules (such as anti-angiogenic factors and anti-tyrosine kinase inhibitors) being used in various phases of clinical trials.

In this chapter, eleven papers have been selected from a variety of clinical and basic science journals that it is hoped are to some degree representative of the trend and direction in which research in cancer biology of urological tumours has gone, although it is obviously beyond the scope of this chapter to include every seminal and significant discovery.

As prostate cancer is the commonest urological cancer, five papers related to this subject have been included, ranging from expression studies between different racial groups and the emerging importance of lymphangiogenesis to sophisticated *in vitro* and *in vivo* experiments in an effort to determine the molecules and pathways involved in progression to hormone-refractory status. At the other end of the disease spectrum, protein profiling of serum offers the promise of detecting localized disease and is the focus of large collaborations in Europe, such as the P-Mark project [1]. It may also herald the discovery of novel biomarkers to challenge prostate-specific antigen (PSA).

Moving on to renal cell carcinoma (RCC), our knowledge of the downstream interactions of the *VHL* gene that plays such a central role in the disease continues to grow together with the search for prognostic factors in advanced cases. The use of antisense oligonucleotide technology to switch off genes also offers the potential for delivering very specific targeted therapy, not only in RCC but also in other cancers.

In transitional cell carcinoma (TCC), differences in the clonal origins of multiple bladder tumours are apparent, indicating that, perhaps in future, molecular profiling of these tumours can help in individualizing treatment strategies. DNA hypermethylation is an important epigenetic mechanism whose reversibility offers an attractive target in controlling downstream events. Finally, the bladder is unique in that it is easily accessible to intravesical treatment. The use of gene therapy is therefore a particularly promising modality as an adjunct to more conventional treatment.

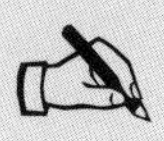

Differential inhibition of invasion and proliferation by bisphosphonates: anti-metastatic potential of zoledronic acid in prostate cancer

Montague R, Hart CA, George NJ, Ramani VA, Brown MD, Clarke NW. *Eur Urol* 2004; **46**: 389–402

BACKGROUND. Prostate cancer (CaP) has a tendency to metastasize to bones, with those developing metastases having a median survival of only 18 months. Furthermore, 84% of those dying from CaP will have bone metastases, with a significant proportion suffering considerable morbidity. In order to metastasize, the prostate cancer cells have to bind to bone marrow endothelial cells, migrate through them and then proliferate to form colonies of metastases. Bisphosphonates are drugs that decrease bone resorption and reduce skeletal morbidity in benign and malignant diseases. Recent work has shown that the more potent of these, such as zoledronic acid, also has anti-cancer properties |2,3|. The aim of this collection of *in vitro* experiments is to determine the mechanisms by which zoledronic acid inhibits and reduces bone metastases from CaP.

INTERPRETATION. The authors found that zoledronic acid significantly reduced the ability of the PC-3 prostate cancer cell line to invade matrigel, a synthetic basement membrane, compared with controls and other less potent bisphosphonates such as pamidronate and clodronate. Zoledronic acid also had a significant impact on reducing the colony size of malignant and non-malignant prostate epithelial cells within cocultures of bone marrow cells, especially when compared with the other bisphosphonates (Fig. 14.1). In addition, it resulted in a marked reduction in the expression of matrix metalloproteinase (MMP)-7 while inducing overexpression of the tissue inhibitors of matrix metalloproteinase (TIMP)-2. However, zoledronic acid had no significant impact on the binding of the prostate cancer cell line PC-3 to bone marrow endothelial cells (BMEC) nor on the permeability of the bone marrow endothelial layer.

Comment

There has been renewed interest in the last few years in the clinical application of bisphosphonates, especially following the positive outcome of studies such as that showing the efficacy of zoledronic acid in prolonging the time to development of

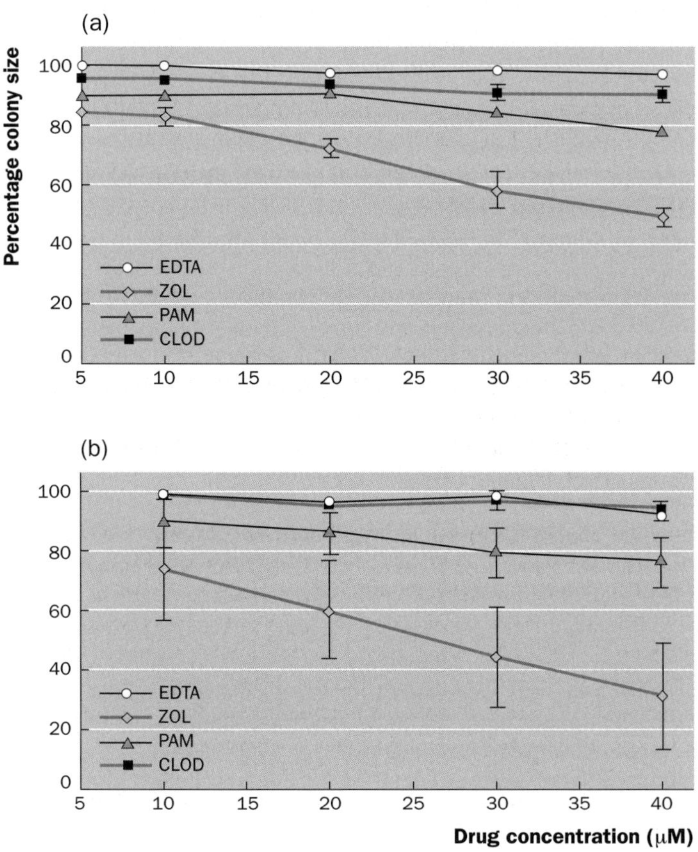

Fig. 14.1 Effect of zoledronic acid on prostate epithelial colony formation in primary human bone marrow coculture compared with other bisphosphonates. Source: Montague *et al.* (2004).

skeletal metastases, as well as reducing the frequency of skeletal-related events **4**. This work by Montague *et al.* has shed more light on the mechanisms by which CaP cells bind, migrate and proliferate in bone marrow and the mode of action of zoledronic acid. Some of the results, such as the lack of impact of zoledronic acid on binding and permeability, are in contrast to other studies, but may be explained by differences in methodology. Of note, clodronate and pamidronate were less effective in reducing the invasive ability and proliferation of prostate cancer cells, underlining how the future may lie in the nitrogen-containing bisphosphonates. The side effects of zoledronic acid on red cell precursors also seemed to occur at concentrations that are above the therapeutic window, thus further supporting its clinical utility. In fact, there are currently prospective, randomized, controlled trials to evaluate further the preventive effects of zoledronic acid in patients with high-risk CaP, highlighting the potential clinical impact of this paper.

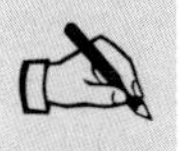

Expression of vascular endothelial growth factor receptor-3 (VEGFR-3) in human prostate

Li R, Younes M, Wheeler TM, *et al. Prostate* 2004; **58**: 193–9

BACKGROUND. The five members of the vascular endothelial growth factor family (VEGF A–E) are associated with angiogenesis and lymphangiogenesis, two processes that contribute to tumour growth and metastasis. VEGF-C promotes the growth of lymphatic vessels in tumours by binding to VEGFR-3. In this retrospective study, the authors use tissue microarray technology to develop a database of radical prostatectomy specimens (paraffin-embedded tissues) operated on by a single surgeon and analysed by one pathologist. Suitable specimens were mapped into three areas: the index tumour (defined as the largest and/or highest Gleason score); normal prostate (peripheral zone away from tumour); or benign prostatic hyperplasia (BPH). Immunostaining was then carried out to compare the expression of VEGFR-3, which was also correlated with clinico-pathological parameters.

INTERPRETATION. Immunoreactivity was assessed using a 0–3 semi-quantitative score for both intensity of staining and percentage of cells stained. A sum index was thus obtained for each specimen, and expression level was defined as low (sum index 0–3) or high (4–6). Of the 554 patients, 49.5% of those with CaP showed high-level VEGFR-3 expression compared with 25% in normal tissue and 22% in BPH. The difference between normal and CaP and between BPH and CaP was statistically significant ($P < 0.001$) but not that between normal and BPH ($P > 0.5$). In addition, there was a statistically significant correlation between VEGFR-3 expression and Gleason score, pre-PSA level and lymph node metastasis, with higher Gleason, PSA and lymph node-positive cases showing more frequent high-level expression. The 5-year biochemical recurrence-free rates in those with low-level expression were significantly higher than in those with high-level expression (77.3 vs 69.6%; $P = 0.037$). However, multivariate analysis failed to identify VEGFR-3 as an independent prognostic indicator.

Comment

Angiogenesis has been in the spotlight in the last decade as a critical factor in the growth and spread of cancer, although lymphangiogenesis may play a more specific role in lymphatic metastasis. This is a large and well-conducted study with sound methodology. However, as with many experiments on differential expression of factors, it is retrospective and included only those specimens containing prostate cancer that was large enough to be cored for microarrays.

The data showed an upregulation of VEGFR-3 in prostate cancer when compared with internal controls, suggesting a possible mechanism by which CaP metastasizes. Previous work has demonstrated the possibility of an autocrine loop as prostate cancer cells also produce VEGF-C, the ligand for VEGFR-3. Interestingly, Jackson *et al.* |5| found that VEGFR-1 and VEGFR-2 are expressed more in well- and moderately differentiated prostate cancers, whereas the authors found that increased VEGFR-3 expression was found in higher Gleason score tumours. VEGFR-3 may therefore be involved in the progression of CaP, and its signalling pathway could become a potential therapeutic target for CaP patients with higher Gleason scores.

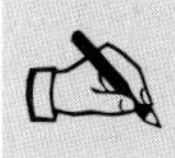

Molecular determinants of resistance to anti-androgen therapy

Chen CD, Welsbie DS, Tran C, *et al.* *Nature Med* 2004; **10**: 33–9

BACKGROUND. Hormone therapy has had a major impact on the treatment of advanced prostate cancer ever since Huggins and Hodges' work in 1941 |6|. Unfortunately, although androgen ablation is initially effective (i.e. hormone sensitive; HS), it eventually becomes resistant to these therapies, and patients develop androgen-independent or hormone-refractory (HR) disease. A number of mechanisms have been postulated, including androgen receptor (AR) mutations, development of ligand-independent AR and alternative pathways that bypass the AR. This study combines a number of *in vitro* and *in vivo* experiments using prostate cancer cell lines and microarray-based profiling of isogenic prostate cancer xenograft models. Their objective was to determine the molecular mechanism that results in the progression from the HS to the HR state.

INTERPRETATION. The authors first set out to analyse the gene expression profiles of seven pairs of HS and HR prostate cancer xenografts. The HR cells were derived from the HS parental lines. Out of more than 12 000 probes used to detect differences in mRNA expression between the HS and the HR group, only one – targeting the AR cDNA – was overexpressed in all seven HR compared with the corresponding HS cells. LNCaP and LAPC4 cell lines were infected with AR-expressing lentivirus, which were then implanted into severe combined immunodeficiency disease (SCID) mice. They observed that tumours formed more quickly in this group compared with mice implanted with normal LNCaP and LAPC4. In addition, using two models of AR mutations and a radiolabelled ligand-binding assay, it was found that AR must bind to its ligand in order to confer HR growth. Furthermore, by comparing LNCaP and LAPC4 cell lines with their counterparts that overexpress AR, it appears that the increase in AR expression converts AR antagonists (in this case bicalutamide) to weak agonists, leading to the induction of the most androgen-sensitive genes. Finally, they examined how the bicalutamide becomes an agonist when AR levels are increased. A slight change in AR protein level changes the balance of corepressors and coactivators on the AR target genes with subsequent effects on transcriptional activity.

Comment

This important paper is actually a series of experiments that help to elucidate the role of ARs in the development of hormone resistance and provide a useful insight into the potential mechanisms involved. It gives compelling evidence that increased expression of AR may be a common pathway in progression from HS to HR status, and that the binding of androgens to the AR is required to confer hormone resistance. It is also interesting to consider the clinical scenario in which the withdrawal of anti-androgen during combined androgen blockade can sometimes paradoxically reduce the PSA levels |**7**|. The findings in this study would suggest that anti-androgen withdrawal syndrome probably occurs in those with the highest level of upregulation of AR. As to why AR antagonists become weak agonists in the presence of AR overexpression, the authors are unable to provide a satisfactory hypothesis.

However, almost all the HS xenograft models have been derived from men with HR disease that has been explanted into male mice. Newer transgenic or knockout models would be necessary to study the progression of truly hormone-naïve prostate cancer cell lines. Nevertheless, despite the remaining questions as to what the exact mechanisms are that result in the upregulation of AR and how they then cause hormone resistance, these results will have significant implications in the development and design of new anti-androgens.

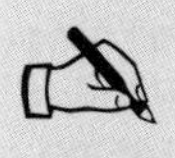

Racial disparity of epidermal growth factor receptor expression in prostate cancer

Shuch B, Mikhail M, Satagopan J, *et al. J Clin Oncol* 2004; **22**: 4725–9

BACKGROUND. The epidermal growth factor receptor (EGFR) is a family of receptors that mediates cellular growth and can promote tumour development and progression through the stimulation of angiogenesis and inhibition of apoptosis |8,9|. Increased EGFR expression has been associated with the ability to metastasize, and is implicated in a number of human solid tumours including prostate carcinoma. Inhibition of EGFR is therefore an attractive target for anti-cancer therapy. The incidence of prostate cancer shows marked variation in different ethnic groups, with US blacks having rates 60% higher than whites. This retrospective study looks at the expression of EGFR in these two groups and offers a molecular basis for this difference.

INTERPRETATION. Immunohistochemistry on 202 radical prostatectomy samples (142 African-American and 60 white men) from two centres in the US was carried out using monoclonal EGFR antibody. Scores ranging from 0 (undetectable) to +3 (strong staining in >10% of tumour cells) were used to assess the level of EGFR expression, which was categorized as negative (scores 0 and 1) and positive (scores 1 and 2). The results showed a significant association between EGFR overexpression and African-American race (Table 14.1).

Comment

The large variation in the incidence of prostate cancer among different ethnic groups highlights the importance of genetic and environmental factors in its

Table 14.1 Association of race and EGFR expression

	EGFR negative	**EGFR positive**	***P*-value**
African-American	78 men (54.9%)	64 men (45.1%)	0.0006
White	49 men (81.2%)	11 men (18.3%)	

Source: Shuch *et al.* (2004).

development. African-American men have one of the highest rates and tend to have more aggressive disease. Several theories have been proposed to account for this, including dietary factors and the hormonal milieu, such as circulating levels of androgens and insulin-like growth factor (IGF)-1. The vast number of genomic studies have been faced with fundamental research challenges presented by the multifocal nature of the disease and heterogeneity between different foci within the same prostate.

The authors have shown a significant difference in EGFR expression, although the functional significance of this remains to be proven. They have also postulated that this may be related to differences in the allelic frequency of (CA)n repeats in the intron 1 part of the *EGFR* gene |**10**|. Increasingly, the secondary end-point also showed a significant association between EGFR overexpression and high pre-treatment PSA (≥10 ng/ml) and stage (both with $P = 0.02$), although not Gleason score ($P = 0.33$) or PSA recurrence ($P = 0.07$). Furthermore, after controlling for confounding factors (such as grade, stage and PSA), the association between EGFR overexpression and African origin remained significant.

This study is limited by its retrospective nature, and additional prospective investigations on a larger cohort of patients and tissue samples would be needed to characterize the relationship between differential expression of EGFR, EGFR gene mutations and their responses to anti-EGFR agents. Nevertheless, these observations shed more light on the molecular determinants that underlie interethnic differences in prostate cancer and will have an important impact on the future design of clinical trials of anti-EGFR agents.

Serum proteomic profiling can discriminate prostate cancer from benign prostates in men with total prostate specific antigen levels between 2.5 and 15.0 ng/ml

Ornstein DK, Rayford W, Fusaro VA, *et al. J Urol* 2004; **172**: 1302–5

BACKGROUND. Given that most diseases are due to abnormal regulation of protein function, serum protein profiling of blood offers the promise of a minimally invasive, quick and easy means of diagnosis. Mass spectrometry refers to a variety of

techniques whereby a sample of analyte (e.g. blood, urine or saliva) is converted to gas phase and ionized, resulting in a mixture of particles with different mass to charge ratios (m/z). These are then analysed to determine their m/z and detected by, for example, the time of flight (TOF) it takes for the particle to travel from the ionizer to the detector plate. A unique profile consisting of a series of peaks can therefore be constructed, but without actually knowing the identity of all the proteins as such.

In this study, the authors use surface-enhanced laser desorption ionization time of flight (SELDI-TOF) mass spectroscopy to compare serum from men with biopsy-proven prostate cancer with those with benign prostatic hyperplasia. The data were analysed using a computer program that is based on an artificial intelligence pattern recognition algorithm, which can evolve with experience.

INTERPRETATION. Serum was obtained from 154 men with total PSA between 2.5 and 15.0 ng/ml undergoing prostate biopsies. This range was chosen as it represents the grey area in which the specificity of PSA is low, and is thus the population that may potentially benefit most from a more specific diagnostic tool. Sixty-three men (30 with prostate cancer; 33 with negative biopsies) were used as the 'training group' to develop several models of algorithm programs. Each program was then used blindly to analyse serum from the other 91 men (28 with cancer; 63 without). The best model was found to have a sensitivity of 100% and a specificity of 67%. The authors therefore conclude that, if proteomic profiling was used to determine the need for prostate biopsies in men with PSA between 2.5 and 15.0 ng/ml, 67% would have avoided unnecessary biopsy, without missing any cancer cases.

Comment

The search for new biomarkers to replace PSA in the detection of early prostate cancer continues, with vast amounts of resources poured into research such as the European collaboration in the P-Mark project. There is, however, little evidence to suggest that detection of early disease will have any impact on long-term survival. On the contrary, we do not as yet have a complete picture of the natural history of prostate cancer. Moreover, the impact on quality of life from diagnosis and treatment of early disease has to be considered carefully. Nevertheless, by using a powerful technique such as mass spectroscopy, a complex profile of serum protein expression can help to discriminate those with prostate cancer from those without it. However, only low-molecular-weight peptides (<20 kDa) were collected in this study. Another limitation was that the performance of the test was assessed on blinded data, generating the specificity of the test but not its predictive value for negative cases. Larger training sets in the general population would have to be carried out before this innovative technology could be applied clinically. Financial costs and reproducibility will also have to be taken into account.

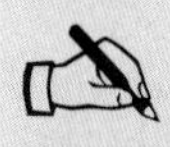

Multifocal transitional cell carcinoma of the bladder and upper urinary tract: molecular screening of clonal origin by characterizing CD44 alternative splicing patterns

Miyake H, Hara I, Kamidono S, Eto H. *J Urol* 2004; **172**: 1127–9

BACKGROUND. The exact mechanism for the multifocal nature of TCC remains controversial. Traditionally, it has been thought to be due to either field change (resulting in independent clones of TCC) or intraluminal seeding (monoclonal tumours). CD44 is a cell surface adhesion molecule with various biological activities including cell–matrix interaction and tumour growth. It is overexpressed in a number of malignant tumours and has been shown to have multiple isoforms expressed in urothelial cancers that may be used as a biomarker to identify its clonal origin. The authors utilized reverse transcription polymerase chain reaction (RT-PCR) to analyse 24 patients (52 tumour samples) with multifocal TCCs of the bladder and upper urinary tract. They used the differential expression of CD44 isoforms and p53 mutations by direct gene sequencing to assess the clonality of these tumours.

INTERPRETATION. The ratios of three major isoforms (CD44s, CD44v10 and CD44v8–10) of CD44 to one another were used to determine whether tumour tissue had the same clonal origin as another within the same patient. Eighteen cases showed similar CD44v10 to CD44s and CD44v8–10 to CD44s ratios among the multiple tumours within each case. However, six patients had markedly different ratios among the tumours. Furthermore, p53 mutations were found in five patients, two of whom had different types of mutations among the multiple tumours. These two cases also showed different patterns of CD44 alternative splicing, indicating that the multiple tumours arose from different clones within the same case.

Comment

If the field defect hypothesis were true, one would expect different tumours within the same patient to have different clonal origins, as the common carcinogen gives rise to different primaries in the urothelium. Conversely, the seeding/implantation theory would result in multiple tumours with the same molecular profile, as they all arose from the same progenitor cell. Molecular methods for investigating these differences are mostly limited to the study of chromosomal inactivation, specific gene mutation and microsatellite analysis (i.e. studies of repetitive nucleotide sequences in the DNA that serve as markers of genetic instability). In this study, 75% of cases (18/24) had similar ratios of CD44 isoforms, three of whom also had p53 mutations among the multiple tumours. Only two cases had both differing CD44 isoform ratios and dissimilar p53 mutations, which could be explained by the field defect hypothesis.

Despite the small sample, these findings support the theory that some multiple TCCs do seem to arise independently and that the expression profile of CD44 isoforms may serve as a biomarker for clonality. This would, of course, have important implications in implementing the best management strategy for the patient in terms of treatment and surveillance for recurrence. However, further investigation is required with a much larger sample size, and it would also be interesting to use normal urothelium from different areas of the genitourinary tract to serve as a control.

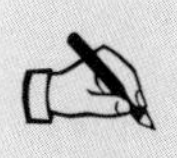

Carbonic anhydrase IX expression predicts outcome in interleukin 2 therapy for renal cancer

Atkins M, Regan M, McDermott D, *et al. Clin Cancer Res* 2005; **11**: 3714–21

BACKGROUND. Immunotherapy for RCC is now well established, with interferon (IFN)- and interleukin (IL)-2 being the most common agents. However, published results of their use have shown very variable response rates that are affected by both the genotype and the phenotype of the RCC, being uniformly low at 7–15%. Given the toxicity and expense of this treatment modality, being able to select those patients most likely to respond would clearly be advantageous. Factors such as performance status, grade and stage are easily assessed and are no doubt of importance, but the genotype of the tumour is possibly one of the most significant factors responsible for the varied effects of immunotherapy.

INTERPRETATION. Carbonic anhydrase IX (CAIX) has been identified as a molecular marker that may be predictive of prognosis in RCC. CAIX expression is controlled via the hypoxia inducible factor (HIF) complex, which in turn is regulated by the von Hippel–Lindau (VHL) protein in response to hypoxia. CAIX maintains extracellular pH in the face of hypoxic and acidotic stress. Sixty-six patients on IL-2 therapy had tumour tissue stained for the presence of CAIX, which was then quantified according to their response to treatment. Additional stratification was carried out by pathological features. Using these data, a model has been suggested that allows prediction of the response to IL-2 therapy based on CAIX expression and pathological risk group (Fig. 14.2).

Comment

Measuring response to immunotherapy is a difficult issue and one that confounds the study of immunotherapy in renal cancer. Despite there being no mention of what the authors have defined as a response, this paper promotes the notion that pre-therapy tumour analysis may be useful in selecting those patients who will benefit most from costly treatment that has significant side effects. But as to whether CAIX is the actual predictive molecule or just a downstream marker of other molecules such as the VHL protein remains to be elucidated.

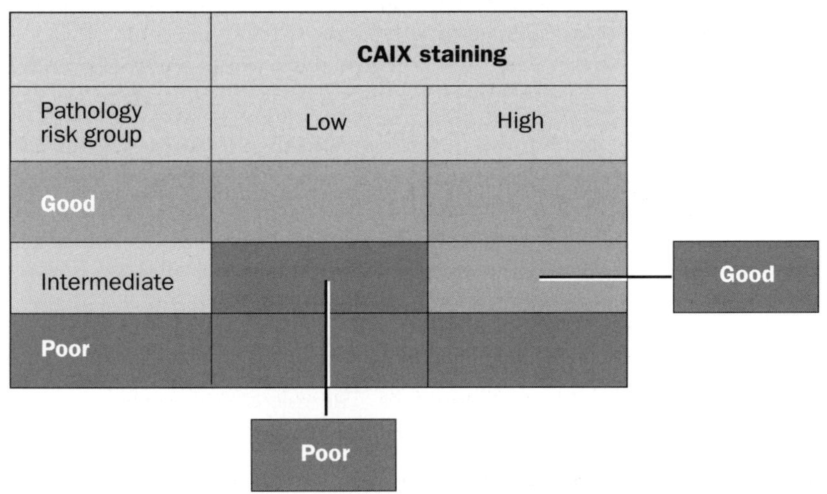

Fig. 14.2 The proposed new model for combining pathology predictive group with CAIX staining. Source: Atkins *et al.* (2005).

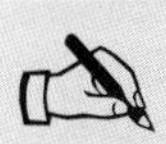

Identification of membrane type 1 matrix metalloproteinase as a target of hypoxia-inducible factor 2 in von Hippel–Lindau renal cell carcinoma

Petrella B, Lohi J, Brinckerhoff C. *Oncogene* 2005; **24**: 1043–52

Background. The role of the *VHL* gene in controlling HIF-1 and HIF-2 in response to hypoxia is now understood, but targets for the HIF complex are still being discovered. The extended role of the VHL protein in addition to controlling HIF is also a growing area of interest. The VHL protein is known to shuttle between the nucleus and the cytoplasm of cells and to be involved in fibronectin and the extracellular matrix. For renal tumours to invade and for metastasis to occur, MMPs are important in the destruction of the extracellular matrix. Increased levels of MMPs in tumours have been correlated with invasiveness and angiogenesis. Membrane type 1 MMP (MT1-MMP) is a membrane-bound MMP that degrades several components of the extracellular matrix and is involved in cell to extracellular matrix contact. It is localized on the leading edge of invasive cells. MT1-MMP has been shown to be significantly increased in RCC tumours of higher stage.

Interpretation. The expression of MMP genes was compared between two cell lines with and without functional VHL protein. This revealed that MMP-2, MT1-MMP and MMP-9 were overexpressed by the VHL null cell line (pRc-9). Using quantitative real-time RT-PCR and transfection vector techniques, the MT1-MMP RNA and protein levels were shown to be dependent on VHL expression via HIF-2. A binding site for HIF-2 in the promoter of MT1-MMP was identified and confirmed using multisite-directed mutagenesis and promoter assay transfection techniques.

Comment

The ability of a cell to become immortal, replicate and then to spread and invade defines a cancerous cell and has been the focus of extensive research over the last 10 years, mostly concentrated on the control and silencing of genes that are involved in the cell cycle and apoptosis (p53/Bcl2/Bax/Fas/Fas-l). The genes involved in angiogenesis and invasion are now being elucidated, allowing a more complete picture of the many different genetic changes that need to occur for a 'successful' cancer cell to become established and invasive. The capacity for cellular invasion undoubtedly involves other molecules apart from MMPs, including selectins, cadherins, cytokines and chemokines. The role of MT1-MMP in early invasion makes it a particularly attractive target for new therapies, especially as it is not expressed by normal epithelial cells.

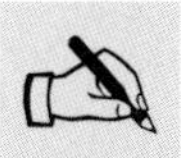

Inhibition of Ki-67 in a renal cell carcinoma severe combined immunodeficiency disease mouse model is associated with induction of apoptosis and tumour growth inhibition

Kausch I, Jiang H, Ewerdwalbesloh N, *et al. BJU Int* 2005; **95**: 416–20

BACKGROUND. Ki-67 is a marker of proliferating cells. The fraction of Ki-67-positive cells in RCC correlates with tumour grade and is an independent factor predicting outcome. Ki-67 protein has a role in the control of higher order chromatin structure, although this role has yet to be completely elucidated. Antisense oligonucleotides (asON) are short (10–50 bp) lengths of complementary nucleotides specifically designed to hybridize to a target mRNA. Once bound, they inhibit the normal translation of the mRNA to protein, and this in turn may induce cellular apoptosis. Conveniently, kidneys accumulate phosphorothioated oligonucleotides, and this may represent a possible therapeutic target for treating RCC with antisense technology.

INTERPRETATION. Three different RCC models were used for investigation—a monolayer, a three-dimensional spheroid culture and a SCID mouse with a RCC xenograft. A SCID mouse allows the use of implanted human xenografts without rejection or immunosuppressive drugs as the mouse has no functioning immune system. The asON were cultured with the cell line or, in the case of the mouse model, injected intraperitoneally on a daily basis for 2 weeks. The authors assessed cell growth, tumour inhibition, apoptosis, microvessel density (MVD) and Ki-67 positivity using immunostaining. They found that there was inhibition of cell growth in monolayer and three-dimensional culture and that systemic administration in a mouse model decreased tumour growth and caused twice the level of apoptosis.

Comment

The mechanism by which asON caused apoptosis in this experiment is hypothesized to be linked to a decrease in Ki-67 expression, as cells undergoing mitosis with insufficient Ki-67 protein cannot complete mitosis and hence undergo apoptosis instead.

The mouse model used does allow for some understanding of the usefulness of asON *in vivo*, although the results seen were not surprising and did not show any effect on tumour MVD. Further work looking at the duration and timing of administration, and the duration of effects as well as overall survival are required before any extrapolation of these *in vivo* data can be applied clinically.

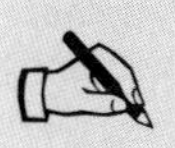

Promoter hypermethylation is associated with tumour location, stage and subsequent progression in transitional cell carcinoma

Catto J, Azzouzi A, Rehman I, *et al. J Clin Oncol* 2005; **23**: 2903–10

BACKGROUND. Despite the histopathological similarity between upper tract and bladder TCC, there is growing evidence that these two diseases have a different genetic basis. This is supported by hereditary diseases that are prone to the development of TCC in a particular location, such as the occurrence of upper tract disease in HNPCC (hereditary non-polyposis colorectal cancer; Lynch syndrome 2). Genetic microsatellites are lengths of genomic DNA that contain repeat nucleotides (e.g. CG CG CG CG CG CG CG CG). Although the length of such repeating regions is variable, they are accurately passed on to the daughter cells during mitosis. Microsatellite instability refers to errors in the copying of these regions and is a common feature in many cancers, representing a failure of normal DNA repair mechanisms. Hypermethylation of such areas controls the expression of the downstream gene and has been shown to be a mechanism by which tumour suppressor genes are inactivated in malignancies such as TCC, RCC and colon cancer.

INTERPRETATION. The methylation status of 11 microsatellites in 116 patients with bladder TCC and 164 patients with upper tract TCC was analysed. The regions chosen included genes involved in DNA repair (*h*MLH1 and *h*MSH2) as well as others previously implicated as playing an important role in TCC and other solid tumours (Table 14.2). The patients' tumour phenotypes were known and grade and stage used in the analysis. The greatest statistical difference was seen in two genes, *hMLH1* and *MINT31*, suggesting that these two loci are involved in upper tract TCC but not in bladder TCC.

Hypermethylation of other loci (RARB, DAPK, E-cadherin and RASSF1A) was associated with increased tumour stage, but only RASSF1A appears to be associated with tumour grade.

Comment

The mechanism by which aberrant methylation occurs in tumours is not known. However, once it has occurred, its role in silencing tumour suppressor genes is well

Table 14.2 Frequency of methylation at cytosine–guanine dinucleotide (CpG) islands in TCC

	GSTP1	**hMLH1**	**hMSH2**	**RARB**	**DAPK**	**p16**	**p14**	**E-cadherin**	**MGMT**	**RASSF1A**	**MINT31**
Bladder											
no.	82	117	117	94	106	102	93	101	93	106	117
no. met	0	1	0	23	8	9	7	61	9	57	1
% met	0	1	0	24	8	9	8	60	10	54	1
UTTs											
no.	163	163	163	159	162	158	161	152	153	159	163
no. met	0	19	0	59	8	34	20	120	13	100	24
% met	0	12	0	37	5	22	12	79	8	63	15
χ *P**		0002		038		01		002			0001
Total											
no.	245	280	280	253	268	260	254	253	246	265	280
no. met	0	20	0	82	16	43	27	181	22	157	25
% met	0	7	0	32	6	17	11	72	9	59	9

UTT, upper tract tumour; no., number of successfully assessed tumours; no. met, number methylated for each island in that TCC population; % met, percentage methylated for each island in that TCC population.
*The methylation at each locus in bladder and UTT is compared using χ^2 test (significant *P*-values are shown).
Source: Catto *et al.* (2005).

recognized. If aberrant methylation could be reversed, normal functioning of the gene should in theory be restored. This certainly offers a promising treatment strategy, which deserves further investigation.

The observation that methylation is seen more frequently in invasive disease may also be of use in the future as a means of genotyping an individual patient's tumour, thereby enabling the clinician to choose the most appropriate treatment and follow-up specific for that patient. However, further confirmatory studies are needed before the data can be used clinically.

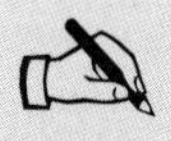

Vaccina virus-mediated p53 gene therapy for bladder cancer in an orthotopic murine model

Fodor I, Timiryasova T, Denes B, Yoshida J, Ruckle H, Lilly M. *J Urol* 2005; **173**: 604–9

BACKGROUND. Over the last few years, our understanding of the genetic basis of many cancers has increased exponentially. However, the conversion of this knowledge to clinical application is still in its infancy. Targeted monoclonal antibodies are already

in clinical use, but gene therapy has been hampered by problems of delivery. Recombinant viruses are an attractive vector for the insertion of specific DNA into cells, and much research has been focused in this area. Advanced TCCs have been shown to have mutations in their *p53* gene. This has the effect of limiting cell apoptosis and decreasing the efficacy of chemotherapy and radiotherapy treatments. If the tumour could be infected with a virus that would express normal p53 protein, it may in theory be more susceptible to such treatments.

Interpretation. Several viral vectors have been used to infect bladder TCC, but infection rates have been limited due to the urothelium not expressing viral receptors and the natural glycosaminoglycan (GAG) barrier of the bladder. The vaccinia virus has a rapid and wide range of infection and is also efficient at expressing inserted genes. This preliminary *in vitro* study of the effects of a p53-expressing vaccinia viral vector were encouraging, showing a 50% expression of p53 in cultured cells. This was then used on a live *in vivo* mouse model. The mice were inoculated with a bladder cancer cell line and treated intravesically with a single dose of p53-expressing vaccinia virus. The results between the p53-infected mice and control virus-infected mice were the same (36 days' survival), but not when compared with a control population of mice (21 days). Only limited expression of the *p53* gene was seen in those tumours that had been exposed to the p53-expressing vaccinia virus.

Comment

The *in vivo* results of this study suggest that it is the virus vector and not the contents of the vector that are producing a difference in survival in this experiment. It is not clear why this is, although direct viral lysis and immune surveillance would be likely causes. With this in mind, viral instillation may be a promising intravesical treatment regardless of the insert of the viral vector, and may complement existing treatments such as intravesical bacillus Calmette–Guéérin (BCG) instillation.

Conclusion

Therefore, despite the huge advances in technology and the ever-increasing body of literature, the search for a cure for cancer remains elusive. In the field of prostate cancer, there are a number of fundamental challenges facing the scientist. These include the multifocal nature of the disease, heterogeneity between different tumour foci and the inherent difficulties in accurately obtaining fresh tissue samples without the help of expensive techniques such as laser microcapture dissection. Even the seemingly straightforward question as to which genes are responsible is not easily answered to the same degree as in other cancers such as RCC. Nevertheless, it may be more important to focus efforts on identifying high-risk cases and studying progression to hormone resistance. By preventing such progression, the concept of cure may become redundant if long-term control can be achieved.

On the other hand, with regard to RCC, basic scientific research has led to the development of novel molecular therapies that are now being assessed in phase III trials. Further work is being done to characterize further the precise pathways.

The potential for the success of gene therapy and antisense oligonucleotide technology is exciting, but many more *in vivo* studies need to be done and delivery systems refined before these techniques can be transferred to the patient.

References

1. van Gils MP, Stenman UH, Schalken JA, Schroder FH, Luider TM, Lilja H, Bjartell A, Hamdy FC, Pettersson KS, Bischoff R, Takalo H, Nilsson O, Mulders PF, Bangma CH. Innovations in serum and urine markers in prostate cancer: current European research in the P-Mark project; *Eur Urol* 2005; **48**(6): 1031–41.
2. Lee MV, Fong EM, Singer FR, Guenette RS. Bisphosphonate treatment inhibits the growth of prostate cancer cells. *Cancer Res* 2001; **61**: 2602–8.
3. Corey E, Brown LG, Quinn JE, Poot M, Roudier MP, Higano CS, Vessella RL. Zoledronic acid exhibits inhibitory effects on osteoblastic and osteolytic metastases of prostate cancer. *Clin Cancer Res* 2003; **9**: 295–306.
4. Saad F, Gleason DM, Murray R, Tchekmedyian S, Venner P, Lacombe L, Chin JL, Vinholes JJ, Goas JA, Chen B; Zoledronic Acid Prostate Cancer Study Group. A randomized, placebo-controlled trial of zoledronic acid in patients with hormone refractory metastatic prostate carcinoma. *J Natl Cancer Inst* 2002; **94**: 1458–68.
5. Jackson MW, Roberts JS, Heckford SE, Ricciardelli C, Stahl J, Choong C, Horsfall DJ, Tilley WD. A potential autocrine role for vascular endothelial growth factor in prostate cancer. *Cancer Res* 2002; **62**(3): 854–59. Erratum in: *Cancer Res* 2002; **62**(7): 2200.
6. Huggins C, Hodges CV. Studies of prostatic cancer: I. Effect of castration, estrogen, and androgen injections on serum phosphatases in metastatic carcinoma of the prostate. *Cancer Res* 1941; **1**: 293–7.
7. Schellhammer PF, Venner P, Haas GP, Small EJ, Nieh PT, Seabaugh DR, Patterson AL, Klein E, Wajsman Z, Furr B, Chen Y, Kolvenbag GJ. Prostate specific antigen decreases after withdrawal of antiandrogen therapy with bicalutamide or flutamide in patients receiving combined androgen blockade. *J Urol* 1997; **157**(5): 1731–5.
8. de Jong JS, van Deist PJ, van der Valk P, Baak JP. Expression of growth factors, growth-inhibiting factors and their receptors in invasive breast cancer II: correlations with proliferation and angiogenesis. *J Pathol* 1998; **184**: 53–7.
9. Karnes WE Jr, Weller SG, Adjei PN, Kottke TJ, Glenn KS, Gores GJ, Kaufmann SH. Inhibition of epidermal growth factor receptor kinase induces protease-dependent apoptosis in human colon cancer cells. *Gastroenterology* 1998; **114**: 930–9.

10. Liu W, Innocenti F, Chen P, Das S, Cook EH Jr, Ratain MJ. Interethnic difference in the allelic distribution of human epidermal growth factor receptor intron 1 polymorphism. *Clin Cancer Res* 2003; **9**(3): 1009–12.

15

Cryotherapy

ULRICH WITZSCH, ANTHONY KOUPPARIS

Introduction

In a recent literature search for the term 'cryotherapy' in PubMed, 1079 articles were identified. The term was found in papers covering several specialties, including ophthalmology (retinoblastoma), surgery (liver), orthopaedics (arthritis, ankle disorders), dermatology (keratosis), neurosurgery (encephalopathy) and gynaecology (cervical cancer). Thirty-seven articles were found on prostate cryotherapy, 60 articles on renal cryotherapy and 195 articles on cryobiology. This chapter will focus on applications in urology, i.e. renal and prostate.

Cryoablation of the prostate, as primary therapy for adenocarcinoma and as salvage therapy in cases of remission, is an established procedure for the treatment of localized prostate cancer. In Europe, the percentage of procedures performed in relation to all procedures performed for localized prostate cancer is less than 1%. Approximately 30 centres have been established for the latest (third-generation) technology; the low number of centres in Europe may be due to the fact that in most countries there is no proper reimbursement. An important publication in 2005 was the positive statement issued by the National Institute for Health and Clinical Excellence (NICE) for both primary (www.nice.org.uk/IPG145guidance) and salvage (www.nice.org.uk/IPG119guidance) cryotherapy. However, although both have important implications for the further development of cryoablation of the prostate, these two papers will not be discussed in detail here.

Cryotherapy for renal tumours adheres to the principle of tumour excision with a wide margin. More recently, new ablative technologies have also provided other management options for patients with small renal masses.

The final papers in this chapter present outcome data for these new ablative techniques. The use of magnetic resonance imaging (MRI) is examined as an imaging modality to guide percutaneous cryotherapy and also as a follow-up technique after percutaneous radiofrequency (PRF) ablation of renal cell carcinoma (RCC). The last paper presents the 3-year follow-up data from a laparoscopic cryoablation programme.

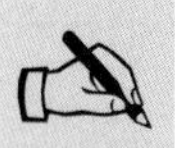

The molecular basis of cryosurgery

Baust JG, Gage AA. *BJU Int* 2005; **95**, 1187–91

BACKGROUND. It has been known for more than a century that freezing and thawing are the destructive forces in cryosurgery. The role of apoptosis and its induction remains unclear. This paper describes possible modifications of the freeze–thaw cycle to intensify these effects.

INTERPRETATION. Cell destruction in cryosurgery is induced by intracellular ice, its shear forces while thawing, and water inflow from extracellular into intracellular space. The failure of the microcirculation also adds to cell kill. Apoptosis is recognized in the peripheral zone of freezing where moderate temperatures are achieved. This can happen at any time from hours to days in experimental settings. The central zone of freezing is characterized by coagulative necrosis, whereas the peripheral zone is oedematous and heterogeneous compared with dead cells, surviving cells and apoptotic cells. Close to the probe/needle, the cooling rate is high. In the periphery it is lower and so the rate of creating intracellular ice is reduced. Nevertheless, a deleterious effect of slow cooling rate is recognized, but for practical reasons the cooling rate should be as fast as possible. A tissue temperature of between –40°C and –50°C is definitely lethal. Duration of freezing should be longer than 5 min although no exact definition can be given. Thawing should be as slow as possible to allow formation of big ice crystals, which create greater shear forces. Repetitive freeze–thaw cycles are necessary especially in prostate cancer. Increased time between freezing cycles increases the chance of post-thaw cell death. Temperature monitoring and imaging of ice formation are essential. MRI might provide better imaging in the future. Limiting the side effects but freezing the entire prostate is the challenge in cryosurgery of the prostate. Additional administration of chemotherapeutic drugs either systemically or locally during thawing might optimize the lethal effect. Due to post-operative microcirculation failure concentrations might remain high.

Comment

This paper provides a good summary of the biological effects of cryosurgery. It explains why European centres tend to have better results when using longer freezing times and do not speed up thawing by actively warming the tissue. The fact that the influence of freezing speed is still controversial **1** leads to the conclusion that more research is needed. Although the aim of the paper is to suggest a plan to allow optimization of apoptosis induction, only trends and potential strategies are given.

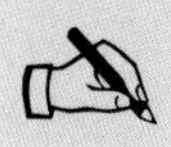

Eiskalter Zelltod, Kryotherapie der Prostata—aktueller Stand

Witzsch U. *Uro-News* 2005; **6**: 48–55

BACKGROUND. Present status of cryoablation of the prostate from a German perspective is shown.

INTERPRETATION. Historically, results show increased effectiveness and reduced side effects with improving technological development and standardization of the procedure. The placement of needles is started 5 mm apart from the capsule with 1 cm distance between the needles.

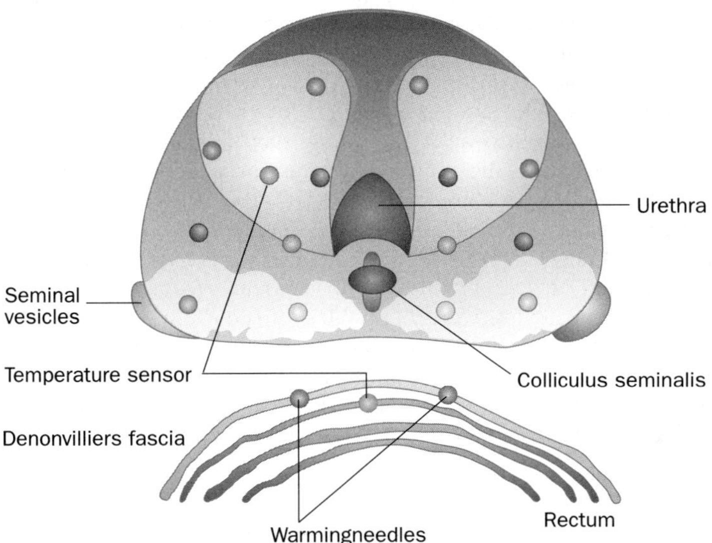

Fig. 15.1 Active rectal wall protection needles are used as described by Cytron *et al.* |**2**|. Freezing is defined by keeping the temperature for 10 min after reaching target temperature. Thawing is done passively and then actively when a plateau is reached. Pull back is performed if the prostate is longer than 35 mm. Source: Witzsch (2005).

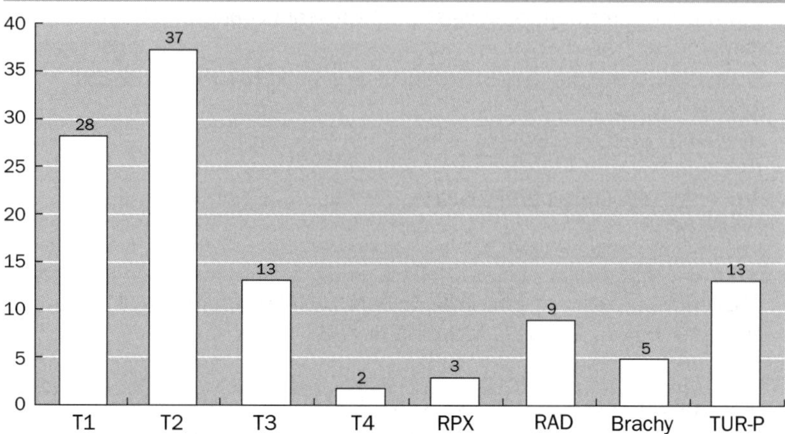

Fig. 15.2 Tumour stages and pre-treatments. Source: Witzsch (2005).

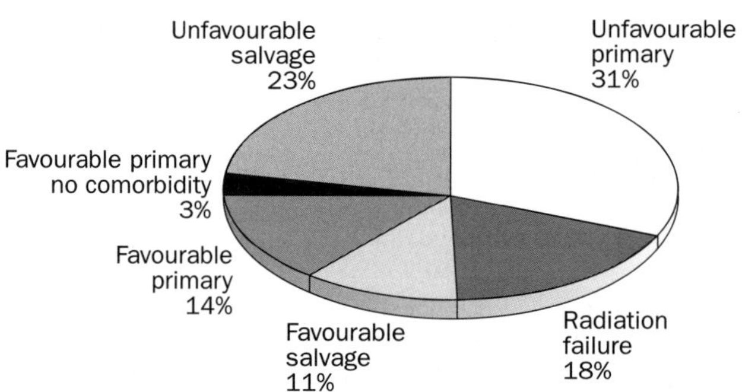

Fig. 15.3 Distribution of the clinical T1 and T2 stages after primary and salvage therapy. Source: Witzsch (2005).

The prostate-specific antigen (PSA) results are demonstrated in Table 15.1 below.

There were no major complications. Transurethral resection of the prostate (TURP) was necessary in 15% 6 weeks after the cryoablation. Fifty-four per cent of the patients suffered post-operative macroscopic haematuria, which ceased the next day without requiring any special intervention.

Table 15.1 Prostate-specific antigen (PSA) results

PSA, *n* = 80	**<0.1 ng/ml**	**0.1–0.5 ng/ml**	**>0.5 ng/ml**
3 months	50%	12%	38%
12 months	34%	13%	53%
24 months	42%	29%	29%

Source: Witzsch (2005).

The cryotherapy training programme consists of a workshop, hands-on training, nurses' training, proctoring and re-proctoring.

Comment

This paper proves that a standardized protocol and technique led to good results even when there is a negative patient selection.

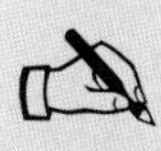

Managing the complications of prostate cryosurgery

Ahmed S, Davies J. *BJU Int* 2005; **95**: 480–1

BACKGROUND. Cryotherapy has developed significantly over the last few decades. Further acceptance of the procedure may be influenced by the impact on quality of life caused by complications.

INTERPRETATION. Stress incontinence (defined by 'using pads') will occur in approximately 5% of primary and 10% of salvage patients. Treatment can include pelvic floor exercises and the injection of bulking agents, as well as artificial sphincters and urinary diversion in rare cases. Erectile dysfunction is most common in cryosurgery of the prostate due to damage of the cavernosal nerves and influence of arterial blood flow. Recovery might occur in 13–34% of patients with the use of standard available therapies for erectile dysfunction. Nerve-sparing techniques should be considered as experimental. Urethral sloughing is caused by necrosis of the prostatic urethra and has been reduced with the inauguration of transurethral warming devices. If sloughing or lower urinary tract symptoms occur and are sufficiently bothersome, TURP might be considered, although it can be technically difficult and with high rates of incontinence. The rate of urethro-rectal fistulas has decreased with the use of transrectal ultrasound (TRUS) and thermocouples. If they occur, antibiotics should be given and urinary as well as faecal diversion considered. Conservative treatment should be attempted because surgical repair might be complex and fail, especially in post-radiation patients. Perineal pain may occur in 0.4–11% of these cases with a higher risk after radiation therapy failure. Non-steroidal anti-inflammatory drugs and warm baths as well as nitroglycerine suppositories may be considered. Urethral or bladder neck strictures due to scarring are rare and need transurethral intervention. Penile numbness occurs in up to 10% but, on the whole, tends to resolve spontaneously.

Comment

A helpful summary of possible complications and their management. Even though the authors have considerable experience in the management of complications after cryoablation of the prostate, it is odd that the avoidance of urinary tract infection by suprapubic catheter (SPC), perioperative antibiotic prophylaxis and repetitive urine cultures is not mentioned. Also it is questionable whether rectal manipulations are allowed or strictly should be avoided due to the higher risk of fistula creation, especially in radiation therapy failures.

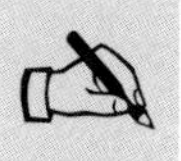

Current status of local salvage therapies following radiation failure for prostate cancer

Touma N, Izawa J, Chin J. *J Urol* 2005; **173**: 373–9

BACKGROUND. Failure of radiation therapy ranges from 15% to 25% in low-risk patients, from 35% to 48% in intermediate-risk patients and from 62% to 65% in high-risk patients. Risk is assessed by PSA, Gleason grade and clinical stage. A literature search was undertaken to compare outcomes and complications of salvage radical prostatectomy and salvage cryoablation of the prostate.

INTERPRETATION. PSA nadir below 0.5 ng/ml, time to PSA nadir >24 months and PSA doubling time >6 months seem to be predictors for absence of distance metastasis in radiation failures. Severe comorbidity, life expectancy <10 years and PSA (initial and post-radiation) above 10 ng/ml are relative contraindications for salvage radical prostatectomy. Salvage cystoprostatectomy has no benefit in survival. There is no consensus regarding pelvic lymph node dissection due to increased comorbidity (lower extremity oedema) and questionable outcome benefit to patients. These results are correlated with rectal injury rates of between 0% and 50% and incontinence rates of between 0% and 80%. Modern cryotherapy has been performed safely as a salvage procedure. Outcomes are not easy to judge because there is no clear definition of failure. Post-cryotherapy presence of vital benign tissue is no predictor for the outcome. Even though the follow-up periods are short, results so far have been good, with positive biopsy rates of between 14% and 37%. Complication rates of salvage cryoablation are higher than those of primary cases. Incontinence rates range from 9% to 83%, erectile dysfunction is mostly prevalent, and the fistula rate can be anything between 0% and 11%. Duration and extension of freezing correlates with side effects. Three-dimensional transrectal ultrasound can facilitate probe placement, with a possible reduction of side effects. Salvage brachytherapy (BT) leads to a no evidence of disease (NED) rate of 34% in 5 years. Incontinence rate was 24% and TURP was necessary in 14% of the patients. Salvage radical prostatectomy has the best NED rate at 5 years, but follow-up in the cryotherapy series is mostly short so 5-year data are not yet available. BT seems to be less effective. Side effects are much more common in radical prostatectomy than in cryotherapy. Incontinence seems to be least prevalent in salvage BT, even though the database is still small.

Comment

This paper shows promising results for salvage cryotherapy in radiation failure patients. Side effects are much less severe than in radical prostatectomy. Salvage cryotherapy is a local treatment option for radiation failures, even if the life expectancy is less than 10 years. Reduced comorbidity gives a positive outcome–side effect ratio. It would have been beneficial if the protocols used had been better described.

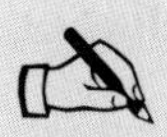

Prostate cryotherapy: more questions than answers

Merrick G, Wallner K, Butler W. *Urology* 2005; **66**: 9–15

BACKGROUND. Because of the absence of prospective randomized trials, comparing the efficacy and safety of local treatments for localized prostate cancer remains controversial. Radical prostatectomy (RP), external beam radiation therapy (EBRT) and BT represent universally accepted local approaches. Cryotherapy is also a potential additional treatment option. Tatsutani demonstrated that cell death is unlikely above –20°C and that cells which are not completely destroyed by initial freezing to –20°C are killed in a second freeze cycle. Recent developments in cryotechnology (17G gas-driven needles) facilitate a more conformal approach. Long-term quality of life and patient outcome data will need another 5 years before they can be interpreted. The answers to the questions regarding optimization, local control, dosimetry and patient selection should then be able to be addressed.

INTERPRETATION. Urethral preservation is essential for reduction of comorbidity. Recent studies have shown that the mean distance of cancer foci from the urethra is 3 mm, and 45–66% of prostate cancers are found within 1–5 mm of the urethra. Urethral warming spares tissue from necrosis at a distance of 5 mm. This might mean that in 84% of patients cancer is also spared. The optimal warming regimen is unknown. Further investigations regarding urethral tissue preservation versus cancer eradication are needed. It is questionable if cryotherapy is an absolute ablative technique when post-operative biopsies show viable benign tissue in 45–70% of cases, with cancer cells demonstrated in only 13–18% of post-operative biopsies. Modifications (perhaps more probes) are needed to increase the percentage of total ablated areas.

Because apex and seminal vesicles are in the periphery of second-generation iceballs recurrences are most likely to be found there. Pull back and increased number of needles in third generation might lead to better results. The hyperechoic edge of the iceball does not visualize the zone of killing. To ensure a sufficient frozen margin around the prostate (99% of extra capsular growth is within 5 mm) precise temperature monitoring is required. For patients with a high risk of lymph node involvement, studies on synergistic effects and comorbidity of neoadjuvant androgen deprivation and pelvic radiotherapy are warranted.

Definitions of biochemical free survival after cryotherapy vary between centres. A cut-off at 0.4 ng/ml or less should be adopted as a standard definition. The relative lack of influence of risk groups in biochemical outcome remains unexplained. The correlation of rising PSA after EBRT and distant growth implies that local therapies might not cure salvage patients. Older studies on salvage cryotherapy showed a biopsy proven local control in 25%. Recent studies showed 59% biochemical free survival (<0.5 ng/ml). PSA trends in the first 30 months after radiation therapy might be misleading: eight patients after BT with rising PSA levels of 2.6–8.4 ng/ml were positive on post-treatment biopsies; all of them refused further therapy and their PSA level normalized to 0.2 ng/ml in time without additional therapy. This implies better definition of recurrence after EBRT by imaging and/or biochemical markers.

It is clear that recent cryosurgical technology advances have resulted in a dramatically decreased complication rate in third-generation cryosurgery compared with second and first generation. Erectile dysfunction is mostly prevalent and might regain in 13% 'without' versus 34% 'with' erectile aids.

Comment

The authors conclude that cryotherapy has not been demonstrated to be as effective or less morbid than RP, EBRT or BT in treatment of localized prostate cancer. This contradicts some of the statements made in this paper and other studies published in the last year. Even so, the conclusion that this review highlights the limitations and sources of improvement in cryoablation of the prostate is questionable.

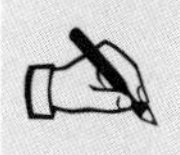

Prostate cancer: gadolinium-enhanced MR imaging at 3 weeks compared with needle biopsies 6 months after cryoablation

Donnelly SE, Donnelly BJ, Saliken JC, Raber EL, Vellet AD. *Radiology* 2004; **232**: 830–3

BACKGROUND. The aim of this paper was to determine if non-enhancing tissue on gadolinium-enhanced magnetic resonance (MR) images obtained 3 weeks after cryoablation of the prostate helps to reliably and accurately predict non-viable cryoablated tissue at 6-month biopsy. Fifty-four consecutive patients with prostate cancer who underwent cryoablation were followed up prospectively. Fifty-one underwent gadolinium-enhanced MR imaging at 3 weeks (three had gadolinium allergy); 49 underwent biopsy at 6 months (three refused and two had other primary malignancies); and all had PSA tests at 6 weeks, 3 months, and every 3 months thereafter. MR images were evaluated and scored according to the degree of signal void and were correlated with the 6-month biopsy reports and, to a lesser degree, PSA levels. The biopsy reports were examined for the presence or absence of cancerous tissue, viable tissue, and non-viable tissue. A one-way analysis of variance was used for statistical and regression analyses.

INTERPRETATION. The correlation of MR imaging scores with PSA levels and MR imaging scores with biopsy findings resulted in *P*-values of 0.337 and 0.780, respectively. A slight statistically significant trend existed for the relation of biopsy results with PSA levels, with a *P*-value of 0.041, which was expected. Findings of post-operative gadolinium-enhanced MR imaging are not predictive of 6-month biopsy results or follow-up PSA levels.

Comment

This study was performed after second-generation cryotherapy. A modified technique such as a 1.5T imager and rectal coil might have improved the results, but this is not discussed (a 0.5T imager and body coil were used). No absolute numbers

Table 15.2 Results of statistical analysis

Test	No. of patients	Response variable	Independent variable	*P*-value
ANOVA	46	MR imaging score	Biopsy results (1, 0, –1 scores)	0.934
Mann-Whitney	46	MR imaging score	Biopsy results (0 and 1 with –1 score)	0.780
Mann-Whitney	51	PSA level	MR imaging score	0.337
χ^2	49	PSA level	Biopsy results	0.041

ANOVA, one-way analysis of variance.
Source: Donnelly *et al.* (2004).

for vital prostate tissue and vital cancer are mentioned. Again, this study shows a demand for better imaging in correlation to cryoablation.

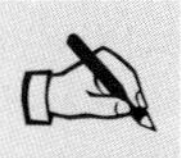

The effects of intentional cryoablation and radio frequency ablation of renal tissue involving the collecting system in a porcine model

Janzen N, Perry K, Han K, *et al. J Urol* 2005; **173**: 1368–74

Background. Cryoablation and RF ablation (RFA) of renal tissue are two evolving techniques allowing minimal invasive treatment of renal masses. The effects on peripheral and deep renal tissue were demonstrated.

Interpretation. Eleven female farm pigs were used in this study. RFA,17G needle cryoablation and 3-mm cryoprobe ablation were assessed. Cryoprobes were placed either with 4-MHz transcutaneous or 8-MHz laparoscopic guidance. Cryoprobes were placed at an edge of an individual calyx without puncturing the collecting system. Two freeze (10 min)–thaw (5 min) cycles were applied. Cryolesions showed uniform coagulative necrosis. RFA lesions showed haemorrhagic and ischaemic necrosis. Cryoablation showed preservation of the collecting system, whereas RFA demonstrated rarely preserved collecting systems. Using 17G needles, the diameters of the cryolesions were 2.0, 2.6 and 3.8 cm with one, three and five needles, whereas one and two 3-mm probes created 2.5- and 4.5-cm lesions respectively. All cryolesions were homogeneous. Laparoscopic ultrasound (US) slightly underestimated the lesion size, whereas transcutaneous US under- and overestimated lesion size in pathology. Deep areas in the parenchyma might be incompletely ablated, so only peripheral kidney tumours should be treated.

Comment

Cryoablation seems beneficial versus RFA with regard to the homogeneity of the lesion and preservation of the collecting system. There was no significant difference in efficacy of 17G needles versus 3-mm probes. Preservation of the collecting system is only prevalent in cryoablation. These data gives hints for differential indications. Deep parenchymal masses are better treated surgically. RFA might be limited only to very small lesions with uncertain outcome.

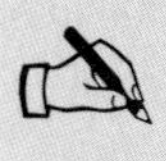

Laparoscopic partial nephrectomy versus laparoscopic cryoablation for the small renal tumour

Desai M, Aron M, Gill I. *Urology* 2005; **66**(Suppl 5A): 23–8

BACKGROUND. Laparoscopic partial nephrectomy and laparoscopic cryoablation are both options for minimally invasive nephron-sparing surgery. Morbidity and oncological outcome should be compared. The main difference is the removal of tissue in partial nephrectomy compared with local ablation in cryosurgery.

INTERPRETATION. Patients who underwent partial nephrectomy had double the blood loss and were 5 years younger overall than cryoablation patients. Recurrence was seen in 0.6% of the partial nephrectomy group versus 3% in the cryoablation group.

There were three deaths in the cryoablation group versus none in the operative group. Creatinine was slightly raised in both groups post-operatively. Mean follow-up was 6 months in the partial nephrectomy group versus 25 months in the cryoablation group. Laparoscopic cryoablation is judged to be simpler than laparoscopic partial nephrectomy.

Comment

Two laparoscopic techniques are compared. Both are not standard in nephron-sparing surgery. It is questionable if both groups are really similar owing to differences in numbers and follow-up. Also, the cryoablative group appears to be biased as a result of a negative selection caused by two patients dying of metastatic disease. Cryoablation seems to produce less morbidity but also seems to be less effective.

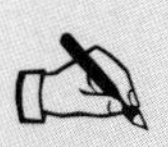

A cost comparison of nephron-sparing surgical techniques for renal tumour

Lotan Y, Cadeddu JA. *BJU Int* 2005; **95**: 1039–42

BACKGROUND. Although open surgery is still widely used for renal tumours, nephron-sparing approaches to managing small renal masses have been shown to yield similar tumour control rates as radical nephrectomy. Laparoscopic approaches for partial nephrectomy (LPN) clearly offer reduced treatment-related morbidity and similar outcomes to date, compared with open surgery. Furthermore, ablative technologies, e.g. PRF and cryotherapy, also offer promising alternatives to surgical approaches. This study recognizes that new technologies are frequently associated with higher costs, often resulting in close scrutiny by hospitals and third-party payers, and examines the real costs associated with open surgery—LPN and PRF in consecutive patients undergoing nephron-sparing surgery at their institution.

INTERPRETATION. The authors reviewed the charts and costs for 46 patients undergoing nephron-sparing partial nephrectomy from March 2003 to March 2004.

Table 15.3 Complications

	Laparoscopic partial nephrectomy	Laparoscopic renal cryoablation	*P*-value
Intra-operative	*n* = 8 (5.2%)	*n* = 1 (1.1%)	0.1
	5 renal haemorrhage	1 pleural injury	
	1 ureteral injury		
	1 inferior epigastric artery injury		
	1 tumour capsule breach		
Post-operative (during hospital stay)	*n* = 16 (11.1%)	*n* = 3 (3.3%)	0.54
	3 atelectasis	1 pneumothorax	
	1 pleural effusion	1 prolonged ileus	
	1 pneumonia	1 atelectasis	
	2 pulmonary embolism		
	2 haemorrhage requiring transfusion		
	2 prolonged ileus		
	1 atrial fibrillation		
	1 gluteal compartment syndrome		
	1 urinoma		
	1 internal jugular vein thrombus		
	1 rhabdomyolysis		
Late complications (after hospital discharge)	*n* = 25 (16.3%)	*n* = 2 (2.2%)	0.01
	1 wound dehiscence	1 pneumonia	
	3 haemia	1 perirenal haematoma	
	8 renal haemorrhage*		
	4 urinary leak		
	1 perinephric abscess		
	2 deep vein thrombosis		
	1 pulmonary embolism		
	1 delayed nephrectomy†		
	2 congestive heart failure		
	2 pneumonia		
Open conversions, *n*	1	0	

*Of the 8 patients, 5 required blood transfusion only and 3 required percutaneous angioembolization.
†Patient required nephrectomy because of expanding haematoma.
Source: Desai *et al.* (2005).

Clinical characteristics, operative techniques, and radiographic and pathological information were recorded. Detailed information on costs was also obtained. The hospital stay was significantly shorter for PRF than with LPN and open surgery. PRF was statistically less costly than LPN and open partial nephrectomy (OPN). There was no significant difference in cost between LPN and open surgery. Surgical supply costs were significantly higher for LPN and PRF than open surgery. LPN had less than one-third

Table 15.4 The patient and tumour characteristics, and the cost components for nephron-sparing procedures

Variable	PRF	LPN	OPN
n patients mean (SD)	16	14	16
Age, years	66 (10.9)	48.9 (19.2)	58.1 (11.3)
Tumour size, cm	2.63 (0.74)	2.18 (1.01)	3.90 (1.28)
Stay, days	0.5 (0.63)	1.86 (0.77)	4.94 (1.12)
Cost components (US$)			
Total	4454 (938)	7013 (934)	7767 (1605)
Surgical supplies	1400	2310 (799)	238 (273)
Operating room	95 (193)	1139 (339)	1397 (405)
Room and board	145 (184)	645 (344)	1978 (658)
Pharmacy	134 (79)	576 (220)	837 (196)
Laboratory/pathology	193 (130)	609 (185)	950 (345)
Radiology	209 (114)	21 (41)	228 (175)
Professional fees	1482	1395	1274

All differences were significant at $P < 0.001$, Kruskal–Wallis test, except professional fees, and as stated in the text.

Source: Lotan *et al.* (2005).

of the room and board costs of open surgery. Decreases in room and board were also associated with lower pharmacy and laboratory costs.

Comment

This is an American study, and as such the costs may differ from the National Health Service (NHS) in the UK. However, financial issues are becoming increasingly important in the UK, especially with the well-publicized hospital budget overspends. The present study indicates that PRF is significantly less costly than LPN and OPN. Although LPN is associated with significantly higher surgical supply costs than open procedures, this is compensated for by the shorter hospital stay. When new technologies have been evaluated for safety and efficacy, data from such studies are useful when justifying their use to those in charge of hospital budgets.

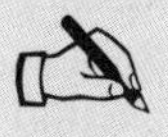

Pain control requirements for percutaneous ablation of renal tumors: cryoablation versus radiofrequency ablation—initial observations

Allaf ME, Varkarakis IM, Bhayani SB, Inagaki T, Kavoussi LR, Solomon SB. *Radiology* 2005; **237**: 366–70

BACKGROUND. Thermal ablative technologies, such as RF ablation and cryoablation, provide targeted therapy for renal tumours with the objective of

improving the morbidity associated with laparoscopic and open surgery. In many cases, PRF ablation and cryoablation of renal lesions can be performed without general anaesthesia and in an outpatient setting. This study retrospectively compares pain control requirements of patients undergoing computerized tomography (CT)-guided PRF ablation with those of patients undergoing CT-guided percutaneous cryoablation of small (4-cm) renal tumours.

Interpretation. Medical records of patients who underwent RF ablation and cryoablation of renal tumours from June 2003 to February 2004, were retrospectively reviewed for clinical data, tumour characteristics, and anaesthesia information. During the study period, ten men underwent cryoablation of eleven renal lesions, and 14 patients (eleven men, four women) underwent RF ablation of 15 renal tumours. Cryoablation was associated with use of significantly less intravenous fentanyl and midazolam. No patients in the cryoablation group required any additional or alternate anaesthetics, however, in the RF group one patient required general anaesthesia, one required supplemental narcotics and sedatives, and one became apnoeic for a brief interval after receiving additional narcotics, and one patient had their treatment terminated prematurely due to excessive pain.

Comment

Increasing use of abdominal imaging has led to an increase in the detection of incidental small asymptomatic renal tumours. Open and laparoscopic partial nephrectomy requires general anaesthesia and is associated with a hospital stay. Furthermore, laparoscopic partial nephrectomy often requires a period of warm ischaemia in addition to substantial surgical skill. Percutaneous thermal ablative alternatives, such as RF ablation and cryoablation, are attractive because they circumvent many of the issues that limit current surgical approaches. The current study indicates that image-guided percutaneous cryoablation appears to require less analgesia than RF ablation. Such data may provide useful information when guiding patients toward the appropriate therapy.

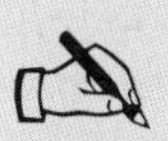

Renal tumours: MR imaging-guided percutaneous cryotherapy—initial experience in 23 patients

Silverman SG, Tuncali K, vanSonnenberg E, *et al.* *Radiology* 2005; **236**: 716–24

Background. Percutaneous thermal ablation therapies have been advocated for the treatment of small renal tumours. Several imaging modalities have been employed for thermal ablation. However, despite the fact that both US and CT are feasible, only MRI allows the procedure to be monitored in real time. This paper evaluates the use of MRI in guiding percutaneous cryotherapy of renal tumours.

Interpretation. Twenty-six renal tumours were successfully ablated, with 23 requiring only one session. Of the patients included in the study, two had a

Table 15.5 Demographics, tumour characteristics, and drug requirements of patients undergoing CT-guided RF ablation or cryoablation for the treatment of small renal tumours

Parameter	**RF ablation**	**Cryoablation**	***P*-value***
No. of patients	14	10	
No. of treatment sessions	15	11	
Age (years)			
Mean	68.1	66.5	0.86†
Range	39–86	36–84	
Sex			
Male	11	10	0.24
Female	3	0	
ASA score			
3	4	4	0.67
4	10	6	
Tumour side			
Right kidney	8	7	0.70
Left kidney	7	4	
Tumour location			
Non-central	9	5	0.69
Central	6	6	
Lesion diameter (cm)			
Mean	2.0	2.3	0.34†
Range	1.3–3.3	1.0–4.0	
No. of electrodes or cryoprobes used per session			
1	15	5	0.002
>1	0	6	
Fentanyl used (μg)			<0.001†
Mean	165	75	
Median	150	50	
Range	125–300	50–150	
Midazolam used (mg)			
Mean	2.9	1.6	0.026†
Median	2.5	1.0	
Range	1.0–6.0	1.0–5.0	

* *P*-values were calculated with Fischer exact test unless otherwise noted.
† *P*-values calculated with Student *t* test.
Source: Allaf *et al.* (2005).

post-procedure complication: haemorrhage requiring transfusion and abscess formation, which was treated with percutaneous drainage.

Comment

This study documents the author's initial experiences with MRI-guided percutaneous cryotherapy and suggests that it is a successful technique for renal tumours of the appropriate size. MRI enables the effects of the freezing process to be monitored during the procedure, which is not possible with CT-guided RF ablation. As a result, the cryoprobes can be repositioned as necessary and the operator is more confident that the tumour is treated successfully. Further advantages of MRI over CT are the ability to reliably predict the amount of tissue necrosis and also the absence of ionizing radiation. With a greater number of renal tumours being treated with percutaneous approaches, urologists need to be aware of the advantages and disadvantages of new procedures in order that they can appropriately counsel their patients. The results of longer-term follow-up studies will be interesting.

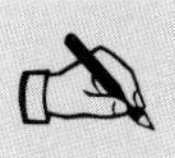

MR imaging follow-up after percutaneous radiofrequency ablation of renal cell carcinoma: findings in 18 patients during first 6 months

Merkle EM, Nour SG, Lewin JS. *Radiology* 2005; **235**: 1065–71

BACKGROUND. Data on the incidence of RCC from the United States indicate a 30% increase over the last 10 years. The majority of these cases have occurred in light of the incidental diagnosis of small localized tumours. In a similar way to open and laparoscopic surgery for such tumours, new percutaneous techniques require adequate follow-up protocols for patients. Follow-up after PRF ablation usually involves contrast-enhanced CT. However, a significant number of patients are unable to tolerate contrast agents owing to renal impairment and contrast allergy. The current study prospectively evaluates MRI findings after RF ablation of RCC.

INTERPRETATION. Eighteen patients who underwent RF ablation between 1999 and 2003 were included in the study. Their follow-up included unenhanced T2-weighted MR images and unenhanced and gadolinium-enhanced T1-weighted MR images immediately after ablation and at 2 weeks, 3 months and 6 months later. The authors found that the renal RF ablation zones increased in size in the first 2 weeks and then gradually involuted. They found that residual tumour was best demonstrated on unenhanced T2-weighted and gadolinium-enhanced T1-weighted MR images.

Comment

Many of the studies published recently on percutaneous techniques for treating small renal tumours describe initial experiences of different institutions. Follow-up protocols following open nephrectomy for RCC are well established; however, those following RF ablation are not. The current study provides important information regarding the normal appearances following RF ablation and also identifies the most appropriate MR images for detecting residual tumour.

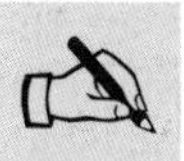

Renal cryoablation: outcomes at 3 years

Gill IS, Remer EM, Hasan WA, *et al. J Urol* 2005; **173**: 1903–7

BACKGROUND. In 1997 the authors initiated a laparoscopic renal cryoablation programme for which the 3-year results are published. Since September 1997, 115 patients have been treated; out of those, 56 have reached a minimum follow-up of 3 years.

INTERPRETATION. Indication was considered to be 4 cm or less peripheral mass of the kidney. Depending on the tumour location, retroperitoneal approach (75%) or transperitoneal approach was used. A laparoscopic ultrasound probe was used for visualization of the tumour. One 4.8-mm diameter cryoprobe was used to apply a double freeze–thaw cycle. The aim was to extend the tumour edge by 1 cm. For follow-up, MRI scans and CT-directed needle biopsies were performed at 6 months. A size reduction of 75% at 3 years was observed. Thirty-eight per cent of lesions were undetectable at 3 years. At 6 months, two out of 39 patients had biopsies that were positive for RCC. Three patients had *de novo* lesions remote to the initial location. Three-year overall survival was 89%, with cancer-specific survival of 98%. Mean creatinine levels increased from 1.2 to 1.4 mg/dl.

Comment

This study shows the feasibility of cryoablation of renal masses in a specialized centre with good results. The results seem to be nearly equivalent to results of nephron-sparing surgery in specialized centres. Even so, medium-term follow-up data are needed.

Conclusion

In 2005 it became obvious that the technological developments in the previous two decades enabled improved Joule–Thompson effect-driven probes or needles and standardized protocols |**2,3**|, which led to better results in cryoablation of the prostate than earlier liquid nitrogen-driven technology |**4**|. However, although encouraging results are reproducible and training is standardized, reimbursement and acceptance by health insurers seem to be a problem |**5**|. Several papers |**6**| demonstrate good results of salvage cryoablation of the prostate and a clear trend of possibly superior results but definitely reduced side effects in correlation with salvage radical prostatectomy; salvage radical prostatectomy must therefore be considered as second-line salvage therapy only after cryosurgery failure. Further improvements may become evident in imaging and monitoring the procedure and administration of drugs or modification of protocol for increased apoptosis induction.

The level of discussion for cryoablation of the prostate is different from that for renal cryoablation. In therapy of localized prostate cancer, the role of cryoablation and optimization of the method is discussed. Larger studies are conducted and medium- or long-term results are published. In renal cryoablation, effectiveness and standardization of protocols remains to be proven and several papers are published on early results. Some authors do treat only peripheral lesions; others are also treating hilar lesions. In general, comorbidity of cryoablation seems to be lower but oncological outcome is not clear. Between the papers, definition of freeze–thaw cycles differs considerably with respect to target temperature, time of freezing and mode of thawing (active, passive). This means that studies should be performed to evaluate the optimal protocol for renal cryoblation. There seems to be a clear trend also in renal cryoablation to use more needle-like cryoprobes rather than single thicker probes. Benefits of longer rather than shorter iceballs have not been identified.

Results from studies on minimally invasive and ablative techniques for treating renal masses are encouraging |**7**|. The observations that many small renal tumours are often incidentally detected, asymptomatic and sometimes benign in nature means that this innovative area will continue to develop. The obvious direction for further research is the confirmation of oncological efficacy with 5- and 10-year follow-up data. These results will undoubtedly form the basis of future chapters in *The Year in Urology.*

References

1. Tatsutani K, Rubinsky B, Onik G, Dahiya R. Effect of thermal variables on frozen human primary prostatic adenocarcinoma cells. *Urology* 1996; **48**: 441–7.
2. Cytron S, Paz A, Kravchick S, Shumalinski D, Moore J. Active rectal wall protection using direct transperitoneal cryo-needles for histologically proven prostate adenocarcinomas. *Eur Urol* 2003; **44**: 315–21.
3. Witzsch UKFr. Cryotherapy as primary therapy for prostate cancer. In: Kirby R, Partin A, Feneley M, Parsons J (eds). *Prostate cancer principles and practice.* London: Taylor and Francis, 2005; pp 875–80.
4. Aus G, Pileblad E, Hugosson J. Cryosurgical ablation of the prostate: 5-year follow-up of a prospective study. *Eur Urol* 2002; **42**: 133–8.
5. Thüroff S, Berges R, Blana A, Braun M, Brehmer B, Häcker A, Muschter R, Neubauer S, Witzsch U, Chaussy Ch. Energy applications in non-surgical therapies: consensus. In: Chaussy Ch, Haupt G, Jocham D, Köhrmann K, Wilbert D (eds). *Therapeutic Energy Applications in Urology Standards and Recent Developments.* Stuttgart: Thieme, 2005; pp 92–4.

6. Ahmed S, Lindsey B, Davies J. Salvage cryosurgery for locally recurrent prostate cancer following radiotherapy, *Prostate Cancer Prostatic Dis* 2005; **8**(1): 31–5.
7. Hruby G, Reisiger K, Venkathesh R, Yan Y, Landman J. Comparison of laparoscopic partial nephrectomy and laparoscopic cryoablation for renal hilar tumors. *Urology* 2006; **67**: 50–4.

16

New minimal invasive techniques in urology

EVANGELOS LIATSIKOS, JENS-UWE STOLZENBURG

Introduction

The continuing technological amelioration of engineering technology has achieved the never-ending production of instruments and minimally invasive techniques. When searching the literature, we found a plethora of very interesting and intriguing scientific papers pertaining to minimally invasive techniques in urology. Unfortunately, not all of them can be included in this 'pantheon'. The selection was based upon the originality and the clinical relevance of the manuscripts. Certainly, there could also be other original papers of extreme clinical importance not included in this chapter. We apologize in advance to their authors.

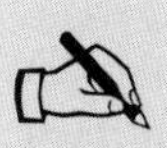

Treatment of complete staghorn stones: a prospective randomized comparison of open surgery versus percutaneous nephrolithotomy

Al-Kohlany KM, Shokeir AA, Mosbah A, *et al.* *J Urol* 2005; **173**: 469–73

BACKGROUND. Staghorn stones represent a troublesome therapeutic challenge to urologists. Currently, most borderline and partial staghorn stones are treated with percutaneous nephrolithotomy (PCNL) alone or with extracorporeal shock wave lithotripsy (ESWL). There is no consensus regarding the treatment of complete staghorn stones. Some studies have compared open surgery versus new treatment modalities. In this study, the authors examined the role of open surgery versus PCNL in the treatment of complete staghorn stones in a prospective randomized manner.

INTERPRETATION. A total of 79 patients with 88 complete staghorn stones were prospectively randomized for PCNL (43) or open surgery (45). Patients with significant residuals in both groups were subjected to ESWL on an outpatient basis. Follow-up was completed for all cases with a mean duration ± SD of 4.9 ± 2.5 months (range 3–14 months). Renal function was evaluated by ^{99m}Tc-mercaptoacetyltriglycine renogram before and after treatment in both groups. Intra-operative complications were recorded in seven patients (16.3%) in the PCNL and 17 (37.8%) in the open surgery groups, a significant difference (P <0.05). Major post-operative complications were observed in eight patients (18.6%) in the PCNL group and in 14 (31.1%) in the open surgery group, a difference of no significant value. PCNL was associated with shorter operative time (127 ± 30 vs 204 ± 31 min; P <0.001), shorter hospital stay (6.4 ± 4.2 vs 10 ± 4.2 days; P <0.001) and earlier return to work (2.5 ± 0.8 vs 4.1 ± 1 weeks; P <0.001). Both treatment groups were comparable with regard to stone-free rates at discharge home (49% vs 66%) and at follow-up (74% vs 82%). At follow-up, renal function improved or remained stable in 91% and 86.7% in the PCNL and open surgery groups respectively.

Comment

Although treatment recommendations for staghorn stones have been proposed, the preferred treatment option for such stones remains unsettled. Studies comparing open surgery with endourological procedures for the treatment of complete staghorn stones are lacking in the literature. The available reports are retrospective comparing these two treatment options in different periods with different follow-up. The present prospective study suggests that PCNL is a valuable treatment option for complete staghorn stones, with a stone-free rate approaching that of open surgery. Moreover, it has the advantages of lower morbidity, shorter operative time, shorter hospital stay and earlier return to work.

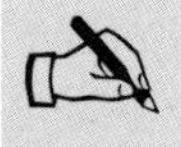

Three-dimensional planning of percutaneous renal stone surgery in a horseshoe kidney using 16-slice CT and volume-rendered movies

Ghani KR, Rintoul M, Patel U, Anson K. *J Endourol* 2005; **19**: 461–3

BACKGROUND. Horseshoe kidney is characterized by the aggregation, usually at the lower pole, of the two kidneys over the spine across the midline. Its incidence is 1 in 400–1000 births, with a slight male predominance, making it the most common renal fusion anomaly. Most patients with horseshoe kidneys are asymptomatic, but the presence of stone disease may change its clinical course and is one of its most common complications. The management and surgical indications for treating these patients follow the same criteria as for patients with normal kidneys. Minimally invasive techniques were developed in the 1980s and applied in these particular patients with good results. Percutaneous management of calculi within horseshoe kidneys can be difficult because of the abnormal renal anatomy. The main concept of this paper was to facilitate pre-operative planning and minimize intra-operative complications.

INTERPRETATION. The authors report the use of 16-slice computerized tomographic (CT) scans to obtain three-dimensional volume-rendered (VR) movies of the pelvicaliceal system and stone for planning percutaneous renal stone surgery. The movie is formatted onto a disk, which can be played on a personal computer without additional software.

Comment

Imaging methods are evolving continuously. Urologists no longer gain blunt access to the pelvicaliceal system as they did many years ago. The conventional access is gained with the aid of renal tract ultrasonography and retrograde contrast injection within the pelvicaliceal system. Lately, three-dimensional CT reconstructive techniques have been developed, ascertaining a more accurate depiction of the pelvicaliceal system for planning percutaneous procedures. The three-dimensional images provide the location, number and size of the stones, but also the anatomical configuration of both the pelvicaliceal system and surrounding structures (i.e. bowel, vessels, direction of branches and the angles between these branches). The authors suggest that this technique allows user-friendly three-dimensional planning in the operating theatre. Unlike conventional two-dimensional images, the three-dimensional VR movie provides a global appreciation for planning.

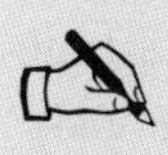

Comparison of flexible ureteroscopes: deflection, irrigant flow and optical characteristics

Abdelshehid C, Ahlering MT, Chou D, *et al. J Urol* 2005; **173**: 2017–21

BACKGROUND. New generation flexible ureteroscopes are significantly better technically than the previous generations. The reduction in tip/shaft size and the increase in deflection ability has launched their widespread application. However, there are many problems that need to be overcome, such as endoscope fragility, less than optimal optical on-camera resolution and suboptimal deflection during therapeutic instrumentation, particularly in the lower pole. The authors measured and compared the deflection, irrigation flow rates, distortion, resolution and light transmission of new generation flexible ureteroscopes.

INTERPRETATION. Multiple characteristics of five flexible ureteroscopes (ACMI DUR-8 Elite, Olympus URF-P3, Storz 11278AU1 [Flex-X], Wolf 7330.072 and Wolf 7325.172) commonly available in the market were measured and compared. Measured data included active deflection, irrigation flow rates and optical characteristics. Each ureteroscope was evaluated with an empty working channel and with various accessories. Optical characteristics, specifically resolution and distortion, were measured using test targets (Edmund Optics, Barrington, NJ, USA). Light transmission was also measured from the ureteroscope tip at 50% and 100% intensity. All five flexible ureteroscopes were tested in a laboratory setting using a Storz OR 1 system to capture the images. For all five ureteroscopes, the angle of deflection was most impaired by a 365-μm laser fibre probe and least impaired by a 2.2-Fr nitinol basket. Among all five ureteroscopes, irrigation flow rate was most impaired with a 3.0-Fr basket and least impaired with 200-μm laser fibre. The Wolf 7325.172 had the highest observed resolution of 25.39 lines/mm, and the Wolf 7330.072 had the lowest distortion at 11.9%. The Karl Storz Flex-X and the ACMI DUR-8 Elite had the highest light output at 374 and 364 mV respectively.

Comment

The continuous evolution of endoscopic technology will have to further improve scopes in the future, thereby facilitating the introduction of flexible ureteroscopy into the everyday practice of urologists worldwide. In the present study, the authors have concluded that the various flexible ureteroscopes differ with regard to flow rates as well as degree of deflection with either an empty or an occupied working channel. The Wolf flexible ureteroscope with a slightly larger working channel and a fused quartz bundle provided superior flow and better optical performance. However, the greatest amount of tip deflection and highest light output were found in the ACMI and Karl Storz flexible ureteroscopes.

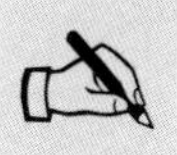

Shock wave lithotripsy success determined by skin-to-stone distance on computed tomography

Pareek G, Hedican SP, Lee FT Jr, Nakada SY. *Urology* 2005; **66**: 941–4

BACKGROUND. The aim of this study was to evaluate whether the skin-to-stone distance (SSD), body mass index (BMI) and Hounsfield unit (HU) density can be used as independent predictors of stone-free (SF) status after shock wave lithotripsy (SWL) of lower pole kidney stones. No studies have evaluated the SSD by non-contrast-enhanced computerized tomography (NCCT) as a predictor of SWL success. Studies have suggested that the BMI and HU density of urinary calculi on NCCT may predict the SF rate after SWL.

INTERPRETATION. The radiographs of 64 patients with lower pole kidney stones measuring 0.5–1.5 cm on NCCT treated with SWL (DoliS lithotripter) were reviewed from March 2000 to April 2004. The average SSD was calculated by measuring three distances from the centre of the stone to the skin (0°, 45° and 90° angles) on NCCT. The BMI and HU density were determined, and chemical analysis was performed on all stones. Radiographic assessment of the kidneys, ureter and bladder at 6 weeks categorized patients into the SF or residual stone group. Logistic regression was fitted, using SSD, BMI and HU density as predictors, to assess the SF rates after SWL. Of 64 patients, 30 were SF and 34 had residual stones. The mean SSD was 8.12 ± 1.74 cm for the SF group versus 11.53 ± 1.89 cm for the residual stone group (P <0.01). Logistic regression analysis revealed only SSD to be a significant predictor of outcome (odds ratio 0.32; 95% confidence interval [CI] 0.29–0.35; P <0.01). An SSD greater than 10 cm predicted treatment failure.

Comment

NCCT has become the radiographic modality of choice in the management of urinary stone disease. Recently, many studies have attempted to correlate the radiographic findings on NCCT with treatment success. Various studies have demonstrated that the consistency, size, shape, location and attenuation value of urinary calculi measured in HU density and BMI may be predictors of SWL success, as determined by the SF rate. In an effort to characterize better the predictability of SF rates after SWL, the SSD's effect on the success of SWL was thus analysed. In addition, the BMI and the attenuation value of calculi (HU density) were measured in the hope of predicting the SF rate after SWL. The authors attempted to formulate a predictive model of SWL outcome, based on the SSD, BMI and HU density, to counsel patients better on the various treatment options (SWL or endourology) for lower pole kidney stones. The authors conclude that the SSD may predict the outcome of lower pole kidney stones after SWL. SWL in patients with an SSD greater than 10 cm is likely to fail. The use of the SSD may be transferable to the treatment of all urinary stones, regardless of location.

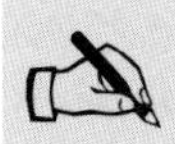

Dismembered percutaneous endopyeloplasty: a new procedure

Sharp DS, Desai MM, Molina WR, *et al.* *J Endourol* 2005; **19**: 210–17

BACKGROUND. Minimally invasive alternatives have largely replaced open pyeloplasty as the initial treatment of choice in most patients with primary and secondary ureteropelvic junction obstruction. Various techniques currently available include percutaneous endopyelotomy, retrograde ureteroscopic endopyelotomy, cutting wire balloon incision techniques and laparoscopic pyeloplasty. The authors have recently developed a novel technique of percutaneous non-dismembered endopyeloplasty (Fenger type). Here, they extend this transrenal technique further and report percutaneous dismembered endopyeloplasty (Anderson–Hynes type).

INTERPRETATION. In five pigs with unilateral ureteropelvic junction (UPJ) obstruction created 3–6 weeks earlier, percutaneous dismembered endopyeloplasty was performed. Percutaneous transrenal access to the UPJ was obtained, and the UPJ was completely dismembered from within the renal pelvis through the solitary percutaneous tract. The dismembered proximal ureter was circumferentially mobilized and, in two animals, the UPJ segment was completely excised and removed. A spatulated end-to-end endopyeloplasty anastomosis (Anderson–Hynes) was created transrenally with 5–10 interrupted sutures using a novel nephroscopic suturing device (Sew-Right SR-5; LSI Solutions, Rochester, NY, USA). In two animals, the entire percutaneous procedure was performed with CO_2 insufflation instead of fluid irrigation.

The technique was developed in three pigs. Subsequently, two pigs were treated and sacrificed at 2 and 5 weeks. All UPJs were dismembered successfully, and a precisely sutured mucosa-to-mucosa anastomosis was created. Intra-operative bleeding was negligible, and the operative time ranged from 3 to 5 h, with the majority of the time dedicated to transrenal retroperitoneal dissection of the scarred, fibrotic UPJ. Carbon dioxide insufflation was efficacious because it minimized fluid extravasation and tissue oedema and also enhanced visibility. Post-operative pyelograms revealed an adequately funnelled UPJ, with good flow into the distal ureter. The two surviving animals had minimal apparent morbidity from the procedure, and retrograde pyelograms at euthanasia revealed a patent anastomosis without extravasation. A 6-F catheter easily crossed the reconstructed UPJ at autopsy in all animals.

Comment

The authors suggest that dismembered percutaneous Anderson–Hynes endopyeloplasty is technically feasible and promising. Further technical experience and additional functional outcome analysis in the survival model are necessary. With the technique described here, the authors introduce the concept of percutaneous intrarenal reconstructive surgery (PIRS), in which advanced intrarenal and retroperitoneal dissection with reconstruction can be performed endourologically, further broadening the horizons of conventional percutaneous techniques.

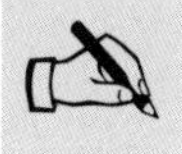

Therapeutic options for proximal ureter stone: extracorporeal shock wave lithotripsy versus semirigid ureterorenoscope with holmium:yttrium-aluminum-garnet laser lithotripsy

Wu CF, Chen CS, Lin WY, *et al. Urology* 2005; **65**: 1075–9

BACKGROUND. Extracorporeal SWL has a high success rate and is the least invasive method for treating calculi in the whole urinary tract. Although SWL has been recommended as the first-line treatment for proximal ureter calculi smaller than 1 cm, it has a variable success rate for large upper ureteral calculi. Large upper ureteral calculi often result in obstructive uropathy and consequent deterioration of renal function. The optimal treatment of these calculi remains under debate, although various treatments have been applied. The main goal of this study was to determine the optimal therapeutic modality in patients with upper ureter stones. The authors analysed the treatment outcomes in patients undergoing semi-rigid ureterorenoscope holmium:yttrium–aluminium–garnet (YAG) laser lithotripsy (URSL) and SWL.

INTERPRETATION. This investigation assessed 220 patients with upper ureteral stones. Those in the SWL group were treated on an outpatient basis using the Medispec Econolith 2000 (Medispec, Germantown, MD, USA) under intravenous sedation. URSL was performed with a 6/7.5-F semi-rigid tapered ureterorenoscope and holmium:YAG laser under spinal anaesthesia on an inpatient basis. A successful outcome was defined as the patient being stone free on radiography 1 month after treatment. The stone size, success rate, post-operative complications and cost were evaluated in each group.

A total of 220 patients were enrolled in this study. Haematuria and flank pain were the most common complaints in each group. The mean stone burden ± SD was 58.7 ± 3.1 mm^2 in the SWL group and 108.4 ± 10.0 mm^2 in the URSL group ($P = 0.000$). The accessibility of the semi-rigid ureterorenoscope for upper ureteral stones was 98.1% (101 out of 103), and the stone-free rate achieved after one treatment was 83.2% (84 out of 101). The initial stone-free rate of *in situ* ESWL was 63.9% (76 out of 119). Significantly, the initial stone-free rate of the URSL group was superior to that of the SWL group ($P = 0.001$). The average cost in the URSL group appeared to be lower than that in the SWL group ($P = 0.000$).

Comment

The authors suggest that miniaturized ureterorenoscopes and improved laser lithotriptors facilitate effective and safe retrograde treatment of urinary tract calculi, regardless of stone size and location. The results of this study have demonstrated that URSL is the favoured endourological treatment for patients with upper ureter calculi with dimensions exceeding 1 cm. Considering the stone-free rate and cost together, URSL should remain the recommended first-line treatment for proximal ureter calculi smaller than 1 cm, although no statistically significant difference was found in the stone-free rate between URSL and SWL.

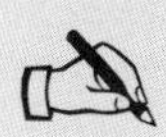

'Angular percutaneous renal access'; multiple tracts through a single incision for staghorn calculous treatment in a single session

Liatsikos EN, Kapoor R, Lee B, Jabbour M, Barbalias G, Smith AD. *Eur Urol* 2005; **48**: 832–7

BACKGROUND. Percutaneous nephrolithotomy (PNL) is a safe and minimally invasive approach when compared with open surgery for patients with complete staghorn calculi. A superior caliceal approach is considered ideal for approaching the renal system in the management of staghorn calculi. An intercostal puncture above the twelfth rib carries a 2.8–12% risk of pleural injury and chest complications. Additional middle or lower pole caliceal punctures may be required for complete clearance of stones. These additional punctures require separate subcostal accesses at either the same or different sessions and separate nephrostomy tubes for drainage through all the access routes. The multiple tracts with multiple nephrostomy tubes add to increased post-operative patient discomfort, increased hospital stay and multiple skin scar formation. All these factors ultimately add to the morbidity and cost of the treatment. The purpose of this study was to present the technique of a single subcostal skin incision with multiple angular punctures to approach the superior, middle and lower pole of the kidney for the management of staghorn calculi.

INTERPRETATION. One hundred patients with staghorn calculi were managed between January 1997 and June 2000. The superior calyx was approached by a subcostal triangulation technique, and the middle and lower calices were approached by angular punctures (Fig. 16.1). Correct advancement of the needle was monitored by biplane fluoroscopy. Maximum effort was made for complete stone clearance in a single session. Eighty-seven per cent of patients were rendered stone free in a single session. The average number of tract dilations per renal unit was 2.4 with an average anaesthesia time of 110 min and an average blood loss of 450 ml. The average hospital stay duration was 4.6 days. The secondary procedures required were 0.11 per patient, and the complication rate totalled 7% with one case of excessive haemorrhage requiring embolization.

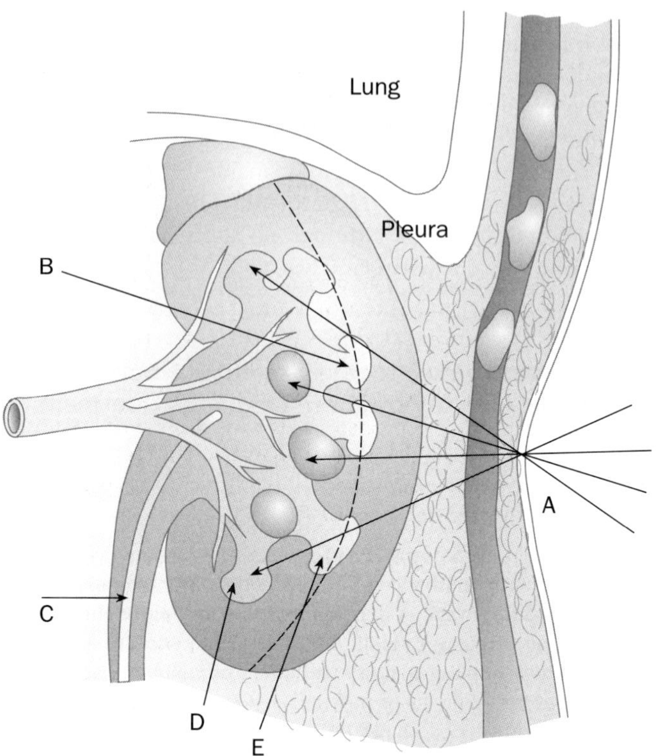

Fig. 16.1 Angular percutaneous puncture through a single skin incision. A. Skin site with angular access tracts to various calyces; B. anterior calyx; C. ureteral catheter; D. posterior calyx; E. posterolateral avascular plane. Source: Liatsikos *et al.* (2005).

Comment

In the management of patients with stone disease, it does not matter how much stone burden the surgeon has cleared, the real question from the perspective of patient satisfaction is how much is left behind and at what cost. The authors propose the triangulation technique as a safe and appealing method for the percutaneous management of staghorn calculi.

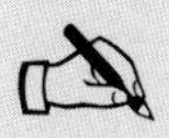

Laparoscopic pyeloplasty versus antegrade endopyelotomy: comparison in 100 patients and a new algorithm for the minimally invasive treatment of ureteropelvic junction obstruction

Ost MC, Kaye JD, Guttman MJ, Lee BR, Smith AD. *Urology* 2005; **66** (5 Suppl): 47–51

BACKGROUND. Minimally invasive therapies, including laparoscopic pyeloplasty and endopyelotomy, have proved to be equally efficacious in treating primary ureteropelvic junction obstruction (UPJO), with the benefits of shorter hospital stays, reduced post-operative pain treatment requirements and faster convalescence. While endopyelotomy has been used regularly and effectively for close to 20 years, a plethora of series on laparoscopic pyeloplasty have amassed over the last decade, with excellent results. The aim of the present article was to assess the treatment efficacy of percutaneous endopyelotomy and laparoscopic pyeloplasty to establish a new algorithm in the minimally invasive treatment of UPJO.

INTERPRETATION. Hospital records, office charts and radiographic studies of patients with UPJO treated endoscopically ($n = 50$), laparoscopically ($n = 50$) or by endopyeloplasty ($n = 5$) were reviewed. All percutaneous endopyelotomies were performed with a cold hook-knife technique, and all laparoscopic pyeloplasties were performed transperitoneally using an Anderson–Hynes dismembered anastomosis. Successful outcomes were defined as relief of obstruction as quantified by diuretic renal scans and/or relief of obstructive symptoms. All patients were followed for an average of 16.0 months (range 2–42 months). In the endoscopically treated group, the average age was 44.6 ± 15.6 years, estimated blood loss (EBL) was 152.1 ± 112.8 ml, and the hospital stay was 2.5 ± 1.0 days. There was no significant change from pre-operative to post-operative creatinine (1.2 ± 0.7 to 1.2 ± 0.7 mg/dl [106 ± 62 to 106 ± 62 μmol/l]). Success rates included 92% (35 out of 38) for primary percutaneous antegrade endopyelotomy and 58% (7 out of 12) for secondary percutaneous antegrade endopyelotomy. All the primary percutaneous antegrade endopyelotomy failures ($n = 3$) had either grade 3 or grade 4 hydronephrosis. In the laparoscopic pyeloplasty group, the average age was 37.9 ± 14.8 years, EBL was 108.3 ± 109.4 ml, and the average hospital stay was 2.6 ± 0.9 days. There was no significant change from pre-operative to post-operative creatinine (1.1 ± 0.4 to 1.0 ± 0.4 mg/dl [97 ± 35 to 97 ± 35 μmol/l]). Success rates included 100% (29 out of 29) for primary repair and 95.2% (20 out of 21) for secondary repair.

Comment

The authors suggest that, in skilled hands, highly successful outcomes can be expected when either antegrade endopyelotomy or laparoscopic pyeloplasty is used to treat a primary UPJO. In the instance of a UPJO associated with a high degree of hydronephrosis, patients may be better served with a laparoscopic pyeloplasty. To maximize an efficacious outcome, minimally invasive UPJO treatment decisions should be based on patient and surgeon preference, as directed by the presented algorithm.

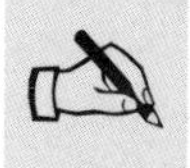

Endoscopic extraperitoneal radical prostatectomy: oncological and functional results after 700 procedures

Stolzenburg JU, Rabenalt R, Do M, *et al. J Urol* 2005; **174**: 1271–5

BACKGROUND. Minimally invasive surgery for localized prostate cancer provides certain advantages compared with open surgery, i.e. an excellent magnified view of the pelvic anatomy, a shorter catheterization time and low intra-operative and post-operative complication rates in terms of blood loss, transfusion rates, re-intervention, urethrovesical stricture and incontinence. Currently, the procedural complexity necessitating considerable learning experience is being discussed as a challenging part of the laparoscopic approach. In this study, the authors review their experience with endoscopic (totally) extraperitoneal radical prostatectomy (EERPE) as first-line therapy for localized prostate cancer.

INTERPRETATION. A total of 700 consecutive patients underwent EERPE. Mean patient age was 63.4 years (range 42–77 years). Mean pre-operative prostate-specific antigen was 10.7 ng/ml. After preparation of the pre-peritoneal space, the technique of EERPE duplicates the steps of classic open descending retropubic radical prostatectomy including a nerve-sparing EERPE when indicated. Mean operative time was 151 min. There was no conversion, and the transfusion rate was 0.9% in six. A total of 14 patients (2%) required early and three patients (0.4%) required late post-operative re-intervention. Pathological stage was pT2a in 89 patients (12.7%), pT2b in 54 (7.7%), pT2c in 245 (35%), pT3a in 229 (32.7%), pT3b in 79 (11.2%) and pT4 in four patients (0.6%). Positive surgical margins were found in 10.8% (42 out of 388) of patients with a pT2 tumour and in 31.2% (96 out of 308) of patients with a pT3 tumour. Mean catheterization time was 6.2 days. Six months after surgery, 83.8% of the patients were completely continent, 10.4% needed one or two pads daily, and 5.8% of patients needed more than two pads daily. Of all patients who underwent nerve-sparing procedures, 100 patients had a post-operative follow-up of 6 months. Of the 66 patients with the unilateral nerve-sparing approach, eight (12.1%) had erections sufficient for intercourse, and 16 out of 34 patients (47.1%) with the bilateral nerve-sparing procedure had erections sufficient for intercourse with or without the help of phosphodiesterase type 5 inhibitors.

Comment

Based on the results of this study, the authors suggest that EERPE can be performed with equal efficacy and results compared with laparoscopic transperitoneal radical prostatectomy, while providing the ease and safety of a totally extraperitoneal approach, completely avoiding intraperitoneal complications.

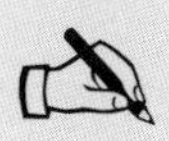

Laparoscopic partial nephrectomy: contemporary technique and outcomes

Haber GP, Gill IS. *Eur Urol* 2006; **49**: 660–5

BACKGROUND. Technical evolution of radiographic imaging has led to increased detection of incidental small renal lesions. Laparoscopic partial nephrectomy (LPN) has emerged as a viable alternative to open partial nephrectomy while minimizing patient morbidity. With increasing laparoscopic experience, the indications of LPN have been carefully expanded to include larger, central, hilar and infiltrating tumours. The authors describe their technique and review their outcomes in specific patient subsets.

INTERPRETATION. Since September 1999, more than 500 laparoscopic partial nephrectomies have been performed by the senior author. Data were collected prospectively. All patients underwent a three-dimensional CT scan prior to the operation. The technique involves pre-operative ureteral catheterization, laparoscopic renal ultrasonography to delineate the tumour, *en bloc* clamping of the renal hilar vascular pedicle, tumour excision with cold endoshears, pelvicaliceal suture repair and parenchymal closure over Surgicel bolsters with biological haemostatic agent (Fig. 16.2). Renal hypothermia was achieved laparoscopically with ice slush in selected cases with anticipated long warm ischaemia time. Mean tumour size was 2.9 cm (1–10.3 cm), 31% of the tumours were greater than 3 cm, 5% occurred in a solitary kidney, and tumour location was central in 40% and hilar in 6% of patients. The transperitoneal approach was employed in 65% of cases. Mean warm ischaemia time was 32 min. Intra-operative complications occurred in 5.5%. Pathology confirmed renal cell carcinoma in 75% of the tumours. In the initial 100 patients with a 3-year minimum follow-up, overall survival was 86% and cancer-specific survival was 100%.

Comment

The authors state that laparoscopic partial nephrectomy is a technically challenging procedure because of its intra-operative complexity and potential complications. It should be reserved for those with adequate prior laparoscopic experience. Initially, it should be employed in selected patients with a small tumour in an anatomically favourable location. With increasing experience, one can move a step forward to treat more advanced and challenging tumours, which hitherto were the exclusive preserve of open partial nephrectomy. Long-term (>5 years) functional and oncological outcomes are currently being confirmed.

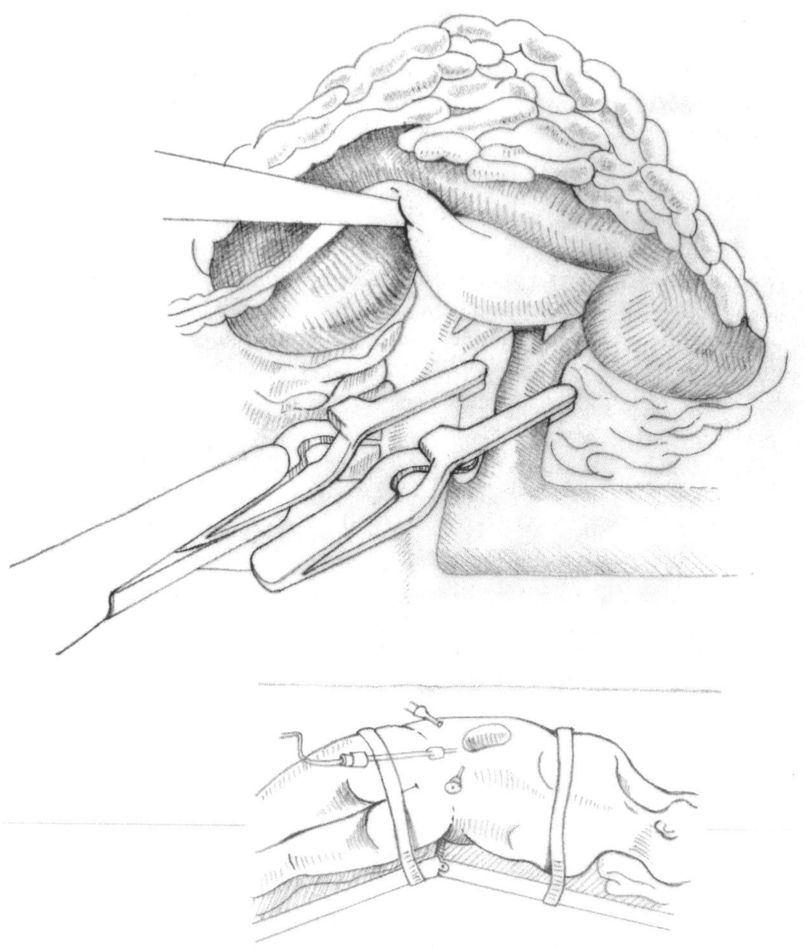

Fig. 16.2 Retroperitoneal laparoscopic partial nephrectomy. Renal artery and vein are dissected separately and laparoscopic bulldog clamps are applied. Source: Haber and Gill *et al.* (2006).

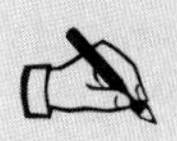

Modular training for residents with no prior experience with open pelvic surgery in endoscopic extraperitoneal radical prostatectomy

Stolzenburg JU, Rabenalt R, Do M, Horn LC, Liatsikos EN. *Eur Urol* 2006; **49**: 491–8

Background. Introducing laparoscopy to urologists who did not receive this type of training during their residencies, is indeed a difficult task. Transfer of skills based on techniques learned performing open surgery is neither appropriate nor effective. There have been a plethora of workshops during postgraduate education courses attempting to provide basic concepts and more advanced notions of laparoscopic techniques. A variety of simulators, ranging from mirrored boxes to costly virtual reality interfaces, have appeared in the literature claiming to be effective in the acquisition and amelioration of laparoscopic skills. The aim of this study was to establish a teaching programme for the performance of EERPE that would ensure the safe and efficacious training of residents with no previous experience of open pelvic surgery.

Interpretation. The technique of EERPE was divided into twelve segments with five levels of difficulty (Table 16.1). During each educational EERPE, the trainee only performed the operative steps corresponding to his/her acquired skill level. The mentor performed the remaining parts of the EERPE, with the trainee assisting. The first 50 and subsequent 100 cases performed by the residents were compared with the first 50 and last 100 cases (cases 521–621) performed by the mentor. Two residents with no prior experience in open pelvic surgery participated in the study and required 43 and 38 procedures, respectively, until they were considered to be competent. The initial 50 procedures performed completely independently by the residents had mean operative times of 176 and 173 min. There were two intra-operative rectal injuries (one patient developed recto-urethral fistula) and one haemorrhage and one lymphocoele post-operatively. The positive margin rate for pT2 disease was 14.3% and 11.5%, and for pT3 tumours 38.8% and 29.1%, respectively. After an additional 100 procedures performed by the same residents, mean operative times were 142 and 146 min. There was one patient who needed a transfusion. Post-operative complications requiring re-intervention were one haemorrhage, two anastomotic leakages and four symptomatic lymphocoeles. The positive margin rate for pT2 disease was 12.8% and 6.5%, and for pT3 tumours 33.3% and 26.3%, respectively. No statistically significant differences were observed compared with the mentor's cases.

Comment

The authors conclude that their proposed training scheme for teaching EERPE is feasible, safe and effective. Based on a highly standardized technique, this concept offers a short learning curve, and it makes it possible to start this complex procedure as a beginner or without experience in open pelvic surgery. While

Table 16.1 The twelve segments of EERPE, with five levels of difficulty

No. of step	Description of surgical procedure	Module level of difficulty
1	Trocar placement and dissection of the pre-peritoneal space	I
2	Pelvic lymphadenectomy	II
3	Incision of the endopelvic fascia and dissection of the puboprostatic ligaments	I
4	Santorini plexus ligation	III
5	Anterior and lateral bladder neck dissection	II
	Dorsal bladder neck dissection	III
6	Dissection and division of vasa deferentia	III
7	Dissection of the seminal vesicles	III
8	Incision of the posterior Denonvillier's fascia – mobilization of the dorsal surface of the prostate from the rectum	III
9	Dissection of the prostatic pedicles	III
10	Nerve-sparing procedure	V
11	Apical dissection	IV
12	Urethrovesical anastomosis	
	Dorsal circumference (4, 5, 6, 7, 8 o'clock stitches)	IV
	3 and 9 o'clock stitches	II
	Bladder neck closure and 11 and 1 o'clock stitches	III

Source: Stolzenburg *et al.* (2006).

training residents is of paramount importance to the future of urology, it cannot come at the expense of patient safety.

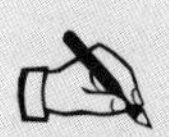

Robot-assisted versus pure laparoscopic radical prostatectomy: are there any differences?

Joseph JV, Vicente I, Madeb R, Erturk E, Patel HR. *BJU Int* 2005; **96**: 39–42

BACKGROUND. Laparoscopic surgery for localized prostate cancer has become the standard of care in many institutions. The combination of lower post-operative morbidity, improved cosmesis, shorter convalescence and comparable oncological outcome has paved the way for the wide acceptance of the technique. In numerous institutions, laparoscopic skills are transferred to perform robotic-assisted prostatectomies (RAP), now used in the USA and Europe, with early results still being reported. The aim of the present study was to compare the authors' experience of pure laparoscopic radical prostatectomy (LRP) with RAP.

INTERPRETATION. The two techniques were compared retrospectively in 100 patients with localized prostate cancer who had LRP or RAP (50 each). Both groups were similar in age, serum prostate-specific antigen level, Gleason score and clinical stage. Their charts were reviewed, collating intra-operative data and early functional outcome. The mean surgical time for LRP and RAP was 235 and 202 min (P >0.05), and mean (95% CI) blood loss was 299 (40) and 206 (63) ml (P = 0.014), with no transfusions in either group. The positive margin rate did not differ significantly (14% LRP and 12% RAP), and there was no biochemical recurrence in either group. Early functional outcomes were similar.

Comment

The authors' findings suggest that both LRP and RAP are technically demanding, but feasible, with the patient clearly benefiting. There were no major surgical differences between the techniques, but RAP is more costly. If a surgeon wishes to use RAP, he should have appropriate experience with laparoscopy. The authors emphasize that the current disadvantage is the enormous cost of the robot-assisted approach compared with pure laparoscopy.

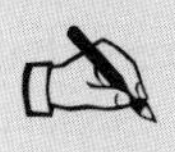

Photoselective vaporization (PVP) versus transurethral resection of the prostate (TURP): a prospective bicentre study of perioperative morbidity and early functional outcome

Bachmann A, Schurch L, Ruszat R, *et al. Eur Urol* 2005; **48**: 965–71

BACKGROUND. Transurethral electroresection of the prostate (TURP) has proved to be the standard surgical treatment for patients with benign prostate hyperplasia (BPH). In an attempt to minimize perioperative morbidity of TURP, various minimally invasive alternatives were introduced to clinical practice. The aim of this study was to compare the early follow-up and perioperative morbidity of photoselective vaporization (PVP) and TURP in patients suffering from lower urinary tract symptoms (LUTS) secondary to BPH.

INTERPRETATION. One hundred and one patients underwent PVP (n = 64) and TURP (n = 37) in a prospective, non-randomized, bicentre trial. Inclusion criteria were identical at both centres. Primary outcome parameters were maximum urinary flow rate (Qmax), post-void residual volume (Vres) and International Prostate Symptom Score (IPSS). Secondary outcomes included intra-operative surgical parameters and perioperative and post-discharge morbidity. The baseline characteristics of both groups were similar. Operating time was slightly shorter in the TURP group (P = 0.047). During TURP, significantly more irrigation solution was used (P <0.001). The decrease in serum haemoglobin (P = 0.027) and serum sodium (P = 0.013) was larger after TURP. Catheter drainage was removed significantly earlier after PVP than after TURP (P <0.001). Outcomes of Qmax and IPSS were similar in both groups within 6 months. The sort of perioperative complications were different in both groups; however, overall cumulative perioperative morbidity was comparable (PVP 39.1% vs TURP 43.2.1%; NS).

Comment

The authors suggest that photoselective laser vaporization is a safe and efficient procedure for the treatment of patients with BPH. PVP is associated with a virtually bloodless real time tissue removal. Objective and subjective outcomes after PVP and TURP are comparable over an early follow-up period of 6 months. PVP results in early relief from obstructive voiding symptoms comparable to TURP. PVP offers advantages over TURP with regard to intra-operative safety. In the future, these results have to be confirmed by a prospective randomized trial between TURP and PVP. Furthermore, the authors state that healthcare economic studies need to compare the costs of both modalities.

Conclusion

Writing a chapter regarding the 'new minimally invasive techniques in urology', one faces a plethora of scientific manuscripts and finally needs to make a decision. The studies presented here were most intriguing to the authors of this chapter. That does not mean that they were better or worse than other published studies. We have attempted to give readers a flavour of what is 'glittering' on the horizon for the future and stimulate further literature research. We hope to have accomplished this difficult task.

Abbreviations

5-ALA	5-aminolaevulinic acid
5-HT	5-hydroxytryptamine
A&E	Accident and Emergency
AChE	acetylcholinesterase
AD	androgen deprivation
AD	antenatal diagnosis
ADT	androgen deprivation therapy
AEU	arbitrary enzymatic unit
AI	arterial insufficiency
AJCC	American Joint Committee on Cancer
AMS	American Medical Systems
APC	antigen-presenting cells
AR	androgen receptor
asON	antisense oligonucleotides
AST	androgen suppression therapy
ASTRO	American Society for Therapeutic Radiology and Oncology
AUA	American Urological Association
AUC	area under the curve
AUR	acute urinary retention
BAUS	British Association of Urological Surgeons
BCF	biochemical or clinical failure
BCG	bacillus Calmette-Guérin
bd	twice a day
BMEC	bone marrow endothelial cell
BMI	body mass index
BOO	bladder outlet obstruction
BP	blood pressure
BPE	benign prostatic enlargement
BPH	benign prostatic hyperplasia
BPO	benign prostatic obstruction
BT	brachytherapy
BTA	botulinum toxin A
CAD	coronary artery disease
CAIS	complete androgen insensitivity syndrome
CAIX	carbonic anhydrase IX
CaP	prostate cancer
CaPSURE	Cancer of the Prostate Strategic Urological Research Endeavor
cGMP	cyclic guanosine monophosphate
CIS	carcinoma *in situ*
CNS	central nervous system
COX	cyclooxygenase enzyme
CPA	cyproterone acetate
CPPS	chronic pelvic pain syndrome
CRP	C-reactive protein
CSA	cross-sectional area
CT	computed tomography
CTKUB	computed tomography scanning of the renal tract
CTU	computed tomographic urography
CVSMC	corpus cavernosal smooth muscle cell
DC	dendritic cell
DHT	dihydrotestosterone
DO	detrusor overactivity
DUA	detrusor underactivity
EAU	European Association of Urology
EBL	estimated blood loss
EBRT	external beam radiotherapy
ED	erectile dysfunction
EDV	end diastolic velocity
EE	end-to-end
EERPE	endoscopic extraperitoneal radical prostatectomy
EEVE	end-to-end vasoepididymostomy

EF	erectile function
EGFR	epidermal growth factor receptor
ELISA	enzyme-linked immunosorbent assay
ENG	electroneurographic
EORTC	European Organization for the Research and Treatment of Cancer
EPCIC	Expanded Prostate cancer Index Composite
ER	extended release
ES	end-to-side
ESVE	end-to-side vasoepididymostomy
ESWL	extracorporeal shock wave lithotripsy
ESWL	extracorporeal shock wave therapy
FACT-G	Functional Assessment of Cancer Therapy—General
FDA	Food and Drug Administration
FH	family history
GAG	glycosaminoglycan
GAQ	global assessment questionnaire
GnRH	gonadotrophin-releasing hormone
GnRHa	gonadotrophin-releasing hormone agonist
GST	glutathione S-transferase
HAL	hexaminolaevulinate
HDR	high dose rate
HIF	hypoxia-inducible factor
HIFU	high-intensity focused ultrasound
HNPCC	hereditary non-polyposis colorectal cancer
HPF	high power field
HR	hazard ratio
HR	hormone refractory
HRCaP	hormone-refractory prostate cancer
HS	hormone sensitive
hTR	human telomerase RNA
HU	Hounsfield unit
I/R	ischaemia/reperfusion
IAS	intermittent androgen suppression
ICIQ	International Consultation on Incontinence Questionnaire
IDO	idiopathic detrusor overactivity
IEF	incontinence episode frequency
IELT	intravaginal ejaculatory latency time
IFN	interferon
IGF	insulin-like growth factor
IH	inguinal hernia
IIEF	International Index of Erectile Function
IIQ	Incontinence Impact Questionnaire
IL	interleukin
ILC	interstitial laser coagulation
IMRT	intensity modulated radiotherapy
IPSS	International Prostate Symptom Score
I-QOL	Incontinence Quality of Life
ISC	intermittent self-catheterization
IVP	intravenous pyelogram
IVV	intravesical volume
LDH	lactate dehydrogenase
LDL	low-density lipoprotein
LIVE	longitudinal intussusception vasoepidiymostomy
LNCaP	human prostate cancer cell line developed from a lymph node metastasis
LOH	late-onset hypogonadism
LPN	laparoscopic partial nephrectomy
LPP	leak point pressure
LRP	laparoscopic radical prostatectomy
LUTD	lower urinary tract dysfunction
LUTS	lower urinary tract symptoms
MCC	maximum cystometric capacity

MCDK	multicystic dysplastic kidney
MDA	malondialdehyde
MDCT	multidetector computed tomography
MDP	maximum detrusor pressure during bladder contraction
MH	microscopic haematuria
MMP	matrix metalloproteinase
MR	magnetic resonance
MRI	magnetic resonance imaging
MSF-4	male sexual function questionnaire
MSV	microsurgical varicocelectomy
MT1-MMP	membrane type 1 MMP
MTD	maximal tumour diameter
MTOPS	Medical Therapy of Prostatic Symptoms
MTT	3-(4,5-dimethylthiazol-2-yl)-2,5-diphenyltetrazoli-umbromide
MUI	mixed urinary incontinence
MVD	microvessel density
NAD[P]H	nicotinamide adenosine dinucleotide phosphate (reduced form)
NASHA/Dx	non-animal stabilized hyaluronic acid dextranomer
NCCT	non-contrast-enhanced computerized tomography
NDO	neurogenic detrusor overactivity
NED	no evidence of disease
NICE	National Institute for Health and Clinical Excellence
NIH-CPSI	National Institutes for Health Chronic Prostatitis Symptom Index
NNT	number needed to treat
NO	nitric oxide
NSAID	non-steroidal anti-inflammatory drug
NTSBM	non-malignant tumour surrounding bladder mucosal
OAB	overactive bladder
OPN	open partial nephrectomy
OR	odds ratio
PA	primary amenorrhoea
PBMC	peripheral blood mononuclear cell
PBSCT	peripheral blood stem cell transplantation
PCNL	percutaneous nephrolithotomy
PCR	polymerase chain reaction
PCSM	prostate cancer-specific mortality
PD	Peyronie's disease
PDDU	penile duplex Doppler ultrasound
PDE	phosphodiesterase
PDT	photodynamic therapy
PE	premature ejaculation
PFE	progression-free survival
PFMT	pelvic floor muscle training
PFS	pressure flow data
PGE2	prostaglandin E2
PIRS	percutaneous intrarenal reconstructive surgery
PIVOT	Prostate Cancer Intervention versus Observation Trial
PNL	percutaneous nephrolithotomy
PpIX	protoporphyrin IX
PRF	percutaneous radiofrequency ablation
PSA	prostate-specific antigen
PSADT	PSA doubling time
PSNT	proximal sciatic nerve transaction
PSV	peak systolic velocity
PTFE	polytetrafluoroethylene
PUF	peak urinary flow
PVP	photoselective vaporization
Qmax	maximum flow
QNG	quantitative grading of nuclei
QoL	quality of life
RAP	robotic-assisted prostatectomy
RBC	red blood cell
RC	renal colic
RCC	renal cell carcinoma

RCT randomized controlled trial
RDV reflex detrusor volume
RF radiofrequency
RFA radiofrequency ablation
RFLP restriction fragment length polymorphism
RI resistive index
ROC receiver operating characteristic
ROS reactive oxygen species
RP radical prostatectomy
RPLND retroperitoneal lymph node dissection
RR relative risk
RT radiotherapy
RT-PCR reverse transcription polymerase chain reaction
SCID severe combined immunodeficiency disease
SD standard deviation
SELDI-TOF surface-enhanced laser desorption ionization time of flight
SF stone-free
SF-36 Short Form 36
SIS small intestine submucosal
SOD superoxide dismutase
SPC suprapubic catheter
SPCG Scandinavian Prostate Cancer Group
SSD skin-to-stone distance
SSIGN Stage, Size, Grade and Necrosis
SSRI serotonin reuptake inhibitor
SUI stress urinary incontinence
SWL shock wave lithotripsy
TCC transitional cell carcinoma
tds three times a day
TIMP tissue inhibitors of matrix metalloproteinase
TIVE triangulation intussusception vasoepididymostomy
TNM Tumour size-lymph Nodes-Metastases
TOF time of flight
TPQ treatment preference questionnaire
TRAP telomeric repeat amplification protocol
Treg T regulator cell
TRUS transrectal ultrasound
TUMT transurethral microwave therapy
TUNA transurethral needle ablation
TUR transurethal resection
TURB transurethral bladder resection
TURBT transurethral bladder tumour resection
TURP transurethral resection of the prostate
TUVP transurethral vaporization
TVT tension-free vaginal tape
TWOC trial without catheter
UCLA-PCI University of California, Los Angeles—Prostate Cancer Index
UDI Urogenital Distress Inventory
UI urinary incontinence
UPJ ureteropelvic junction
UPJO ureteropelvic junction obstruction
URSL ureterorenoscope laser lithotripsy
US ultrasound
USI urodynamic stress incontinence
UTI urinary tract infection
UUTT upper urinary tract tumour
VE vasoepididymostomy
VEGF vascular endothelial growth factor
VHL von Hippel–Lindau
VLAP visual laser ablation
VOD veno-occlusive disease
VR volume-rendered
Vres post-void residual volume
VUR vesicoureteric reflux
VV vasovasostomy
WW watchful waiting
YAG yttrium–aluminium– garnet

Index of papers reviewed

refractory metastatic prostate cancer. *Urology* 2005; **66**(3): 571–6. **94**

D'Amico AV, Chen MH, Roehl KA, Catalona WJ. Identifying patients at risk for significant versus clinically insignificant post-operative prostate-specific antigen failure. *J Clin Oncol* 2005; **23**(22): 4975–9. **96**

D'Amico AV, Moul J, Carroll PR, Sun L, Lubeck D, Chen MH. Surrogate end-point for prostate cancer specific mortality in patients with non-metastatic hormone refractory prostate cancer. *J Urol* 2005; **173**(5): 1572–6. **97**

D'Amico AV, Renshaw AA, Sussman B, Chen MH. Pre-treatment PSA velocity and risk of death from prostate cancer following external beam radiation therapy. *JAMA* 2005; **294**(4): 440–7. **97**

Dannull J, Su Z, Rizzieri D, Yang BK, Coleman D, Yancey D, Zhang A, Dahm P, Chao N, Gilboa E, Vieweg J. Enhancements of vaccine-mediated antitumour immunity in cancer patients after depletion of regulatory T cells. *J Clin Invest* 2005; **115**: 3623–33. **75**

Datta MW, Dhir R, Dobbin K, Bosland MC, Melamed J, Becich MJ, Orenstein JM, Kajdacsy-Balla AA, Patel A, Macias V, Berman JJ. Prostate cancer in patients with screening serum prostate specific antigen values less than 4.0 ng/dl: results from the cooperative prostate cancer tissue resource. *J Urol* 2005; **173**(5): 1546–51. **103**

Davison BJ, Elliott S, Ekland M, Griffin S, Wiens K. Development and evaluation of a prostate sexual rehabilitation clinic: a pilot project. *BJU Int* 2005; **96**(9): 1360–4. **212**

Dearnaley DP, Hall E, Lawrence D, Huddart RA, Eeles R, Nutting CM, Gadd J, Warrington A, Bidmead M, Horwich A. Phase III pilot study of dose escalation using conformal radiotherapy in prostate cancer: PSA control and side effects. *Br J Cancer* 2005; **92**(3): 488–98. **117**

de Crevoisier R, Tucker SL, Dong L, Mohan R, Cheung R, Cox JD, Kuban DA. Increased risk of biochemical and local failure in patients with distended rectum on planning CT for prostate cancer radiotherapy. *Int J Radiat Oncol Biol Phys* 2005; **62**(4): 965–73. **121**

Deeb A, Hughes IA. Inguinal hernia in female infants: a cue to check the sex chromosomes? *BJU Int* 2005; **96**: 401–3. **4**

Denham JW, Steigler A, Lamb DS, Joseph D, Mameghan H, Turner S, Matthews J, Franklin I, Atkinson C, North J, Poulsen M, Christie D, Spry NA, Tai KH, Wynne C, Duchesne G, Kovacev O, D'Este C; Trans-Tasman Radiation Oncology Group. Short-term androgen deprivation and radiotherapy for locally advanced prostate cancer: results from the Trans-Tasman Radiation Oncology Group 96.01 randomised controlled trial. *Lancet Oncol* 2005; **6**(11): 841–50. **110, 114**

de Reijke TM, Kurth KH, Sylvester RJ, Hall RR, Brausi M, van de Beek K, Landsoght KE, Carpentier P; European Organization for the Research and Treatment of Cancer-Genito-Urinary Group. Bacillus Calmette–Guerin versus epirubicin for primary, secondary or concurrent carcinoma *in situ* of the bladder: results of a

General index